# PRAISE FOR JOY BAUER AND *JOY BAUER'S FOOD CURES*

"If you think of food as the enemy, then you need to devour this book. Joy has compiled the total guide to 'eating yourself healthy.' It's no surprise I call her the patron saint of no-nonsense nutrition."
—Meredith Vieira, former cohost of the *Today* show

"Joy Bauer is the best nutritionist in the world!"
—Shaquille O'Neal

"Joy Bauer, a fabulous nutritionist, has produced a great resource for understanding the relation of specific components of healthy diet to fighting common diseases of our Western civilization—diseases largely caused by our toxic lifestyle."
—Arthur Agatston, MD, bestselling author of *The South Beach Diet*
and *The South Beach Heart Program*

"I have nothing but the utmost respect for Joy and her work. For many years she has helped me and my family with dieting and nutrition. She is forever searching for new ways to improve health and wellness. She is a star in my eyes."
—Tommy Mottola, music mogul and former chairman of Sony Music Entertainment

"When it comes to questions about nutrition, Joy Bauer is your go-to source. She's got all the facts, with great tips for healthy eating and living with a totally sensible and, more importantly, realistic outlook on all of it. In my experience, this is the woman—and now the book—with the answers."
—Bobby Flay, TV personality and chef/owner of Mesa Grill, Bar Americain, and
Bobby Flay Steak, and author of *Bobby Flay's Throwdown!*

"While reading *Joy Bauer's Food Cures,* I felt like I was visiting with Joy at her office. The book captures her real-life persona . . . one of encouragement, humor, resiliency, support, genuine concern . . . and, above all, her ability to present realistic and practical options in achieving your personal goals and objectives!"
—Paul Carlucci, publisher of the *New York Post*

"Joy Bauer has somehow made the impossible, possible. She makes smart eating, weight loss, and now, in this book, preventive and curative health a reality. Joy's simple and practical steps are easy to follow, even for those who feel challenged in this area. Our family knows firsthand that success is inevitable when you listen to Joy."
—Jessica Seinfeld, author of *Deceptively Delicious*
and founder/president of Baby Buggy, Inc.

"In a world crammed with crackhead nutritionists, Joy Bauer is a beacon of sanity. No joke—she saved my life."     —Dany Levy, founder of *Daily Candy*

"Joy Bauer is an amazing food coach! *Food Cures* will connect the dots between eating well, feeling healthy, and really enjoying your life."
—Vicki Wellington, publisher of *Food Network Magazine*

"Joy Bauer has written a remarkable book. It outlines with clarity and caring professionalism a road map to better health. It is easy to read and amazingly easy to live by—all one needs is a touch of discipline—and that seasoning is under your control."
—Maurice Tempelsman, chairman of the board
and director at Lazare Kaplan International, Inc.

# PRAISE FROM THE MEDICAL COMMUNITY

"This is an easy-to-read, absolutely comprehensive, medically accurate guide to food as a body fuel. This book is a real contribution to the field—it explains the principles of nutrition and lays out the practices of eating for health and well-being. It is a gem."

—Orli R. Etingin, MD, professor of clinical medicine, Weill Cornell Medical College, New York–Presbyterian Hospital

"Joy has written a superb, readable, and tremendously useful book that distills all her expertise into a volume I will use personally and give to all my patients. It's uniquely valuable."

—Marianne J. Legato, MD, founder and director of the Foundation for Gender-Specific Medicine, Inc.; professor of clinical medicine, Columbia University; and adjunct professor of medicine, Johns Hopkins

"Wow! Joy has finally given us what we need. She has written a comprehensive, well-researched, easy-to-use nutritional guide for people who want to protect their vision from cataracts and macular degeneration."

—Paul T. Finger, MD, FACS, clinical professor of ophthalmology, New York University School of Medicine, and author of *The Macular Degeneration Network* (www.macular-degeneration.org)

"Joy Bauer has been the 'go-to' nutritionist in New York for many years. This easy-to-read book captures her warmth, her humor, her clinical wisdom, and her vast experience, and gives sensible advice about managing your diet and staying healthy. It is a most welcome resource!"

—B. Timothy Walsh, MD, Ruane Professor of Psychiatry, College of Physicians & Surgeons, Columbia University; and director, Eating Disorders Research Unit, New York Psychiatric Institute

"Joy's book serves up heaping portions of useful nutritional and general health information, coupled with lots of common sense advice and guidance. She spices it up with great anecdotes and recipes, written in a conversation style that makes this book a joy to read. I thought I'd just glance at the Weight Loss and Beautiful Skin chapters, but each chapter was filled with so many goodies I could not put it down."

—Marsha Gordon, MD, clinical professor, dermatology, Mount Sinai School of Medicine

"*Joy Bauer's Food Cures* offers a welcome addition to my shelf of trusted books. It is a well-researched guidebook for helping select the foods that will make and keep you healthy."

—Evelyn Attia, MD, director, The Eating Disorders Clinic, New York State Psychiatric Institute; and clinical professor of psychiatry, Columbia University College of Physicians & Surgeons

"Joy Bauer's new book is well written, easily read, and a great guide for eating properly. Her style and 4-step outlines make it easy for anyone to understand and follow the programs. It is a great recipe for all of us to learn."

—Phillip Bauman, MD, orthopedic consultant for the New York City Ballet

# JOY BAUER'S
# FOOD
# CURES

# JOY BAUER'S
# FOOD CURES

### EAT RIGHT TO GET HEALTHIER, LOOK YOUNGER, AND ADD YEARS TO YOUR LIFE

**JOY BAUER, MS, RD, CDN**

**WITH CAROL SVEC**

RODALE.

Rodale books may be purchased for business or promotional use or for special sales. For information, please write to:
Special Markets Department, Rodale, Inc., 733 Third Avenue, New York, NY 10017

Printed in the United States of America

Rodale Inc. makes every effort to use acid-free ⊗, recycled paper ♻.

Book design by Christina Gaugler

**Library of Congress Cataloging-in-Publication Data**

Bauer, Joy.
    Joy Bauer's food cures : eat right to get healthier, look younger, and add years to your life /
Joy Bauer with Carol Svec.—Rev. ed.
       p.    cm.
    Includes bibliographical references and index.
    ISBN 978-1-60961-312-9 paperback
    1. Diet therapy—Popular works.  I. Svec, Carol.  II. Title.  III. Title: Food cures.
RM217.B38  2011
615.8'54—dc23                                         2011015722

**Distributed to the trade by Macmillan**

8  10  9          paperback

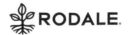

We inspire and enable people to improve their lives and the world around them.
www.rodalebooks.com

*This book is dedicated to health and medical researchers everywhere. Their brilliant behind-the-scenes work allows me and other wellness educators to improve the health of millions of people.*

# CONTENTS

## Part 6—Resources

# ACKNOWLEDGMENTS

Many remarkable people were involved in the creation of this book. I'm especially grateful to the world-class physicians who continuously trust and support my work, and to my extraordinary clients—their successes have made this book possible by teaching me the things readers need and want to know.

I'm indebted to my editorial director, Johannah Sakimura. Johannah, you're the master of all research and thanks to you, this revised edition is filled with robust, cutting-edge, and accurate information.

Tremendous thanks to Carol Svec—appreciation is an understatement. This book is a direct result of your exceptional talent and professionalism.

Sincere thanks to Dystel and Goderich Literary Management. Jane and Miriam, your wisdom, ongoing support, and direction mean the world. And big thanks to Jamie Kandel for helping spread the word of good health!

Thanks to the entire crew at Rodale Inc. Your enthusiasm and dedication to this book are greatly appreciated. Special thanks to my fabulous editors, Pam Krauss and Tory Glerum; to designers Amy King and Christina Gaugler; and to project editor Zachary Greenwald.

Great big thanks to my friends at NBC's *Today* show who enable me to improve the health of America. Heartfelt thanks to Jim Bell, Steve Capus, Elena Nachman-off, Don Nash, Noah Kotch, Dee Dee Thomas, Marc Victor, Tammy Filler, Jaclyn Levin, Rainy Farrell, Debbie Kosofsky, Jayme Baron, Melanie Jackson, Emily Goldberg, Liz Neumann, and the countless producers and assistants who help me each week.

Thanks also to the fabulous *Today* hosts: Matt Lauer, Meredith Vieira, Ann Curry, Al Roker, Natalie Morales, Hoda Kotb, Kathie Lee Gifford, Lester Holt, Tamron Hall, and Amy Robach. Special thanks to medical guru Dr. Nancy Snyderman. Also, thank goodness for everyone in the hardworking stage crew and prop, wardrobe, hair, makeup, and Web site departments.

Many thanks to my colleagues at Waterfront Media and Everyday Health; Mike Keriakos, Ben Wolin, Steven Petrow, Dan Wilmer, Bill Maslyn, Debbie Strong, Brianna Steinhilber, Karim Farag, Eleanor Meyer, and Jennifer Perciballi for understanding the magnitude and many dimensions of *Food Cures*—and making it come to life online.

I'm incredibly grateful to my top-notch editors at *Woman's Day* magazine for giving me the opportunity to spread my health message to their millions of readers; Elizabeth Mayhew, Ellen Breslau, Amy Brightfield, and Barbara Brody.

Special thanks goes to Erica Ilton, for helping with the initial research, and to Jennifer Iserloh, a phenomenal chef with a true passion for health.

Hugs to everyone in my wonderful families: the Beal family (Debra, Steve, Ben, Noah, Becca, Chloe, Jenny, and Dunkin), the Schloss family (Ellen, Artie, Pam, Dan, Charlie, Cooper, Glenn, Elena, Trey, their new baby, and Otis), and the Bauer family (Carol, Vic, Mary, Nat, Jason, Mia, Annabelle, Zach, Harley, and Jimmy).

Infinite, deep, and everlasting thanks to my mom and dad, Ellen and Artie Schloss. You are my lifelines and my touchstones. Your support means the world, and I'm forever grateful for your encouragement, advice, cashews, and wine.

I can't say enough about my husband, Ian, and my three children, Jesse, Cole, and Ayden Jane—you are everything valuable in the world . . . my heart . . . my bliss . . . my home . . . my loves.

# PART 1

# WELCOME TO MY OFFICE

# CHAPTER 1

# WELCOME TO MY OFFICE

My motto is this: Life is hard . . . food should be easy.

But for many people, knowing what to eat, when to eat, and how much to eat is a puzzle they have lost all hope of ever solving.

Anyone who has ever tried to make a commitment to healthy eating knows the obstacles: The dizzying number of choices in grocery stores and restaurants; the crazy, always-on-the-go schedules of nearly every member of the family; the relentless hype and marketing surrounding fatty and sugary snack foods; and the powerful appetites fueled by habits, traditions, and humongous portion sizes. As if that wasn't enough pressure, add in the swirl of conflicting information about specific diets—high-carb versus low-carb, high-fat versus low-fat, calorie-counting versus no-counting, cabbage versus grapefruit versus eggs versus whatever.

Who wouldn't feel overwhelmed and frustrated? And when we're frustrated, we tend to fall back into old, unhealthy eating patterns. Have you ever gone on a diet to lose weight but ended up gaining weight instead? Or did you lose weight only to put it back on again within a year or two? Has your doctor ever put you on a special diet to treat a health problem, but you soon abandoned it because it was just too complicated for real life? If so, you're not alone. These scenarios happen more often than you might think. No one consciously plans to eat her way into a larger dress size or to make himself a candidate for triple bypass surgery. But dietary uncertainty can turn the best intentions sour, even when the stakes are high. When it comes to good nutrition, it is so easy to go from being totally motivated to feeling utterly defeated.

It doesn't have to be that way. Whatever else is going on in your life, food should be the least of your worries. Eating is a piece of cake.

Really.

## HOW FOOD MAKES US NUTS

We have a strange love/hate relationship with food. We want to eat cupcakes but still be as slim as Gwyneth Paltrow. We fantasize about our ideal meal but settle for a burger and fries from a drive-thru window. We buy "skinny jeans" for the body we want to have but then eat comfort foods because those jeans don't fit anything but our dreams. Love/hate—two sides of the same sneaky cookie.

Food does more than nourish us, so it makes sense that it can elicit complex feelings. Of course, its most important role is to give us the vitamins, minerals, energy, and nutrients necessary to keep us alive and healthy—but food is also about love and family traditions. It's how we celebrate and comfort and nurture—which is why food is at the center of weddings and funerals and why it's the first thing we think to bring when we hear a friend is sick. Food is about taking away the pain of hunger, but it also has become about easing our boredom, stress, or depression. We tend to eat too much of almost everything whenever we get the chance. We eat in the car, at work, in front of the TV, or standing over the kitchen sink. We snack before meals, after meals, and sometimes in the middle of the night, sometimes without even waking up. Next to sex, eating is the activity most responsible for making us feel any number of emotions, including happiness, longing, pride, pleasure, shame, weakness, and power.

Food is like that great big proverbial elephant in the room—that also follows you around all day. We try to ignore it, but every time we turn around, there it is. Yet despite the huge (mammoth!) role food plays in our lives, we don't really know how to talk about it, at least not in a way that helps us make the best choices when it comes time to eat.

I believe the reason some diets become wildly popular for a time is that they allow us to understand food and eating in a new way, and they give us a different language to use when trying to sort out our confusion. Think about it: During the past decade, we've all learned the language of "carbs"—what carbs are, what low-carb eating looks like, the difference between net carbs and total carbs, bad carbs and good carbs. Before that, we studied the language of "fats." And before fats, we all knew how to parse calories.

So it's not that people lack information about food and eating. In fact, most of us have more information than we know what to do with. Many of my clients have such sophisticated vocabularies that they sound like third-year nutrition students. The problem is that they don't know how to combine all the disparate pieces of the diet puzzle into a plan that they can use to achieve their individual, highly personal goals. They are eager—desperate, perhaps—to gain control over food. But they can't do it with words alone!

That's where I come in.

## THE POWER OF A STEP-WISE PROGRAM

I've been a nutritionist for more than 2 decades and have helped thousands of people overcome their worst problems with eating. In the process, they have grown stronger and healthier. In many cases, they have added 10, 15, or even 20 years to their lives by controlling or even reversing disease.

How can food turn your life around? Let me tell you about 56-year-old Stephen, a high-powered lawyer who was all but ordered by his doctors to make an appointment with me. To say he was initially resistant to seeing a nutritionist would be an understatement, but in the end, the encouragement (and begging and pleading) of his wife and children persuaded him to come to see me.

He was a nutritional wreck. At 5 foot 9 and 250 pounds, Stephen was significantly overweight. His body mass index (BMI) was 37, officially classifying him as obese. His lab values were high across the board: High cholesterol and triglycerides put him at high risk of heart disease, and, due to his high fasting glucose levels, he was officially diagnosed with type 2 diabetes.

To try to get control over these risk factors, Stephen's doctors put him on three powerhouse medications: a blood pressure drug, a statin to lower his cholesterol, and Glucophage to lower his blood sugar. And then I got ahold of him.

I gave him a food plan to help him lose weight and lower his blood sugar and cholesterol, and when he had an episode of gout, I gave him tips on how to treat that, too. Once he overcame his initial reluctance, Stephen approached his new eating program with the same intensity that he used to succeed in every other aspect of his life. He made a spreadsheet to track his weight loss and his lab numbers, and he memorized and followed his plan religiously. He consulted me whenever circumstances made it more than likely that he would need to deviate from the plan; that way, he made sure he wouldn't do too much harm. He ate cake at his birthday party, he socialized with friends, and he enjoyed holiday celebrations, but he always came back to the guidelines of his food program.

At the end of a year, Stephen had lost more than 60 pounds. His critical blood measurements—triglycerides, cholesterol, and fasting glucose—had all dropped to within normal ranges. He continued to take the statin, but he was able to stop taking the Glucophage and the blood pressure medication. As of this writing, Stephen has maintained his weight loss and health benefits for eight years. His doctor told him that because of the nutritional changes, Stephen has probably added at least ten healthy years to his life.

As amazing as this story sounds, Stephen's results are not unusual, and they're well within anyone's reach. No matter what your personal health aspirations are, I have a terrific food plan for you. I'll even help you figure out exactly what your goals should look like.

My objective is to make reading this book as similar as possible to an in-person, one-on-one consultation with me. I'll tell you everything you need to know to lose weight, look gorgeous, improve your mood and memory, boost your bone density, and stay healthy. I'll even give you a script to follow—a focused 4-Step program that spells out everything you need to know in order to think and eat just like a nutritionist. In short, you'll find all of the tools you need for success.

## STEP INSIDE MY OFFICE

Let's start at the beginning, with the absolute basics. One of the questions I'm asked over and over is: What defines good nutrition? In general, it means eating the right foods in the right combinations throughout the day to optimize your energy and overall health.

Of course, the people who come to see me lead different lives and strive to achieve a wide range of goals. So for some, good nutrition means focusing on increasing energy. I've worked with professional and student athletes, dancers, actors, and business executives who need to maintain a consistent level of performance. For other people who have a strong family history of disease, good nutrition means minimizing their risk of heart disease, diabetes, dementia, migraine headaches, arthritis, osteoporosis, or cancer. For others, it means finding a way to lose the weight they might have been struggling with for years.

A while ago, a man I'll call Bruce called me up and told me that one of his friends had lost a ton of weight after he became my client and that this friend now looked phenomenal. This client of mine said that I worked miracles. Bruce was calling because he had a weight problem, and he knew all the tricks and had been on all the diets, and he had gained and lost 100 pounds more times than he could count. But he was a very busy man and didn't want to bother with an appointment if I couldn't guarantee success. "Tell me," he said, "are you the person who is absolutely going to help me prevail, once and for all?"

The answer to this outright question is what all my clients, and probably you, want to know. Can my programs work immediately, quickly, and forever? The short answer is: Yes, dramatic and long-lasting results are absolutely possible. But the odds of success depend entirely on you. I don't want to give anyone false promises, not in my office and not in this book. I'm only as good as my clients' follow-through, so if you're after the kind of transformation that your friends will call miraculous, I'm here to help. We are a team—I'm your food coach, but ultimately, you're the one who'll be doing the heavy lifting.

## A FEW WORDS ABOUT COMMITMENT

To meet your goals, you absolutely need:

1. The right coach. Well, you've got me, so cross this one off your list. I have a great track record of success with my clients.

2. Rock-solid nutrition and health information. Cross this one off the list, too, because that's what this book is all about.

3. A personal commitment to stay in it for the long haul. This one is up to you!

Personal commitment is a big deal. None of my tenets will work for very long if you're following them only because you're going on vacation or because someone else is on your back about losing weight. You have to be doing this because *you* want to succeed. You have to want results and be willing to work for them, no matter what obstacles get in your way. After the economy took a tumble in 2008 and unemployment skyrocketed, I heard lots of stories about how people ran for comfort foods and the liquor cabinet and gave themselves permission to overeat and drink—for months. My belief is that it's incredibly important, especially in times of intense stress, to stay on top of your nutrition and health.

Think about it: Whenever you say "I'm overwhelmed" or "I'm depressed . . . or too busy . . . or too anxious," what do you do? Many people react by giving up on good nutrition and eating foods that contribute to illness and make them put on weight that they then spend months trying to shed. In the end, they're left feeling depressed, sluggish, and irritable. What they don't feel is healthy—physically or emotionally.

Your commitment to this plan is essential. It is a commitment you'll need to honor when you're home, when you're out, when you're traveling, and when you're socializing. It is a commitment to totally change your lifestyle.

## PREPARE YOURSELF

Changing how you eat is never easy. The first step is to get in the right place mentally. If we're going to try to create a little nutritional magic, there are a few things you need to do to prepare for this adventure.

◆ **Repeat after me: "I can do this!"** The prospect of trying another healthy lifestyle or weight-loss program can feel like staring into a black hole—no joy, no light, no end in sight. It's easy to feel defeated before you even begin, so some degree of nervousness is understandable. But a more appropriate response is enthusiasm and confidence. Trust me. I've done this hundreds and hundreds of times before. No matter what your personal issues are, I've seen worse (and you'll read some of those stories in the chapters to come). I will give you all the secrets for success that I've learned over the years.

◆ **Dare to make the leap.** Pop quiz: Which is more fun, wading into the shallow end of the pool or doing a cannonball off the diving board? When we were kids, all we wanted to do was jump into the deep end. We tend to lose that sense of courage and daring as we get older. Find a way to get back that feeling of "one, two, three, let's go!" And we're talking about nutritional changes, so you can't hurt yourself by making a full, unrestrained leap. This is about your health—not acting is the biggest risk. So go ahead, take a deep breath, and jump in.

◆ **Think big.** As far as I'm concerned, small changes add up to small results. Grand changes equal grand, life-altering results. So you might as well go for it. The payoffs will be larger, and your gratification will come sooner.

◆ **When the going gets tough, remember that it's just food.** That probably sounds crazy coming from a nutritionist, but it's a critically important point to remember. Write it on a piece of paper and tape it up on your refrigerator: "It's just food." If you're in a restaurant trying to stick to your food plan, but you're salivating over the meal that the person next to you is eating, remember to ask yourself: *Is it worth it?* The food is only going to be there for 15 to 20 minutes at most, and then it's gone. Is it worth it? That's a question only you can answer. If, after careful and deliberate consideration, you answer yes, it is worth it, then go for it. We'll consider it your "meal off," like a little vacation day for your tastebuds. But those meals off should be rare and special, just like real vacations.

◆ **Prepare to feel fabulous.** I won't try to fool you into thinking that, once you start following my advice, you'll no longer crave sweet, fatty foods or want to go whole hog at a buffet. We're all magnetically drawn to those yummy temptations on every street corner, at every dinner party, and in all our friends' homes. They will always be there, every day, for the rest of your life. But the payoff for avoiding them is well worth the fight. And when you allow temptation the upper hand and eat poorly, you end up feeling sluggish, lethargic, and unhealthy. What's the point?

So instead of giving in just to end up feeling bad, invest some energy and effort and feel fabulous. In the end, if you feel energetic and healthy, and you're more agile and comfortable, and you've added years and years onto your life, and you smile more often, and you're less moody, and you're more productive at home and at work, isn't it worth putting on the temptation blinders and ducking the doughnuts?

I say revel in your passion for life, not potato chips. And as your coach and nutritionist, I refuse to let you settle for anything less than success. You can do this, and I'm excited to help you.

# CHAPTER 2

# THINK LIKE A NUTRITIONIST

f you were visiting my office, I would ask you for two things. The first is a three-day food diary, essentially a snapshot of how food fits into your life. For three days, you would record everything you ate at every meal, every supplement, every snack, every beverage. I would ask what brand of breakfast cereal you ate, how much pasta you had for dinner, how you prepared your vegetables, what type of spread you ate on your bread, the name of the restaurant where you ate lunch, what you added to your coffee, and what time of day you ate each meal or snack. This information would tell me exactly what changes were necessary to transform your diet.

Even though I won't be able to review it, my advice to you as a reader is similar: I highly recommend that you keep a food diary. Simply write down all the foods you eat for any three days of an average week. Don't worry about brands, but be sure to note what, when, and how much you eat and drink from the minute you wake up until you go to sleep. Everything counts—that "sliver" of cake from the office birthday party, the handful of french fries you grabbed off your son's dinner plate, the finger scoops of cookie dough you "tested" while baking for your family, and, yes, the two margaritas you sipped last night at happy hour. Record it all. This diary will provide us with a baseline indication of where your eating habits are now. We won't use it in the course of the book, but the diary is a terrific way to focus your mind on the details of eating and help you notice patterns you'd like to change. Plus, a few weeks from now, when you've mastered a new way of eating, you'll be able to look back with pride when you see just how far you've come. It's often an incredible comparison, with a remarkable payoff.

The second thing I would ask for is your detailed medical history. My nutrition programs are designed to help you take control of your most pressing health problem first and then tackle the rest. I recommend writing down all diseases, disorders, or diet-related concerns that affect your life. These can include being overweight, having a certain medical condition, or even getting lab results indicating that you're at risk of a specific disease. Beneath that, write down all diseases or disorders that run in your family, particularly those of your parents, grandparents, and siblings. When a biological family member has suffered from something such as macular degeneration or breast cancer, this often puts you in a higher risk category. This list makes up your total universe of health issues, and we're going to take them on, one at a time.

## WHAT TO EXPECT FROM EACH CHAPTER

Each chapter of this book includes information about a particular health issue: how food, the environment, and other factors contribute to it; what foods to eat or avoid; which remedies might offer the best chance for curing or controlling symptoms; and other lifestyle changes you can make to feel better. Whenever possible, I include a story from my practice or personal experience to illustrate how nutrition has helped change someone's life. (Although the details of the stories are accurate, I have changed names and identifying information to protect my clients.)

Each chapter also has its own focused, customized 4-Step program that summarizes all of the advice offered in the rest of the chapter and then goes full force into specific food lists and meal plans. *Step 1: Start with the Basics* is a list of things you can do today, immediately, to take your first steps on the path to better health. *Step 2: Your Ultimate Grocery List* details foods that have been proven to be beneficial, and I've arranged them in convenient grocery-aisle shopping lists. *Step 3: Going Above and Beyond* is a list of next steps, additional activities, supplements worth considering, or lifestyle changes that will improve your chances for success. *Step 4: Meal Plans* includes menus with the right mix of all the best foods—arranged into breakfast, lunch, dinner, and snack options—to help you accomplish your goals. Plus, each chapter contains at least two nutrient-rich (and delicious!) recipes.

Common old-school wisdom says that you should eat breakfast as if you were royalty, lunch as if you were rich, and dinner as if you were flat broke. What this means is that breakfast, which jump-starts your day with energy and nutrition, really is the most important meal. Lunch is also essential to keeping up your strength and stamina. Dinner is much less important because it comes at the end of the day, when you really don't need much fuel to carry you to bedtime. So ideally, you should eat the most calories at breakfast, nearly as many calories at lunch, and very few calories at dinner. Although I'm a health expert, I'm also a realist. I understand that the world doesn't work this way, so I've structured my meal plans to reflect the way people really eat. In each meal plan in every chapter, breakfast options are only 300 to 400 calories, lunch options are 400 to 500 calories, and dinner options are 500 to 600 calories.

So now that you've had a basic tour, it's time to choose where you want to start.

## HOW TO CHOOSE WHICH PROGRAM TO FOLLOW

I bet that you already know which health issue you want—or need—to tackle first. Wait . . . don't tell me . . . could it be weight loss?

Unwanted pounds are the primary concern for about 60 percent of my clients, either because of how that extra weight makes them feel or because it contributes to another health disorder, such as diabetes or heart disease. If weight is an issue for you, begin by reading Weight Loss (page 17). It explains the basic mechanisms of losing weight and reveals some of the secrets used by models, dancers, athletes, and other body-conscious individuals. After more than 20 years spent working with CEOs and store clerks, A-list celebrities and struggling musicians, supermodels and prima ballerinas, Olympic gold medalists and couch potatoes, I know what works. There is no one-size-fits-all plan. However, overweight people share many common struggles, and I present universal tricks that have been tested over and over again by my clients who have successfully lost weight and kept it off. If weight is your primary medical problem, then follow Joy's 4-Step Program for Weight Loss (page 39) from beginning to end.

If you have other health issues in addition to being overweight, I recommend reading the weight-loss chapter first to learn what your daily caloric intake should be and so that you understand how to apply my general principles. Follow one week of my 4-Step Program for Weight Loss. Then look in the table of contents for the chapter that addresses your next most pressing health problem, read that chapter, and follow that 4-Step Program. You won't lose out on weight loss, because the meal plans I provide in every chapter are scaled to help you drop pounds. If you follow the plans precisely, your three meals and one or two daily snacks will amount to 1,400 to 1,900 calories, depending upon the specific foods you choose. That's well below the 2,000 to 5,000 calories most Americans eat every day. So whether you follow the program for beauty, mood, migraines, or celiac disease, you will always have the chance to eat delicious foods and lose weight.

If weight is not an issue for you, congratulations! Either you have been blessed with the kind of metabolism that would make most people envious or you have worked hard to maintain your weight. If you are part of this lucky minority, use the same food lists and meal plans listed in each chapter, but let your hunger cues guide portion size.

No matter which chapter you choose to focus on, the information in the 4-Step Program is your road map to success. But like all maps, it is designed for general navigation—it is not a single strict path. Feel free to make adjustments for your personal taste and circumstances, as long as you stay within the general guidelines. For example, I might recommend a dinner of grilled salmon with a sweet potato and a mixed green salad with tomatoes and walnuts. If salmon isn't your favorite, choose another fish from the options given on the grocery list. Or, if you are eating out and they don't have sweet potatoes, ask for a serving of brown rice or a baked white potato instead. If tomatoes aren't in season, choose any mixed side salad and you'll still be within the general meal plan guidelines. If you only have time to microwave a frozen dinner, choose one that includes a grilled fish, a whole grain, and a vegetable. Similarly, if you are at a diner for an omelet breakfast, the cook certainly won't use a nonstick cooking spray on the griddle. So order an egg white omelet, ask them to fill it with your choice of vegetables, and eat your whole wheat toast dry to compensate (at least somewhat) for the butter or grease used to cook the omelet. I provide the ultimate combinations of foods in calorie-controlled portions, and you provide the creativity to make them work in your life.

## TOP TIPS FOR THINKING LIKE A NUTRITIONIST

Before you begin, let me offer some helpful hints that will help you succeed, even if you've never been able to stick to a diet before.

1. **Preplan meals as much as possible.** Don't wait until you're starving before looking in the pantry. If it's 8:00 p.m. and all you have in there are canned beans and potato chips, chances are you'll opt for the latter. Try to shop on the same days of the week, every week, so you always have healthy, satisfying foods on hand. If you plan your lunch and dinner in the morning, while you're having breakfast, you'll be able to pick up any missing ingredients during the day.

2. **Use the meal plans as a starting place.** The chapter meal plans include the recommended foods in portions and combinations that are nutritionally sound and promote weight maintenance or loss. They are valuable if you want to follow them to the letter, but they also work as examples. Feel free to substitute other foods from your chapter's Ultimate Grocery List.

3. **Purge your home of unhealthy foods.** Get rid of indulgences that you tend to crave and overeat. If you need to buy treats for your kids, choose snacks that you don't enjoy. That way, they can have their goodies and you won't be tempted. Maybe later on, when you are feeling stronger and more in control of your cravings, you can bring whatever your personal "gotta have 'em" foods are back into your life.

4. **Load up on vegetables.** Eat vegetables whenever you can, in almost any quantity. There is no greater source of vitamins, minerals, and disease-fighting phytochemicals than vegetables. Aim to eat three to eight servings of vegetables daily.

5. **Eat two-plus servings of fresh fruits daily.** Fruits are healthy, but they are higher in calories and sugar than vegetables. Aim to eat two to four servings of fresh fruit daily. Calorie-laden fruit juices are another story; you'll want to strictly limit them.

6. **Choose whole over white.** White flour is whole wheat flour, but with the healthy fiber and other nutrients taken out. White rice is the same as brown rice, but also stripped of its nutritional benefits. Whenever possible, go for whole grains over refined white grains.

7. **Account for liquid calories.** High-calorie beverages can undo even the best weight-loss efforts if you forget to figure them into your daily calorie count. Fruit juice and whole milk contain healthy nutrients, but they're also very caloric. Soda is full of sugar and almost nothing else, and wine, beer, and liquor also contain more calories than you may think. To enjoy greater quantities of healthy foods without gaining weight, choose no-cal beverage options, such as water, naturally flavored seltzer, and unsweetened coffee and tea.

8. **Be wary of alcohol.** Besides being caloric, alcohol can lower your inhibitions, which may make it more difficult to stick to your nutritional plan. In some chapters, you'll be advised to avoid alcohol altogether, but unless specifically noted, you can certainly drink in moderation. Most health professionals define *moderate* as one glass daily for women and two glasses daily for men. If you regularly drink more than that, I recommend cutting down for the sake of your overall health.

9. **Don't forget breakfast, and eat within 90 minutes of waking.** You're fasting for as long as you sleep, and your body needs to energize for the day ahead. That's what breakfast is for. It is your best opportunity to start each day on the right nutritional track.

10. **Maintain the right mix of foods.** Try to eat a combination of high-quality proteins and carbohydrates at every meal. You'll be energized throughout the day, and you'll stay fuller longer. In addition, combining foods will help your body maintain optimal levels of brain and other body chemicals. (My plans include high-quality carbs and proteins in all meals, with the exception of the dinners in my Insomnia chapter, where carbs are the focus to help induce sleep.)

11. **Fill up on fiber.** Fiber—which is naturally found in vegetables, fruits, starchy beans, lentils, and whole grains—helps fill you up, lowers your cholesterol, regulates your system, stabilizes your blood sugar, and more. My meal plans are loaded with fiber, so you don't have to worry about counting grams.

12. **Aim for three-plus servings of calcium-rich foods daily.** Calcium does more than just build strong bones: It is also necessary for muscle function and blood pressure management. You can get plenty of it from dairy foods, some leafy green vegetables, fortified juice and milk alternatives, almonds, fortified cereals, and canned fish with bones, like salmon and sardines.

13. **Eat every four to five hours.** Eating regularly will help you maintain a stable blood sugar level, which is important for many health issues in this book and also for general well-being, focus, and energy.

14. **Exercise every day.** Fitness is part of nutrition. It allows us to burn extra calories, use nutrients efficiently, keep our minds active, strengthen our bones and muscles, and much more.

15. **Curb your calories after 8:00 p.m.** If you are hungry after dinner, enjoy a small snack of 200 calories or less. (Nearly all snacks listed in my meal plans fit this bill.) If you have a history of nighttime nibbling, find a way to shut out food as an option after you finish dinner. Perhaps you could have a cup of herbal tea instead—and then close down the kitchen and brush and floss your teeth. Eventually, your body will recognize the tea as a sign that eating is over, and the urge to snack will subside.

16. **Watch out for weekends.** It is easiest to stay with the program during the week, when your time is probably more structured. If you understand in advance that following the eating plans might be more difficult on weekends and vacations, you can make a plan of attack. Make it a point to structure your downtime until the program becomes second nature.

17. **Be patient.** Although a few chapters contain nutrition changes that will have immediate effects on your health and body, most of the fixes here work gradually. Some have invisible results, such as changes in cholesterol, which may not be noticeable until you have blood work done. It is important to give this program at least six weeks. Resist all temptation to stop early. You'll be proud of yourself and thrilled with the results.

## FINAL WORDS OF ADVICE

I don't expect you to eat perfectly 100 percent of the time. Even nutritionists have days when we indulge our food lusts. But I make healthy foods my habit and rich desserts an occasional treat. If you really want to think like a nutritionist, start by becoming mindful of your eating habits. The good ones are your keys for overall health, weight management, and quality of life. Think of the indulgences as luxuries you can only occasionally afford.

I know you can do this. Go ahead, find your starting chapter, and dive in!

Visit Food Cures online at www.joybauer.com for customized nutrition advice, interactive quizzes, printable shopping lists, and much more information on how food affects your health.

# PART 2

# LOSING WEIGHT

# CHAPTER 3

# WEIGHT LOSS

f you are reading this chapter, then you've decided you want to lose weight. Good for you! I'm going to help you do it.

Unwanted pounds are the number one reason people come to see me. Some of my clients are hundreds of pounds overweight; others have been trying for years to drop just 10 pounds. Some people are referred by doctors because their weight puts them at high risk of certain disorders, while others want to fit into a wedding dress or return to their wedding weight in time for an anniversary or a big birthday. I advise actors and actresses who need to look a particular way for a role, athletes who need to boost their strength and energy, and fashion models who need to be thin but not emaciated. No matter what your personal reasons or motivations, I'm thrilled that you have made the commitment to a healthier, slimmer you. Whatever brought you here, welcome to the party!

Yes, you read that correctly: This is a party, not a dreary march down a dark and fruitless dieting path. A plan that has enjoyed as much success as this one is a cause for celebration. Just think: By this time next year, you can be significantly slimmer, several sizes smaller, more active and agile, and feeling happier and healthier than ever. Better still, you'll feel great throughout your entire journey. While losing weight is your overall goal, the process of getting there is incredibly empowering. After just one week following my 4-Step Program for Weight Loss, most people feel more confident and in control, they sleep better and feel more alert during the day, and their clothes are more comfortable. After a month, my clients are reveling in their newfound energy and can't imagine going back to their old ways. After three months, friends start asking them for their weight-loss secrets. Your commitment is the first essential step in this process, and visible results aren't far behind.

## WEIGHT-LOSS BASICS

Most of my clients know quite a bit about the mechanics of weight loss. Chances are you do, too, so I'm not going to go into exhaustive detail. I'll just review enough of the basics so that you understand the reasons behind some of my recommendations. I will also include client stories and weight-loss lessons to help you avoid some potential traps.

## HOW MUCH SHOULD YOU WEIGH?

Are you overweight?

The answer is not as straightforward as you might think. Sure, there are scales and charts and different scientific methods for calculating "fatness," but determining whether a particular person is overweight isn't as easy as saying whether a light is on or off. Contextual factors play a role in judging whether someone is carrying extra pounds. Ballerinas and sumo wrestlers, for instance, have very different definitions of overweight. Physicians and their patients may have different definitions, too. Like judging artwork or the taste of a meal, there is an aspect of weight that is less scientific and more subjective. That's why it's important to give yourself a "weight reality check" using standardized tools, such as body mass index (BMI) and waist circumference.

### Body Mass Index

Ever hear someone say "I'm not fat, I'm just short for my weight"? That is one way to look at it. When doctors decide who is or is not overweight, they rely on charts and calculations that provide a range of healthy weights based on height. It's important for them (and you!) to know if you are overweight, because hundreds of scientific studies confirm that those extra pounds increase the risk of many types of diseases, and losing weight can reduce those risks.

In order to standardize the height-weight relationship to a simple numerical scale, scientists created the body mass index. BMI is a basic calculation that takes into consideration both your height and weight measurements and simplifies them into a single number.

By using this chart, you can compute your BMI and then use it to determine whether you fall into a healthy weight range. There are five BMI categories.

- ◆ Underweight: BMI under 18.5
- ◆ Normal weight: BMI of 18.5 to 24.9
- ◆ Overweight: BMI of 25 to 29.9
- ◆ Obese: BMI of 30 to 39.9
- ◆ Extreme obesity: BMI over 40

Using the BMI calculation, people are considered overweight or obese if they carry more weight than what is usually expected for someone of their height. For example, a 5-foot-8 woman who weighs 155 pounds has a BMI of 23.6 and falls into the "normal weight" category. However, a 5-foot-4 woman who weighs 155 pounds has a BMI of 26.6 and falls into the "overweight" category. At the same weight, a woman who is 5 feet tall is classified as "obese" with a BMI of 30.3.

BMI is not perfect, but it's a pretty reliable—not to mention quick and inexpensive—indicator that can be easily calculated during any physical examination. If you haven't already checked out where you fall on these charts, check now. Do the charts say you are overweight? If so, and you're not overly muscular (i.e., a body builder), chances are the charts are right.

## Waist Circumference

Body mass index provides a quick-and-dirty assessment of total body fatness, but health experts now know that body fat distribution, or where you carry your fat on your body, is just as important, if not more so, than the amount of extra fat you're toting around. Research has shown that fat stored around the midsection is the most dangerous, toxic type of fat. Belly fat is associated with insulin resistance and

### Body Mass Index Table

| | Normal | | | | | | Overweight | | | | | Obese | | | | | | | | | | Extreme Obesity | | | | | | | | | | | | | | |
|---|---|---|---|---|---|---|---|---|---|---|---|---|---|---|---|---|---|---|---|---|---|---|---|---|---|---|---|---|---|---|---|---|---|---|---|---|
| BMI | 19 | 20 | 21 | 22 | 23 | 24 | 25 | 26 | 27 | 28 | 29 | 30 | 31 | 32 | 33 | 34 | 35 | 36 | 37 | 38 | 39 | 40 | 41 | 42 | 43 | 44 | 45 | 46 | 47 | 48 | 49 | 50 | 51 | 52 | 53 | 54 |
| Height (inches) | | | | | | | | | | | | Body Weight (pounds) | | | | | | | | | | | | | | | | | | | | | | | | |
| 58 | 91 | 96 | 100 | 105 | 110 | 115 | 119 | 124 | 129 | 134 | 138 | 143 | 148 | 153 | 158 | 162 | 167 | 172 | 177 | 181 | 186 | 191 | 196 | 201 | 205 | 210 | 215 | 220 | 224 | 229 | 234 | 239 | 244 | 248 | 253 | 258 |
| 59 | 94 | 99 | 104 | 109 | 114 | 119 | 124 | 128 | 133 | 138 | 143 | 148 | 153 | 158 | 163 | 168 | 173 | 178 | 183 | 188 | 193 | 198 | 203 | 208 | 212 | 217 | 222 | 227 | 232 | 237 | 242 | 247 | 252 | 257 | 262 | 267 |
| 60 | 97 | 102 | 107 | 112 | 118 | 123 | 128 | 133 | 138 | 143 | 148 | 153 | 158 | 163 | 168 | 174 | 179 | 184 | 189 | 194 | 199 | 204 | 209 | 215 | 220 | 225 | 230 | 235 | 240 | 245 | 250 | 255 | 261 | 266 | 271 | 276 |
| 61 | 100 | 106 | 111 | 116 | 122 | 127 | 132 | 137 | 143 | 148 | 153 | 158 | 164 | 169 | 174 | 180 | 185 | 190 | 195 | 201 | 206 | 211 | 217 | 222 | 227 | 232 | 238 | 243 | 248 | 254 | 259 | 264 | 269 | 275 | 280 | 285 |
| 62 | 104 | 109 | 115 | 120 | 126 | 131 | 136 | 142 | 147 | 153 | 158 | 164 | 169 | 175 | 180 | 186 | 191 | 196 | 202 | 207 | 213 | 218 | 224 | 229 | 235 | 240 | 246 | 251 | 256 | 262 | 267 | 273 | 278 | 284 | 289 | 295 |
| 63 | 107 | 113 | 118 | 124 | 130 | 135 | 141 | 146 | 152 | 158 | 163 | 169 | 175 | 180 | 186 | 191 | 197 | 203 | 208 | 214 | 220 | 225 | 231 | 237 | 242 | 248 | 254 | 259 | 265 | 270 | 278 | 282 | 287 | 293 | 299 | 304 |
| 64 | 110 | 116 | 122 | 128 | 134 | 140 | 145 | 151 | 157 | 163 | 169 | 174 | 180 | 186 | 192 | 197 | 204 | 209 | 215 | 221 | 227 | 232 | 238 | 244 | 250 | 256 | 262 | 267 | 273 | 279 | 285 | 291 | 296 | 302 | 308 | 314 |
| 65 | 114 | 120 | 126 | 132 | 138 | 144 | 150 | 156 | 162 | 168 | 174 | 180 | 186 | 192 | 198 | 204 | 210 | 216 | 222 | 228 | 234 | 240 | 246 | 252 | 258 | 264 | 270 | 276 | 282 | 288 | 294 | 300 | 306 | 312 | 318 | 324 |
| 66 | 118 | 124 | 130 | 136 | 142 | 148 | 155 | 161 | 167 | 173 | 179 | 186 | 192 | 198 | 204 | 210 | 216 | 223 | 229 | 235 | 241 | 247 | 253 | 260 | 266 | 272 | 278 | 284 | 291 | 297 | 303 | 309 | 315 | 322 | 328 | 334 |
| 67 | 121 | 127 | 134 | 140 | 146 | 153 | 159 | 166 | 172 | 178 | 185 | 191 | 198 | 204 | 211 | 217 | 223 | 230 | 236 | 242 | 249 | 255 | 261 | 268 | 274 | 280 | 287 | 293 | 299 | 306 | 312 | 319 | 325 | 331 | 338 | 344 |
| 68 | 125 | 131 | 138 | 144 | 151 | 158 | 164 | 171 | 177 | 184 | 190 | 197 | 203 | 210 | 216 | 223 | 230 | 236 | 243 | 249 | 256 | 262 | 269 | 276 | 282 | 289 | 295 | 302 | 308 | 315 | 322 | 328 | 335 | 341 | 348 | 354 |
| 69 | 128 | 135 | 142 | 149 | 155 | 162 | 169 | 176 | 182 | 189 | 196 | 203 | 209 | 216 | 223 | 230 | 236 | 243 | 250 | 257 | 263 | 270 | 277 | 284 | 291 | 297 | 304 | 311 | 318 | 324 | 331 | 338 | 345 | 351 | 358 | 365 |
| 70 | 132 | 139 | 146 | 153 | 160 | 167 | 174 | 181 | 188 | 195 | 202 | 209 | 216 | 222 | 229 | 236 | 243 | 250 | 257 | 264 | 271 | 278 | 285 | 292 | 299 | 306 | 313 | 320 | 327 | 334 | 341 | 348 | 355 | 362 | 369 | 376 |
| 71 | 136 | 143 | 150 | 157 | 165 | 172 | 179 | 186 | 193 | 200 | 208 | 215 | 222 | 229 | 236 | 243 | 250 | 257 | 265 | 272 | 279 | 286 | 293 | 301 | 308 | 315 | 322 | 329 | 338 | 343 | 351 | 358 | 365 | 372 | 379 | 386 |
| 72 | 140 | 147 | 154 | 162 | 169 | 177 | 184 | 191 | 199 | 206 | 213 | 221 | 228 | 235 | 242 | 250 | 258 | 265 | 272 | 279 | 287 | 294 | 302 | 309 | 316 | 324 | 331 | 338 | 346 | 353 | 361 | 368 | 375 | 383 | 390 | 397 |
| 73 | 144 | 151 | 159 | 166 | 174 | 182 | 189 | 197 | 204 | 212 | 219 | 227 | 235 | 242 | 250 | 257 | 265 | 272 | 280 | 288 | 295 | 302 | 310 | 318 | 325 | 333 | 340 | 348 | 355 | 363 | 371 | 378 | 386 | 393 | 401 | 408 |
| 74 | 148 | 155 | 163 | 171 | 179 | 186 | 194 | 202 | 210 | 218 | 225 | 233 | 241 | 249 | 256 | 264 | 272 | 280 | 287 | 295 | 303 | 311 | 319 | 326 | 334 | 342 | 350 | 358 | 365 | 373 | 381 | 389 | 396 | 404 | 412 | 420 |
| 75 | 152 | 160 | 168 | 176 | 184 | 192 | 200 | 208 | 216 | 224 | 232 | 240 | 248 | 256 | 264 | 272 | 279 | 287 | 295 | 303 | 311 | 319 | 327 | 335 | 343 | 351 | 359 | 367 | 375 | 383 | 391 | 399 | 407 | 415 | 423 | 431 |
| 76 | 156 | 164 | 172 | 180 | 189 | 197 | 205 | 213 | 221 | 230 | 238 | 246 | 254 | 263 | 271 | 279 | 287 | 295 | 304 | 312 | 320 | 328 | 336 | 344 | 353 | 361 | 369 | 377 | 385 | 394 | 402 | 410 | 418 | 426 | 435 | 443 |

Source: Adapted from *Clinical Guidelines on the Identification, Evaluation, and Treatment of Overweight and Obesity in Adults: The Evidence Report.*

increased levels of inflammation throughout the body. Individuals who carry most of their extra weight around their middle are at increased risk of heart disease, stroke, type 2 diabetes, and dementia, compared with individuals who carry their weight in their hips and thighs.

BMI doesn't take into account body fat distribution, but fortunately, a simple waist circumference measurement succeeds where the BMI fails. Waist circumference is a good indicator of how much abdominal fat is lying under the skin, and therefore it's a reliable predictor of disease risk.

To determine your waist circumference, all you need is an inexpensive flexible tape measure. Wrap the tape measure around your waist just above your hip bone. Make sure the tape is parallel to the floor all the way around. To take your measurement, relax, exhale, and pull the tape measure so it is snug but not squeezing into your skin. (No sucking in or holding your breath allowed!)

For men, a waist circumference higher than 40 inches is considered high risk. For women, a waist circumference over 35 inches is high risk. If your waist circumference falls above these cutoffs, you should make weight loss a priority, even if your BMI is in the normal range.

## Personal Evaluation

In addition to these mathematical formulations and charts, there is another expert you need to consult on the question of fatness—your own gut (pun intended). Do *you* think you are overweight?

Losing weight shouldn't be about pleasing other people or meeting some arbitrary social standard. Losing weight is about feeling great, both physically and emotionally. You know yourself and your body better than anyone else. You know your energy level, how well you're sleeping, whether your appetite is under control, and how your waist size has changed in the past year or two (or ten). You know whether you've been dragging or feeling energetic and fit. And you know whether you are happy with the way you look and feel. That counts for a lot.

Weight loss requires hard work, faith in yourself, and a dream for your future. If it comes down to a battle between numbers on a BMI chart and emotions, emotions win every time. Your doctor can advise you, but he or she can't give you incentive. That's why I always encourage my clients to get in touch with their true motivation for wanting to lose weight: something to keep them going that has nothing to do with the numbers.

Take a moment now and think about your weight-loss motivations. You might be inspired by a milestone event you hope to enjoy with your family, like seeing your child graduate from college. It can be as simple as wanting to fit into a particular designer outfit or as complex as the pure frustration you feel because of a weight issue that has stuck with you since childhood. Whatever your reasons, embrace them. They will carry you forward to success.

## CALORIES COUNT

Calories are a measure of how much energy food provides. We need calories to do chores, run after the kids, make it through a full day of work, or go out with friends. All body processes use energy, too, including breathing, digesting, growing hair and fingernails, and making hormones and enzymes. Even the most inactive sofa sloth needs a certain number of calories to get through the day, and active people need quite a bit more.

Here is the weight-loss formula: If you take in more energy (from food calories) than you use, the excess gets stored as body fat—most noticeably around your waist, hips, or thighs. If you use more energy than you take in, then your body gets the energy it needs by breaking down the stored fat, and you lose weight. Using up more calories than you eat is what it takes to slim down. Of course, you and I and everyone on the planet knows that it is easier said than done.

### Calorie Calculations

If your goal is to burn more calories than you take in, you need to know how many calories your body needs on an average day. There's a mathematical formula I use to make this estimate. Although this calculation can be incredibly helpful, it doesn't take into account genetics, age, and muscular makeup, all of which play an important role in the number of calories you burn each day. As we go along, I'll run through the numbers with a hypothetical 180-pound woman (height doesn't matter here).

1. Take your current weight (in pounds) and multiply it by 10. That's the number of calories your body needs just to keep breathing and digesting and doing all that other maintenance work. This is called your basal metabolic rate (BMR).

*180 pounds × 10 = 1,800 calories (BMR)*

2. Determine your activity level.

   • Average activity level: 0.30 (little to no regular exercise)

   • More active than most: 0.40 (light, planned exercise or sports one to three times per week)

   • Very active: 0.50 (moderate, planned exercise or sports three to five times per week)

   • Extremely active: 0.60 (vigorous, planned exercise or sports five to seven times per week)

For our example, let's say the activity level is average:

*Activity level = 0.30*

3.  Multiply your BMR by your activity level. This is your activity factor. (I'll talk more about this concept later!)

*1,800 (BMR) × 0.30 (activity level) = 540 (activity factor)*

4.  Add your BMR and your activity factor to get your maintenance calories. You need about this many calories to make it through an average day. (Important note: When you lose weight, you'll have to recalculate your numbers.) If you eat this exact number of calories, you will neither gain nor lose weight—you will maintain your current weight:

*1,800 (BMR) + 540 (activity factor) = 2,340 (maintenance calories)*

So, for our 180-pound woman to maintain her weight, she should eat approximately 2,340 calories a day. (Remember, these calculations are not an exact science.) But, of course, you don't want to stay the same weight, do you? If you want to lose weight, you have to eat fewer calories than your maintenance calories. The greater the difference between your maintenance calories and the number of calories you eat daily, the faster you will lose weight. In our example, the maintenance calories are 2,340. Eating 1,800 calories per day will result in weight loss:

*2,340 (maintenance calories) – 1,800 (actual calories) = 540 weight-loss calories*

In order to lose a pound of fat, you need to accrue 3,500 weight-loss calories. In our example, the 540 weight-loss calories "spent" per day adds up to 97,200 weight-loss calories over a six-month period (180 days), which yields a projected weight loss of about 28 pounds in six months.

Reducing calories further to only 1,600 calories per day will result in faster weight loss:

*2,340 (maintenance calories) – 1,600 (actual calories) = 740 weight-loss calories*

These 740 weight-loss calories per day add up to 133,200 weight-loss calories over a six-month period, which yields a projected weight loss of about 38 pounds in six months. Important note: Do not eat fewer than 1,000 actual calories per day. There is no advantage to ultra-low-calorie dieting—your metabolism will slow, you'll be more likely to binge due to ravenous hunger and feelings of deprivation, and you may develop some vitamin and mineral deficiencies from not eating enough healthy food.

Remember, you plug more than just the calories you eat into the equation—there's also your activity level. If you increase your maintenance calories by upping your activity level, you'll also speed up weight loss. For example, if our hypothetical woman increases her activity to the 0.40 level, she will raise her maintenance calories to 2,520:

*1,800 (BMR) × 0.40 (activity level) = 720 (activity factor)*

*1,800 (BMR) + 720 (activity factor) = 2,520 (maintenance calories)*

Eating 1,800 calories per day will result in weight loss:

*2,520 (maintenance calories) – 1,800 (actual calories) = 720 weight-loss calories*

These 720 weight-loss calories per day add up to 129,600 weight-loss calories over a six-month period, which yields a projected weight loss of about 47 pounds in six months.

But eating only 1,600 calories per day will result in faster weight loss:

*2,520 (maintenance calories) – 1,600 (actual calories) = 920 weight-loss calories*

These 920 weight-loss calories per day add up to 335,800 weight-loss calories per year, which yields a projected weight loss of about 96 pounds in a year.

Notice that even at the same calorie levels, weight loss is faster when you bump up the exercise and give your metabolism a boost. In our example, if the same 180-pound woman ate 1,800 calories per day, she could lose 28 pounds in six months with an average activity level—but 37 pounds in six months by increasing her activity level just one notch above average.

## BOOSTING METABOLISM

One of the most frequently asked questions I get from viewers, clients, neighbors, and friends is: How can I boost my metabolism?

Metabolism is simply the total amount of calories burned through all body processes—your basal metabolic rate plus your activity factor. When it comes to improving your metabolism, there's good news and bad news.

First, the bad news: Most of what controls your metabolism isn't under your control. Some people are genetically blessed with a high-burning metabolism. They didn't ask for it, they were born with it. (So don't hate them for it—unless, of course, they rub it in!) On average, men have a metabolism that is 10 to 15 percent higher than women's, mainly because of their larger size and greater muscle mass. Whether you're a man or a woman, your metabolism naturally decreases with age. Scientists have estimated that metabolism slows about 2 percent per decade, beginning at age 30, as we experience physiological changes such as a decrease in muscle mass. Hypothyroidism (underactive thyroid) lowers metabolism and causes weight gain. Fortunately, in this case, if a blood test confirms there's a problem, your doctor will prescribe medication that can boost it back up to baseline.

Now the good news: Your metabolism doesn't have to remain stagnant or take a nosedive. You can burn more calories and lose more weight just by changing the way you eat and move.

## Food Fixes for Metabolism

Remember—our basal metabolic rate includes the energy we need for body processes, including digestion. About 10 percent of our calories are used to process the

## FAQS

**I'm tempted to try one of those metabolism-boosting supplements I see advertised on TV. Do you recommend them?**

If over-the-counter supplements worked, no one would be overweight. The supplements that are supposed to boost metabolism fall into two main categories: those that are simply ineffective and those with stimulant ingredients that may cause a dangerous rise in heart rate and/or blood pressure. When the minor effect of the stimulants wears off, your metabolism soon returns to normal. As much as we wish otherwise, there is no quick fix for weight loss. Even prescription weight-loss medications don't work as well as the scientists who developed them hoped. As of right now, your best bet is healthy food in moderate portions and exercise.

foods we eat. As the calories are burned, our bodies generate heat. This phenomenon, known as the thermic effect of food, is influenced by how much, how often, and what we eat. In addition, food can directly affect metabolism by altering the way the body functions (which changes the amount of energy it needs). Here are my best recommendations for maximizing metabolism.

◆ **Eat at least 1,000 calories per day.** Although it is generally true that eating a low-calorie diet will help you take off weight, if you eat too few calories, your metabolism will get slower and slower as it tries to conserve energy. More important, eating too few calories could backfire and cause you to binge or overeat in response to extreme restriction.

◆ **Eat every four to five hours.** A regular meal schedule helps keep your body working to digest and absorb foods and will prevent you from getting ravenous and overeating. Between breakfast and bed, aim to eat a meal or small snack every four to five hours. And try to eat breakfast within 90 minutes of rising: It helps fire up your metabolism after a full night on a slow simmer. People who regularly eat a healthy breakfast are more likely to control their weight.

◆ **Eat protein with every meal.** All foods contribute to the thermic effect, which means that all macronutrients—carbohydrates, fats, and proteins—help give metabolism a gentle nudge higher when we eat them. But protein has the greatest thermic effect of all. In addition, protein can increase metabolism by helping maintain and build muscle mass. (For more information about good sources of protein, see page 26.)

## Exercise Fixes for Metabolism

A big percentage of your maintenance calories—the amount you burn in the course of a day—comes from your activity level. If you go from having average activity levels to being extremely active, you can double the amount of calories burned (that's activity factor calories, not BMR calories). This is why any activity—every extra step you take—can help boost your metabolism. Part of my recommendation is to move as much as possible: Climb the stairs instead of taking the escalator, park at the opposite end of the mall and walk to your favorite store, garden instead of watching TV . . . anything, as long as it involves extra movement.

In addition, I strongly encourage everyone to work out regularly. The optimal weight-loss fitness program consists of both aerobic exercise and strength training. Regular exercise can increase your activity factor and your metabolism. As you get older and your metabolism slows, you can rebalance your energy needs by increasing the duration or intensity of your workouts.

◆ **Aerobic exercise.** Aerobic exercises (commonly known as cardio) use energy and increase many different metabolic processes (such as your heart rate), all of which burn calories. All aerobic activities—including running, brisk walking, swimming, skating, skiing, and cycling—increase metabolism while you're exercising and also keep your metabolism burning higher for hours afterward. I recommend doing some form of aerobic activity four or five days per week for at least 30 minutes per day.

◆ **Strength training.** Strength-training exercises strengthen and tone your muscles. Try lifting weights, working with resistance bands, or doing yoga, Pilates, circuit training, and calisthenics (including pushups, chinups, and abdominal crunches). These activities directly raise your BMR by increasing muscle mass—which is more metabolically active than fat and helps you burn more calories every minute of every day. I recommend doing some form of strength training two or three days per week. Plan a strength-training regimen that's realistic for you and your schedule. That may mean 15 minutes of calisthenics in the privacy of your bedroom or a more elaborate weight-training regimen at the gym.

## HOW FOOD AFFECTS WEIGHT AND WEIGHT LOSS

You probably know exactly which foods are healthy choices and which are guilty pleasures. With every meal and snack, you have an opportunity to decide which direction to go—you can make the energizing, slimming choice or fall back on one of the choices that brought you to this chapter in the first place. Whenever you choose comforting, familiar junk food instead of healthy meals, that's a fallback choice. Whenever you eat the wrong foods to reduce stress, that's a fallback choice. If you ever sneak food or find yourself thinking *I know it's bad but what the heck,* you're making a fallback choice.

Don't you deserve more than the fallback? Of course you do! Remember this: The taste of food remains in your mouth for a very short time, but the calorie consequences remain *long* after. Before you go with a fallback choice, consider how defeated you'll feel 30 minutes after finishing it. Then consider how fabulous you'll feel 30 minutes after finishing a healthful, nutrient-rich food. Don't make the wrong choice for short-term satisfaction. Instead, make the right choice for long-term results! You deserve foods that can help you lose weight and lower your risk of disease.

### Lean Protein

As I already mentioned, eating protein can help raise metabolism because it has a high thermic effect and because it can help maintain and increase your lean muscle mass. Protein also keeps you feeling satisfied longer, so you are less likely to snack on high-calorie fallback foods between meals. In addition, when eaten as part of a well-rounded nutrition plan (which includes vegetables, high-quality carbohydrates, and healthy fats), protein helps keep your blood sugar at an even level. That means that you'll generally be in a better mood, better able to handle stress, and less likely to reach for comfort foods to get through the day.

The key is to add some protein but not go overboard. Most Americans already eat far too much protein—and usually the wrong kind. The wrong kind contains large amounts of saturated fat. I'm talking about hamburgers, hot dogs, salami, bologna, spareribs, high-fat dairy products (including whole and 2% milk and full-fat cheese), fried foods, and poultry skin. The right kind, the kind you should choose instead, is lean protein, such as skinless chicken and turkey, fish, low-fat or fat-free dairy products, beans, lentils, and whole soy foods. The meal plans in this chapter and throughout this book contain a healthy mix of proteins and other nutrients.

> **BEST FOODS FOR LEAN PROTEIN:** *skinless turkey and chicken, fish and shellfish, pork tenderloin, lean beef, egg whites, yogurt (fat-free, low-fat), milk (fat-free, 1%), cheese (fat-free, reduced-fat), starchy beans (such as black, navy, pinto, garbanzo, kidney), lentils, split peas, tofu, tempeh, soybeans (edamame), soy milk*

## High-Quality Carbohydrates

Just as there are superior protein choices for weight loss and good health, there are good (and poor) carbohydrate choices. Carbs are necessary because your body breaks them down into glucose, the kind of simple sugar used by your cells for energy. When we eat low-quality carbs, we're essentially dumping glucose into our bloodstream, which provides a quick rush of energy, followed eventually by a slump that causes us to eat more. It's a vicious cycle. A smart weight-loss plan limits or avoids low-quality carbs, including sugary baked goods and snacks, anything made with white flour, soda, and fruit juice.

High-quality carbs, on the other hand, are rich in vitamins, minerals, and fiber. Fiber is the unsung hero of weight loss. There are two kinds of fiber, both abundant in vegetables, fruits, and whole grains. The first, soluble fiber, turns gooey when digested and stabilizes your blood sugar, keeping you feeling full. The second, insoluble fiber, is a volumizer—it adds bulk to food, so you can eat a lot more without a lot of extra calories.

Fiber is critical to weight maintenance. Nutrition researchers at the University of Texas at Austin discovered that those who maintain a healthy weight eat 33 percent more fiber and 43 percent more complex carbohydrates than those who are overweight. By including fiber-rich, high-quality carbohydrates with your meals, you'll feel energetic, full, and satisfied as you slim down.

**BEST FOODS FOR HIGH-QUALITY CARBOHYDRATES:** *vegetables, fruits, starchy beans (such as black, navy, pinto, garbanzo, kidney), lentils, brown rice, wild rice, oats, whole grain cereal, whole grain bread, whole grain pasta, whole grain crackers, barley, bulgur, kamut, quinoa, amaranth, wheat berries, millet*

**BEST FOODS FOR SOLUBLE FIBER:** *psyllium seeds (ground), lima beans, starchy beans (such as black, navy, pinto, garbanzo, kidney), Brussels sprouts, oat bran, winter squash, parsnips, turnips, sweet potatoes, lentils, black-eyed peas, split peas, green peas, okra, eggplant, barley, oats, rice bran, guava, oranges, grapefruit, apples, peaches, plums, nectarines, pears, prunes, mangoes, strawberries, blackberries, raspberries, bananas, apricots, raisins, white potatoes, avocados, broccoli, carrots, green beans, spinach, cabbage, kale, wheat germ, ground flaxseed*

## Healthy Fats: Monounsaturated and Omega-3

Along with protein and carbs, fats are an important component of a good nutrition program. But they are not all created equal. Saturated fats (found mainly in full-fat dairy products and fatty meats) and trans fats (found in some stick margarines and packaged foods) are unhealthy fats that raise bad cholesterol levels and initiate inflammation throughout your body. On the other hand, healthy fats like omega-3 fatty acids (found mainly in fatty fish and some nuts and seeds) and monounsaturated fats (found mainly in olive oil, canola oil, avocados, and some nuts and seeds) play an important role in promoting overall health as well as weight loss. Healthy fats can help satiate your appetite and stabilize blood sugar levels. (My Best Foods list includes only the fatty fish that have been shown to be low in mercury, PCBs, and dioxins.)

Fats convey much of the flavor and texture that most people find—and here's the official term for it—yummy. It's natural to want to eat them. But both saturated and unsaturated fats contain more than twice the number of calories as the same weight of carbohydrates and proteins, so eating an ounce of a fatty food will cause you to put on more weight than an ounce of a nonfatty food will. Studies have shown that people who are overweight tend to have diets that are high in fat. In fact, some intervention studies have shown that, over the long run, people who reduce the amount of fat in their diets (especially the bad fats) and increase the amount of fiber they eat lose up to three times more weight than people who follow other types of diets.

The solution? Rid your diet of as much saturated fat as possible, and eat controlled portions of foods rich in healthy unsaturated fats.

**BEST FOODS FOR MONOUNSATURATED FATS:** *olive oil, canola oil, avocados, olives, macadamia nuts, hazelnuts, pecans, almonds, peanuts, cashews, Brazil* *nuts, pistachios, pine nuts, peanut butter, almond butter, cashew butter, maca-damia nut butter, sunflower seed butter*

BEST FOODS FOR OMEGA-3 FATTY ACIDS: *wild salmon (fresh, canned), her-ring, mackerel (not king), sardines, anchovies, rainbow trout, Pacific oysters, chia seeds, ground flaxseed, walnuts, butternuts (white walnuts), seaweed, wal-nut oil, canola oil, flaxseed oil, soybeans (edamame)*

## Juicy Foods

Some foods are mostly water, which is great when it comes to filling you up. Plain water goes right through you—it's absorbed or eliminated very quickly—but water that's integrated into food hangs around your stomach, making you feel full longer. Fortunately, these high-water-content foods are healthy fruits and vegetables. You still need to count the calories, but my successful clients know that making these foods a fixture in their daily menus is a big help in achieving their ideal weight.

BEST JUICY FOODS: *The following foods are at least 75 percent water (by weight): apples, artichokes, asparagus, beets, bell peppers, blackberries, blue-berries, broccoli, Brussels sprouts, cantaloupe, carrots, cauliflower, celery, cher-ries, cucumbers, grapefruit, grapes, honeydew, kale, kiwifruit, lemons, lettuce, limes, mangoes, mushrooms, nectarines, onions, oranges, papayas, peaches, pears, peas, pineapple, plums, potatoes, pumpkins, raspberries, rhubarb, spin-ach, squash, strawberries, tangerines, tomatoes, turnips, watermelon*

## THE PLAN: OVERVIEW

All the meal plans in this book (including the one in this chapter on page 42) have been calculated to provide 1,200 to 1,500 calories per day from meals alone. All of my meals break down like this: Each breakfast option provides 300 to 400 calories, each lunch option provides 400 to 500 calories, and each dinner option provides 500 to 600 calories. The additional calories you consume from snacks will be entirely up to you. You'll notice I provide snack options that are 100 calories or less and snack options that are 100 to 200 calories. Depending on your daily caloric goal, pay close attention to the number and kinds of snacks you consume.

If you want or need to lose weight and have other medical concerns to address, I recommend following my 4-Step Plan for Weight Loss for the first full week. This will show you the basics of a low-calorie meal plan, jump-start your metabolism,

## FAQS

### Is there a way I can lose belly fat first?

Unfortunately, no. When it comes to losing weight, your body has its own agenda, and it's just not possible to target a specific problem spot. But there's good news: When you eat less and move more, you burn fat from all over your body—and that means eventually (if not at first) your belly.

and help you drop a few pounds fast. Then, if you have other health concerns, turn to the appropriate chapter and follow the specific recommendations there. As mentioned earlier, the meal plans in every chapter hold to the same calorie limits, so you can continue to lose weight while addressing other health issues. There are three exceptions: If your primary concern is celiac disease, severe irritable bowel syndrome, or type 2 diabetes, read this chapter through to the end to understand the mechanics of weight loss, but don't follow the weight-loss meal plan. Instead, turn to your appropriate chapter, and begin that program immediately.

If weight loss is your primary concern, feel free to follow the 4-Step Plan for Weight Loss for as long as you like, or until you achieve your goal. The weight-loss meal plan contains custom-designed menus that are delicious and easy to follow. But if you prefer to create your own menus, use the following guidelines. They provide the basic building blocks for constructing healthy meals and snacks that will lead to weight loss while still allowing for personal flexibility. (Keep in mind that the meals listed in my custom-designed menus—in this and all other chapters—do not necessarily follow these guidelines. My calculations take into account many additional factors, but this is a good set of rules for simple meal planning.)

## MAKE-YOUR-OWN WEIGHT-LOSS MEALS

◆ At each meal, eat **ONE SERVING of high-quality starchy carbohydrates,** for a total of three servings per day. (During the first week, skip the dinner starch. It's an easy way to minimize calories during the meal at which people are most inclined to overeat.)

  **One serving** *of high-quality starchy carbs can include your choice of the following: 1 slice whole wheat bread; 2 slices reduced-calorie bread; ½ cup brown or wild rice; ½ cup whole wheat pasta; 1 mini whole wheat pita; ½ regular whole wheat pita; ½ medium baked white potato; ½ medium baked sweet potato; ¾ cup whole grain breakfast cereal; ½ cup dry plain oats; ½ whole grain English muffin; ½ cup peas; ½ cup corn; ½ cup starchy beans or lentils; ½ cup acorn or butternut squash.*

◆ At each meal, eat **ONE SERVING of lean protein.**

  **One serving** *of lean protein can include your choice of the following: 3 to 5 ounces lean meat, poultry, fish, or shellfish; 6 to 8 ounces tofu; 1 cup fat-free or 1% milk; 1 cup fat-free yogurt; 1 cup fat-free or 1% cottage cheese; 1 to 2 ounces fat-free or reduced-fat cheese; 1 whole egg plus 3 egg whites; ½ to ¾ cup starchy beans or lentils.*

◆ At each meal, eat no more than **ONE SERVING of fat.**

  **One serving** *of fat can include your choice of the following: 1 to 2 teaspoons olive oil; 1 tablespoon regular salad dressing; 2 to 4 tablespoons reduced-calorie salad dressing; 1 to 2 tablespoons nuts; 1 tablespoon peanut butter; 1 tablespoon regular cream cheese or 2 tablespoons light cream cheese; 1 tablespoon soft tub, trans-fat-free margarine; 1 to 2 tablespoons guacamole; 1 to 2 tablespoons reduced-fat mayonnaise or 1 to 2 teaspoons regular mayonnaise.*

◆ Every day, you may eat **UNLIMITED SERVINGS of nonstarchy vegetables** (all veggies are unlimited except corn, peas, winter squash, and potatoes).

◆ Every day, eat **TWO SERVINGS of fresh fruit.** These can be eaten at meals or as snacks.

> **One serving** *of fruit can include your choice of the following: 1 medium piece of fruit (apple, pear, peach, nectarine, orange, etc.); ½ banana; ½ mango, papaya, or grapefruit; ¼ cantaloupe; 1 cup berries, grapes, or cut-up melon; ¾ cup fresh fruit salad.*

◆ Before lunch and dinner, drink **TWO 8-ounce GLASSES of water.** Feel free to drink as much additional water as you like with your meals and throughout the day.

◆ Every day, feel free to eat **ONE FUN FOOD** (150 calories or less). This will help satisfy cravings and lessen the feelings of deprivation. If you choose, you may skip the treat and enjoy an additional serving of any of the food categories: fruit, high-quality starchy carbohydrate, protein, or fat.

## BEST LESSONS

To sum it all up, the ideal diet consists of moderate amounts of high-quality carbohydrates, lean protein, and healthy fats. I wish it could be sexier than that, but the information doesn't have to be exciting to work, and my program definitely works.

But human nature can find loopholes in even the simplest program. Some of my favorite weight-loss secrets have come from finding solutions for the problems posed by my unique and wonderful clients. I'm sure you'll find some answers here, too.

**Even very low-calorie foods can add up.** Christina is principal ballet dancer with a national company; she works diligently to perfect her craft and her body, putting in hours and hours at rehearsals every day. She came to see me because she had started gaining weight, despite counting every calorie. Her problem? Christina loved the "I Can't Believe It's Not Butter" spray. As the label says, a single serving of 5 sprays gives foods a buttery taste with zero calories. What Christina (and most people) didn't know was that each aerated spray serving has a little less than 1 calorie, and the label rounds down to zero. However, there are many, many servings per 8-ounce bottle, adding up to about 90 grams of fat and 900 calories. Because she thought the product had no calories, Christina went through an entire buttery bottle every day. When she broke the spray habit, the pounds dropped off. *The lesson: There are few foods you can eat in unlimited quantities. Even a so-called zero-calorie product can cause weight gain if you eat enough of it.*

**There is no reason to be a Sally.** In the movie *When Harry Met Sally,* there is a restaurant scene that shows Sally ordering a salad and pie à la mode. She wants her pie heated with ice cream on the side, strawberry not vanilla, but if there isn't strawberry then whipped cream, but only real whipped cream, and if there isn't real whipped cream then the pie shouldn't be heated. As her list of special demands goes on and on, we begin to understand that Sally is a high-maintenance kind of girl (adorably so, in that Meg Ryan way!). Many of my high-profile clients are understandably afraid of being labeled high maintenance or—even worse—a diva. They ask me about the best way to stick to their meal plans while attending a dinner party or public function without acting like a Sally. Simple. I tell them to eat a single portion of whatever they are served (no matter what it is). They can even eat a dessert (or half a dessert) if it will put them and their hosts at ease. The key is to eat extra carefully for the rest of the week. *The lesson: You can have a social life while trying to lose weight. Follow your meal plan as closely as possible when you are in control of cooking at home or ordering in a restaurant, but relax and allow yourself to be an easy dinner guest.*

**Starvation diets backfire.** Fashion model Rinna was convinced that if she lost just 10 more pounds she would be able to book more jobs, and she resorted to starving herself when nothing else worked. By the time she came to see me, she was depressed and desperate—her self-imposed diet had worked for a little while, but then she regained every pound. Rinna skipped breakfast, exercised in the morning, skipped lunch, drank diet sodas all day long, chewed sugarless gum, and ate a calorie-controlled dinner. Then came what she called her all-night eating orgy—nonstop bingeing on the limited food items she kept in her apartment (things like dry cereal, oatmeal, and toast with peanut butter and jam). Her body craved food! She would wake up the next morning feeling bloated and sluggish and then start the cycle all over again. We figured out that between 9:00 p.m. and midnight, she would eat about 2,200 calories—as much as many people eat all day! I encouraged her to start eating regular meals. She was terrified that she would gain even more weight—that she would eat all day and then eat all night, too! But eventually she trusted my experience and took the leap. She ate breakfast, lunch, an afternoon snack, dinner, and even a small snack before bed. After one week, she lost 4 pounds. All

## FAQS

### My husband and I both went on the same diet at the same time, but he's losing weight so much faster than I am. How come?

Men generally burn more calories than women just by living and breathing. On average, men are taller, heavier, and have more lean muscle mass than women. It takes more energy (in the form of calories) to fuel all the body processes necessary to keep his larger body going than it does to keep your body going. Plus, lean muscle mass increases metabolism, so his testosterone-fed muscles give him an automatic weight-loss advantage. Increasing your muscle mass through resistance training will give you a boost, but his weight loss will always be easier than yours. Try not to make losing weight a competition. Instead, plan a celebration every time one of you loses 10 pounds—with the two of you losing at different rates, you'll be able to celebrate twice as often.

10 pounds were gone after six weeks. *The lesson: You can feel good and look the way you want to, all while eating healthfully. Starvation is never a good choice, and it may even move you further from your goal.*

**Limit or eliminate alcoholic beverages.** Nearly every weekday, Scott—a brilliant CEO of a large, national company—meets with clients for lunch and dinner. These schmoozing fests often involve alcohol, sometimes two or three drinks each. Scott understands the use of alcohol as a social lubricant, but he has no particular craving for it himself. In fact, he would just as soon drink iced tea, but he wants clients to feel comfortable and typically matches them drink for drink. The problem, of course, is that alcohol is loaded with empty calories, and they contributed significantly to Scott's weight problem. Perhaps worse, the alcohol lowered Scott's usual inhibitions; his best-laid plans to make healthy menu choices crumbled after a couple of drinks, and decadent, calorie-rich desserts often followed full meals. We did two things that helped Scott take control while still enabling him to court clients. First, I made him promise that his first drink of the meal would be club soda, and then he would alternate between club soda and his standard vodka. That way, if the client had three drinks and Scott matched him order for order, Scott drank one vodka. He would not only save calories, he would also be sharper, less buzzed, and more aware throughout the meeting. Second, he changed the way he ordered his drink. Scott enjoyed the flavor of vodka straight up, with just a hint of extra flavor from a twist of lemon. We discovered that if he did without the lemon, he drank a little more slowly. The lemon twist made the drink go down easier. By removing the twist, his drinks lasted longer, so he ordered fewer of them. After just one week on his new routine, Scott lost 6 pounds. After four months, he had lost more than 30 pounds, and he was as gracious a host as ever. *The lesson: You can dilute the negative effects of alcohol on weight. Make each drink last as long as possible by removing your personal flavor "incentives." Also, always alternate alcoholic beverages with no-calorie drinks.*

**It is possible to get too much of a good thing.** Many of my most nutritionally knowledgeable clients are athletes. They know that their performances depend on good nutrition, so they do everything right. Emma is an Olympic medalist who was a nutrition fanatic. She ate whole grains, organic fruits and vegetables, fat-free dairy, and lean meats. She never ate sugar or white flour. And yet she still needed to drop about 15 pounds to get to her optimal performance weight. It was a joy to see such stellar eating habits, and I found it painful to nitpick at her diet. It came down to nuts. She loved walnuts and almonds. Nuts are a healthy food choice—rich in healthy fats, vitamins, and minerals—but I don't recommend eating more than a handful at one sitting. Emma ate a generous portion of nuts with breakfast and another as an afternoon snack. In all, she was eating about 1½ cups of nuts per day, or about 1,100 calories. Nuts are portable and bite-size, which makes them easy to overeat. They are also high in calories.

Emma cut back on the nuts, lost the weight she needed, and was back in award-winning form in just seven weeks. *The lesson: Go easy on foods (even healthy foods) that are easy to pop into your mouth—including grapes, olives, sunflower seeds, and dried fruits.*

**Condiments are not always your friends.** Many people forget that condiments contain calories. If you use them sparingly, they can add dimension and a little flavor to your meal. If you eat them in excess, they may be standing in the way of your weight-loss goal. One ounce of ketchup, for instance, contains about 40 calories. (Each tablespoon of ketchup provides 15 calories; barbecue sauce can often be higher.) If you use more, the calories multiply. Other add-ons are worse: 1 tablespoon of mayonnaise contains about 100 calories; 1 tablespoon of French, blue cheese, or other creamy dressing has about 75 calories; a 1-ounce packet of tartar sauce can contain more than 150 calories. I have clients who have finally taken off those last 5 stubborn pounds when they learned that condiments aren't calorie free. For intense taste with minimal calories, I recommend: tomato salsa (¼ cup has only 30 calories—much less than ketchup); mustard (1 tablespoon has 9 to 15 calories, and you typically don't use that much); pickle relish (1 tablespoon has about 14 calories); reduced-sodium soy sauce (1 teaspoon has about 3 calories); and hot-pepper sauce (1 teaspoon has about 1 calorie). *The lesson: Don't forget that condiments aren't just toppings—they are food. Use them wisely and sparingly.*

**Beware of mindless eating—part one.** Sarah never counted calories and never kept a food log because she thought she ate perfectly. She was frustrated that her weight never budged, despite her being a busy mom who never seemed to sit down. I asked Sarah to pay close attention to every mouthful, and she was surprised to discover that she actually did a lot of "tasting" while cooking—enough to add up to a significant number of calories. We fixed that by having her chew sugarless gum whenever she prepared meals so she couldn't mindlessly enjoy these tasting portions before dinner. *The lesson: "Tasting" is eating. If you nosh your way through food preparations, keep your mouth otherwise occupied by chewing sugarless gum, sipping hot tea, or singing along with your favorite CD.*

**Beware of mindless eating—part two.** Kimberly didn't overeat—she just picked off other people's plates. Because it was only a couple of french fries from her son's portion or a cookie from her daughter's snack pack, Sarah didn't think those nibbles could account for the trouble she was having losing those few extra pounds. As an experiment, I asked her to carry a bunch of plastic zippered sandwich bags with her for a day. Every time she picked off someone's food, she was to place it in a bag instead of eating it. Then she brought that single day's worth of pickings to me. We were both surprised to discover that she was grazing through about 1,000 extra calories per day of other people's food! That's a full breakfast and dinner. *The lesson: Be picky about your pickings! If you plan for calories, you can enjoy them more. Be mindful.*

**Choose your sweets for their staying power.** Brenda is a writer who spends most of her days sitting in front of a computer. She kept a jar of hard candies on hand for whenever she got the urge for something sweet. Brenda inevitably crunched the candy instead of sucking it and ate one after the other, racking up calorie upon calorie. Each piece has less than 25 calories, but Brenda could easily eat six (about 140 calories) in just a few minutes. I had her swap her hard candy for large Atomic FireBalls, which are very hot candies. They are hard as rocks, so Brenda couldn't just crunch them away. They give off two waves of "atomic" heat, so she never forgot that she had a candy in her mouth. After just one, Brenda was satisfied and didn't need any more "sweet" for the afternoon. Although each Atomic FireBall has 40 calories—more than a small sucking candy—Brenda still saved herself about 100 calories per day and up to 10 pounds in a year! *The lesson: If you have a sweets habit that you can't break, look for a way around it by substituting similar treats that might last longer or give you fewer overall calories.*

**Avoid the snack traps.** Kevin, a television actor, had done a good job of dropping most of the weight he had put on between seasons, but he had a snack habit that kept him from his weight-loss goal. His determination fell apart when faced with "snacky" foods—especially late in the afternoon. One serving would turn into two, which could turn into three or four before he would finally stop eating. For three weeks in a row, he vowed to me (and to himself) that he would stop after eating just one serving of pretzels or one small bag of baked chips or one granola bar. But vow or no vow, he ate two to three times more than he was allotted. They say that the camera adds 10 pounds, so he was justifiably worried that his extra weight would be magnified on the screen. I suggested that he switch from "snacky" foods to "real food" snacks—calorie-controlled portions of foods that we typically eat at meals. For example, he now snacks on a two-serving container of fat-free cottage cheese or 2 cups of hearty vegetable soup or half a turkey sandwich on whole wheat bread with lettuce, tomato, and mustard. It worked like a charm! The key for Kevin was that the snacky nature of snack foods made him want to continue eating, while the foodlike nature of my substitutes allowed him to feel satisfied sooner. Everyone has certain foods that are, well, let's say problematic. Foods that, once you start eating, trigger a need to keep eating. For Kevin, it was snacks. For other people, it is ice cream or peanut butter or even dry breakfast cereal. *The lesson: It is possible to break away from the never-ending snack without going hungry. If you have a problem controlling snack portions, avoid your triggers. Try a different type of food that you don't usually associate with snacking.*

**Slow difficult transitions.** Long-standing habits can be difficult to break. Bill is a historian whose morning routine has long included a newspaper and two huge mugs of coffee. His weight loss plateaued when he was still about 15 pounds above his goal weight, all due to his coffee habit. Bill liked his coffee very light and creamy—

# JUMPING PAST A WEIGHT PLATEAU

The trickiest time during any weight-loss program is the plateau—that long stretch when the quick drop in pounds you saw at first tapers off and every additional ounce feels hard-won. Frustration can turn to overeating, which leads to weight gain, which will move you off your plateau for sure—but in the wrong direction. Don't give up, and don't lose heart. There's hope.

- **Don't worry about the steady state.** If you're on a plateau, that means you've already lost weight. Enjoy it! Take a few days (or weeks, if necessary) to celebrate your new body. If you keep eating well and exercising, all plateaus end. Of course, it may be that you have reached your body's ideal weight, and striving for any new weight loss will be fighting against nature. If that's the case, acknowledge your great accomplishment and enjoy (and accept) the new body you have.

- **Exercise a little more.** As the weight comes off, metabolism slows down. The only way to rev it back up is by increasing the duration or intensity of your exercise. Just adding an extra ten minutes of aerobic exercise to your daily routine will help you burn an additional 50 to 100 calories per day, which could add up to an extra 10 pounds of weight gone by the end of the year!

- **Change your routine.** Maybe you and your body are becoming bored with the same old program. Vary your food choices, share recipes with a friend, try a new restaurant, or modify your exercise routine. Sometimes little changes are just enough to get you out of a rut.

- **Look for sneaky foods.** Some foods that sound healthy (and some that actually *are* healthy) are weight-loss saboteurs. Granola and granola bars can be chock-full of calories, fat, and sugar. Dried fruit, yogurt-covered nuts or raisins, banana chips, trail mix, and so-called natural potato chips are all diet busters. Eliminate the sneaky foods and see if that doesn't make a big difference.

- **Eliminate starchy carbohydrates with dinner.** Starchy carbohydrates are delicious, no doubt about it. But they are also relatively high in calories and easy to eat in large quantities, and some people even claim they're psychologically addictive. Of all healthy foods, people crave starches the most. So when you want to break a plateau, avoid all pasta, rice, bread, potatoes, corn, and peas for a week or two. Instead, choose dinners that consist of lean protein and nonstarchy vegetables, such as broccoli, carrots, peppers, spinach, cauliflower, zucchini, and green beans.

- **Close the kitchen after dinner.** Eliminate nighttime snacking and alcohol for a few weeks when you need a weight-loss boost. Clean the kitchen, put all of the dishes away, and move away from the pantry. Find a noncaloric way to train your body to understand that eating time is over. Drink a cup of herbal tea (peppermint can be particularly soothing, if you don't have heartburn), floss your teeth, and perhaps apply a tooth whitener . . . anything that keeps your mouth feeling clean and otherwise occupied.

**How can I stick with my weight-loss plan during the holiday season, especially during the month of December? I want to avoid overindulging but enjoy the festivities at the same time.**

First, be selective about your splurges. Choose a few special events or parties that you look forward to all year, and plan to indulge at those celebrations. The rest of the time, try to stick to your normal, healthy eating habits.

Second, for those special times when you do choose to splurge, follow my Rule of One: Stick with just *one* of each deliciously tempting hors d'oeuvre, one plate of food, one alcoholic drink, and one dessert. By keeping your portions in check, you can enjoy every highlight of your favorite holiday meals without going overboard.

specifically, with about $\frac{1}{2}$ cup of half-and-half in each mug—1 cup of half-and-half per day. It was obviously the source of his extra weight. He fought this last change to his diet, but as it became clear that his weight wasn't going to budge unless he broke this habit, he relented. It was a slow transition. Over the course of six months, Bill transitioned from half-and-half to whole milk . . . to 2% milk . . . to 1% milk . . . to fat-free milk. That saved him 232 calories every day and enabled him to drop 12 pounds. *The lesson: You don't have to make difficult changes all at once. Find intermediate steps that can make the process as painless as possible.*

**Make evening hours less threatening.** Busy people sometimes face the "feet up" diet challenge—the minute they stop running around long enough to put their feet up, they binge. As a senior editor at a publishing company, Jillian doesn't have a spare private moment in her day. She is always in meetings or on the phone, planning for the next project or solving some problem with a current book. By the time she got home—often after 9:00 p.m.—she would just want to relax in front of the TV and eat. No matter what she had for dinner or when she finished, Jillian would create a buffet of high-calorie comfort foods—including cookies, cake, ice cream, dry cereal, and crackers. She woke up each morning with the best intentions for the evening, but by the time she reached home, exhausted from the day, her resolve went out the window. Jillian and I drew up a contract: Before starting her nighttime binge, she first had to eat three low-calorie foods that we agreed upon. So before she could spoon out the ice cream, Jillian committed to first eating two handfuls of baby carrots, one container of fat-free flavored yogurt, and one apple. After that, she could eat whatever she wanted. Of course, our strategy worked. She discovered that after she finished her three must-haves, she felt full and in control. Good-bye binges! Even though those snacks added an extra 250 calories to her daily food plan, they saved her from eating thousands of extra calories each night. *The lesson: If you can't stop yourself from eating at the end of the day (or whenever your particular challenging time is), front-load the binge with three healthy foods. If you vow to eat those three healthy snacks first, it gives your body time to feel satisfied while allowing your psyche the pleasure of eating.*

## BONUS POINTS

◆ **Donate your "fat clothes."** Losing weight is a major accomplishment. As soon as an item of clothing is too big for you, give it away. Don't keep it in your closet as part of your "just in case" wardrobe. It is easier to backslide if you have bigger pants to slide into.

◆ **Keep a weight-loss journal.** Write down your food choices and portions, where you eat, why you eat, how much exercise you do, and anything else that allows you to see your healthy (and unhealthy) patterns. That way you can spot areas for improvement and make adjustments as you go along. Use the journal to track your progress as you weigh yourself once or twice a week.

◆ **Consider the buddy system.** Some people do better if they have a friend, spouse, or therapist—someone they can talk to about successes or setbacks. Ideally, this person is nonjudgmental and unconditionally supportive. If you thrive with a little help from your friends, go ahead and ask for their help and guidance.

◆ **Slow your eating.** Strive to make every mouthful a sensual experience. Taste your food. Savor the texture. Put your fork down between every two bites, and sip water during your meal.

◆ **When you eat, focus.** This is not the time for multitasking. Make meal time (and snack time) all about the food. Avoid the mindlessness of eating while checking e-mail, watching television, or performing any other distracting activity.

◆ **Drink water before meals.** Within 30 minutes of lunch and dinner, guzzle two glasses of water. This will help meet your daily fluid quota and remind you to follow through with smart food choices at the upcoming meal. Perhaps it will also fill you up and take the edge off your hunger, but most important, it will keep you thinking about your plan. Also, thirst can mimic the feelings of hunger—if you wait ten minutes after drinking water, you may find you don't want to eat at all.

◆ **Keep sugarless gum on hand.** Sugarless gum can give you a hit of flavor, keep your mouth busy (so you'll be less likely to snack), and clean your teeth when you can't brush. And, contrary to popular belief, sugarless gum won't stimulate your appetite.

◆ **Repackage snacks.** Before you dig into that megasize bag of pretzels, break it down. Divide the large bag into individual portions in snack-size plastic zipper bags so that you'll be ready with appropriate servings when you need them. Also, seek out snacks that are in portion-controlled units—lollipops, fat-free pudding cups, mini bags of microwave popcorn, or other individual snacks that are 150 calories or less per serving. Just remember to only eat one serving!

◆ **Shock your tongue.** Be liberal with spices—chile peppers, curry, hot salsa, wasabi. Hot and spicy flavors encourage slower eating. Hot (temperature-wise) low-calorie beverages can also help you feel satisfied and hydrated. When you're bored, it's possible to nurse a hot skim latte, green or herbal tea, or low-fat hot cocoa for much longer than it would take to eat a snack.

◆ **Forgive slipups.** When dieters give in to temptation and "fall of the wagon" for one meal or one day, they often tell themselves they've blown their diets and throw in the towel for good. To be successful, you have to learn to overcome these temporary setbacks. You can't let one binge or one "off day" turn into a full week—or month—of splurging. Instead, shake it off and get right back on track at your next meal or the following day. And remember, nobody gains weight from one rich dinner or a single slice of cake. The real trouble starts when you allow that one "splurge" to snowball into an all-out eating frenzy. So take it one meal at a time and learn to forgive yourself.

◆ **Get enough sleep.** During sleep, our bodies rest and regenerate so we can be strong and clearheaded the following day—this helps us make wise food choices. What's more, sleep deprivation causes an imbalance in certain hormones, including ghrelin (which causes weight gain) and leptin (which decreases appetite). When we don't get enough sleep, our levels of ghrelin go up (more weight gain) and levels of leptin go down (so we are hungrier). Aim for at least seven hours of sleep each night.

## SUPPLEMENTS

While you are concentrating on the weight-loss part of your program, you may lose sight of your vitamin and mineral needs. As backup, I recommend:

◆ **A multivitamin.** There's no need to go crazy with lots of different pills or mega-doses. A single multivitamin that contains 100 percent Daily Value of most vitamins and minerals is fine. If you are a man or a menopausal woman, choose an adult formula that doesn't contain iron.

◆ **Calcium with vitamin D$_3$.** Some women trying to lose weight skimp on calcium-rich foods. If you fall into this category, consider taking a separate calcium supplement with vitamin D$_3$. (See chapter 10 for more information on appropriate calcium supplementation.) There is some evidence that too much calcium may increase the risk of prostate cancer. Therefore, men should always talk with their doctors before taking calcium supplements.

Visit Joy's online Weight Loss Program at www.joybauer.com to sign up for Joy's comprehensive diet plan, complete with hundreds of recipes, custom meal and fitness plans, one-on-one nutrition coaching, community support, a weight and inch tracker, a calorie calculator, and more.

# JOY'S 4-STEP PROGRAM
## FOR WEIGHT LOSS

Follow this program if you want to lose weight.

## Step 1 ... START WITH THE BASICS

- ◆ Calculate your basal metabolic rate and your maintenance calories.
- ◆ Begin an exercise program that combines aerobic and strength training.
- ◆ Eat regularly—every four to five hours—to keep your metabolism up and hunger controlled.
- ◆ Consider taking a multivitamin to fill in any nutritional gaps.
- ◆ Consider taking a calcium supplement with vitamin $D_3$ if you are a woman who is not eating enough calcium-rich foods.
- ◆ Keep your pantry and refrigerator stocked with healthy foods from the grocery list below.
- ◆ Avoid or limit the worst weight offenders, including high-calorie drinks (such as sodas, fruit juices or drinks, flavored waters, commercial smoothies, and sugary coffee drinks); refined, white carbs; full-fat dairy; and high-fat meats.

## Step 2 ... YOUR ULTIMATE GROCERY LIST

The following comprehensive list provides foods that are healthy and conducive to weight loss, and most are featured in the meal plans on page 42. Find items that are personally appealing and toss them into your grocery cart each week.

### FRUIT

*All* fruit, but especially:

| | | |
|---|---|---|
| Apples | Berries (blackberries, blueberries, raspberries, and strawberries) | Cherries |
| Apricots | | Clementines |
| Bananas | Cantaloupe | Dates |
| | | Figs |

## FRUIT *continued*

Grapefruit

Grapes

Honeydew

Kiwifruit

Lemons

Limes

Mangoes

Nectarines

Oranges

Papaya

Peaches

Pears

Pineapple

Plums

Prunes

Raisins

Tangerines

Watermelon

## NONSTARCHY VEGETABLES

*All* nonstarchy vegetables, but especially:

Artichokes

Asparagus

Beets

Bok choy

Broccoli

Broccoli raab

Brussels sprouts

Cabbage

Carrots

Cauliflower

Celery

Collard greens

Cucumbers

Dark leafy greens (beet, collard, dandelion, kale, mustard, Swiss chard, and turnip)

Eggplant

Fennel

Green beans

Kale

Lettuce (all varieties)

Mushrooms

Okra

Onion

Peppers (all varieties, hot and bell)

Pumpkin (100% canned puree)

Radishes

Rhubarb

Seaweed

Snow peas

Spaghetti squash

Spinach

Squash, summer (yellow)

Sugar snap peas

Swiss chard

Tomatoes (fresh and canned)

Turnips

Watercress

Zucchini

## LEAN PROTEINS

Beef, lean

Cheese, fat-free or reduced fat (full-fat cheese exceptions: Parmesan and Romano)

Chicken, ground (at least 90% lean)

Chicken, skinless

Cottage cheese (fat-free or 1%)

Eggs and egg substitutes

Fish and shellfish, fresh or canned (such as light tuna in water, sardines, and wild salmon)

Ham, lean

Milk, fat-free or 1%

Milk alternatives (almond, rice, and soy)

Pork tenderloin

Tempeh

Tofu

Turkey, ground (at least 90% lean)

Turkey, skinless

Turkey bacon

Turkey burgers, lean

Veggie burgers

Yogurt (fat-free or low-fat)

## HIGH-QUALITY STARCHY CARBOHYDRATES (INCLUDING STARCHY VEGETABLES)

Amaranth

Barley

Beans, starchy (such as black, garbanzo, kidney, navy, and pinto)

Bread, whole grain (reduced-calorie and regular)

Bulgur

Cereals, whole grain (no more than 150 calories per 1-cup serving and at least 3 grams fiber)

Corn (fresh or frozen kernels)

Crackers, whole grain

Millet

Oats

Pasta, whole grain

Peas, green

Peas, split

Pitas, whole grain (mini and regular-size)

Potatoes (sweet and white)

Quinoa

Rice (brown and wild)

Rice cakes

Soybeans (edamame)

Squash, winter (acorn and butternut)

Tortillas, whole grain

Waffles, whole grain

Wheat berries

Wheat germ

## FOODS THAT COUNT TOWARD HEALTHY FATS

Avocados

Canola oil

Nuts:

- ◆ Almonds
- ◆ Butternuts (white walnuts)
- ◆ Cashews
- ◆ Hazelnuts
- ◆ Macadamia nuts

- ◆ Peanuts
- ◆ Pecans
- ◆ Pine nuts
- ◆ Pistachios (in shells)
- ◆ Soy nuts
- ◆ Walnuts

Nut and seed butters (almond, cashew, peanut, and sunflower)

Olive oil

Olives

Seeds:

- ◆ Chia seeds
- ◆ Flaxseed, ground
- ◆ Sunflower seeds (in shell)

## MISCELLANEOUS

Applesauce, unsweetened

Beverages (naturally flavored coffees, seltzers, and teas)

Broth, low-sodium (chicken, beef, and vegetable)

Cream cheese (fat-free or reduced-fat)

Garlic

Herbs and spices (fresh, dried, and ground)

Hot sauce

Hummus

Marinara sauce (60 calories or less per ½ cup)

Mayonnaise, reduced-fat

Mustard (all varieties)

Salad dressing, reduced-calorie

Salsa

Sour cream (fat-free or reduced-fat)

Soft tub spread, reduced-fat and trans-fat-free

Soy sauce, reduced-sodium

Steak sauce

Teriyaki sauce, reduced-sodium

Vinegar (all varieties)

# Step 3 ... GOING ABOVE AND BEYOND

To maximize your weight-loss potential, here are some additional things you can try.

◆ Keep a weight-loss journal.

◆ Be aware of the foods that entice you to enter an eating danger zone. Keep them out of your pantry.

◆ Don't multitask while eating—focus and enjoy.

◆ Get enough sleep.

# Step 4 ... MEAL PLANS

These sample menus include the foods and specific food combinations that will help you lose weight while feeling energized. Each meal is balanced with the right mix of high-quality carbs, protein, fat, and calories to help keep your blood sugar levels stable and hunger at bay. Get ready to lose weight and feel *flabuloss!*

Some things you should know:

1. All 42 meals—that's 14 options each for breakfast, lunch, and dinner (plus one bonus lunch, just because I couldn't decide which yummy option to eliminate!)— are presented at the lower end of the caloric range to accommodate people who have lower caloric needs. For example, although breakfast meals through- out the book range from 300 to 400 calories, breakfast options in this chapter

## DON'T RUSH DINNER

Speed eating through meals could be hurting your waistline. In an interesting experiment, women were invited to eat a pasta lunch on two different days. On one day, the women were given a small spoon and asked to take small bites, put the spoon down between bites, and chew each bite at least 15 times. On the second day, the women were given a large spoon and asked to eat as quickly as possible without stopping between bites. On both occasions, the women ate until they felt comfortably full. When researchers measured how many calories the women had eaten, they found that they ate 67 more calories when they ate quickly than when they ate slowly. Although this may not sound like much, calories add up. If you wolf down both lunch and dinner, it could mean an additional 134 calories per day, or 48,910 calories per year. That's the equivalent of 14 pounds. Once again, the tortoise beats the hare.

are approximately 300 calories each (lunch options are approximately 400 calories, and dinner options are approximately 500 calories). If you have higher caloric needs and/or find yourself too hungry at any one meal, I've also included instructions for adding 100 calories to each meal.

2. Don't feel that you need to be limited to the meal plans. You can enjoy all the recipes in this book in your personal nutrition plan because I've provided caloric information for each. If you find that there are certain meals you love, by all means, repeat them. Although variety will ensure you get a wide range of vitamins and minerals in your diet, it is okay to revisit the meals you enjoy the most. Also, if you sometimes eat frozen entrées, choose brands that fit within your calorie range for that meal. For example, a quick dinner might include a healthy frozen entrée with 400 calories or less and a prewashed bag of salad with a reduced-calorie dressing. When eating out, keep your choices simple—grilled fish with steamed veggies and salad with dressing on the side. If you have some extra calories to play with, you may consider having a glass of wine with dinner or fresh berries for dessert.

3. Every day, choose one option for each of the three meals—breakfast, lunch, and dinner. Then, one or two times per day, choose from my variety of suggested snacks. Snacks are grouped according to their calorie amounts ("100 Calories or Less" and "100 to 200 Calories"). Your job is to strategically pick snacks that fit into your personal program. You may also replace one of your daily snacks with one item on the Fun Foods list. Pay close attention to the number of snacks you choose (and their portions)—when you're trying to lose weight, everything counts. *Carefully note my recommendations for teaspoons and tablespoons. There are three teaspoons in a tablespoon—a mistake could get you three times the calories you counted on!*

4. For the first week, starch is omitted from dinner—all starch, even high-quality starch like sweet potatoes, brown rice, peas, and butternut squash. Instead, your dinner for the first seven days comprises lean protein and nonstarchy vegetables like broccoli, peppers, cauliflower, leafy greens, and more. I use this approach during the first week because many successful clients have found it incredibly effective, and I'm sure you will, too! If you miss eating starch with dinner, rest assured that you'll be seeing it again—moderate amounts are incorporated during week two.

5. Beverage calories are not included. I encourage you to drink plenty of water with your meal and two 8-ounce glasses of water before eating lunch and dinner. (This will help keep you hydrated and thinking about our plan.) If you'd prefer something other than water, stick with any preferred noncaloric beverages. Enjoy coffee and tea plain or with fat-free milk (and optional 1 to 2 teaspoons/packets sugar or sugar substitute).

## BREAKFAST OPTIONS

(300 TO 400 CALORIES)

> *Each breakfast option is approximately 300 calories. If you'd like to increase to 400 calories, follow the instructions for adding 100 calories.*

### Fiesta Vegetable Omelet with Toast

In a heated pan coated with oil spray, sauté ½ cup chopped onion, ½ cup sliced mushrooms, and ½ cup chopped bell pepper (red, yellow, or green) until soft. Beat 1 whole egg with 3 egg whites, pour over the sautéed vegetables, and add preferred seasonings. When the bottom is cooked, gently flip. Fold the omelet over and cook until the egg mixture is firm. Serve with 1 toasted slice whole wheat bread (or 2 slices reduced-calorie bread) and top with 1 teaspoon reduced-fat, soft tub, trans-fat-free spread.

*To add approximately 100 calories:* Add ½ cantaloupe, 1 banana, or 1 cup berries.

### Cold Cereal with Milk and Fruit

Mix 1 cup whole grain cereal (150 calories or less per 1-cup serving and 3 grams or more fiber) with 1 cup milk (fat-free, 1%, or soy milk) and ½ sliced banana (or 2 tablespoons raisins or ½ cup berries).

*To add approximately 100 calories:* Add 1 hard-cooked egg.

### Strawberry-Banana Cottage Cheese with Almonds

Mix 1 cup fat-free or 1% cottage cheese with ½ sliced banana, ½ cup chopped strawberries, and 1 tablespoon slivered almonds. For the cottage cheese, you can substitute 1 cup fat-free plain or flavored yogurt (180 calories or less).

*To add approximately 100 calories:* Add another tablespoon slivered almonds and 1 tablespoon wheat germ or ground flaxseed.

### PB&J English Muffin

Spread each half of 1 toasted whole grain English muffin with 1 level teaspoon peanut butter and 1 teaspoon jam. Serve with ½ grapefruit (or 1 orange, peach, or plum).

*To add approximately 100 calories:* Use a total of 2 level teaspoons peanut butter and 2 teaspoons jam on each muffin half.

### Scrambled Eggs with Turkey Bacon and Fruit

Beat 1 whole egg with 2 egg whites. Cook in a heated pan coated with oil spray, adding any preferred chopped vegetables (onion, red and green bell peppers, or tomato). Enjoy with 2 strips turkey bacon and 1 orange (or ½ grapefruit or ¼ cantaloupe).

*To add approximately 100 calories:* Add 1 egg white (3 total) and 2 strips of turkey bacon (4 total).

### Oatmeal with Berries and Nuts

Prepare ½ cup dry oats with water and top with 1 tablespoon chopped nuts (walnuts, pecans, or slivered almonds) and ½ cup berries (sliced strawberries, blueberries, raspberries, and/or blackberries). Optional: Sweeten with 1 to 2 teaspoons sugar, honey, pure maple syrup, or sugar substitute.

*To add approximately 100 calories:* Enjoy a side serving of 6 ounces fat-free plain or flavored yogurt (100 calories or less).

### Skinny Breakfast Burrito

Beat 1 egg with 2 egg whites. Scramble in a heated pan coated with oil spray. Mix cooked eggs with ¼ cup black beans and 2 tablespoons shredded fat-free or reduced-fat cheese. Wrap in 1 whole grain tortilla (100 calories or less). Add optional onion, bell pepper, salsa, and/or hot sauce.

*To add approximately 100 calories:* Add 2 tablespoons fat-free or reduced-fat cheese and 2 tablespoons reduced-fat sour cream or guacamole.

### Apple Slices with Peanut Butter

Spread 2 level tablespoons peanut butter (or any preferred nut butter) over 1 sliced apple (or banana).

*To add approximately 100 calories:* Add 1 level tablespoon peanut butter (for a total of 3 level tablespoons).

### Toast with Cream Cheese, Tomato, Onion, and Lox

Top 2 toasted slices reduced-calorie whole wheat bread (50 calories or less per slice) with 1 tablespoon fat-free or reduced-fat cream cheese, sliced tomato, onion, and 2 ounces smoked salmon.

*To add approximately 100 calories:* For the reduced-calorie bread, substitute 2 slices regular whole wheat bread or add ¾ cup fresh fruit salad.

### Ham and Cheese Omelet with Toast

Beat 1 whole egg with 2 egg whites. Cook in a heated pan coated with oil spray. Add 2 ounces diced lean ham (or turkey). When the bottom is cooked, gently flip. Top with 2 tablespoons shredded fat-free or reduced-fat cheese. Fold the omelet over and cook until the cheese is melted and the egg mixture is firm. Season with preferred herbs. Enjoy with 1 slice whole wheat toast (or 2 slices reduced-calorie whole wheat toast) topped with 1 teaspoon reduced-fat, soft tub, trans-fat-free spread.

*To add approximately 100 calories:* Add an additional slice of whole wheat toast topped with 1 teaspoon reduced-fat, soft tub, trans-fat-free spread, or have 1 cup grapes.

### Whole Grain Waffles with Yogurt

Toast two frozen whole grain waffles and top with 6 ounces fat-free flavored yogurt (100 calories or less) and 1 tablespoon wheat germ (or ground flaxseed).

*To add approximately 100 calories:* Add 1 cup berries (or 2 tablespoons chopped walnuts, pecans, slivered almonds, peanuts, or soy nuts).

### Rice Cakes with Cottage Cheese and Tomato

Top 3 rice cakes with sliced tomato, onion, and 1 cup fat-free or 1% cottage cheese.

*To add approximately 100 calories:* Add ½ cantaloupe (or 1 apple, 1 banana, or 1 cup grapes).

## Peanut Butter Pita and Yogurt

Spread 1 mini (70-calorie) whole grain pita (or 1 slice whole wheat bread) with 1 level tablespoon peanut butter. Enjoy with 1 cup fat-free plain or flavored yogurt.

*To add approximately 100 calories:* Substitute 1 regular-size whole wheat pita (150 calories or less) for the mini pita and add 1 extra teaspoon (not tablespoon) peanut butter.

## Tomato-Cheddar Melt

Lightly toast 2 slices reduced-calorie whole wheat bread (50 calories or less per slice). Top each slice with sliced tomato, optional onion, and 1 slice reduced-fat Cheddar cheese. Bake in a 350°F oven until the cheese melts. Enjoy with 1 cup fresh berries (or 1 apple or 1 grapefruit).

*To add approximately 100 calories:* For the 2 slices reduced-calorie bread, substitute regular whole wheat bread (or add 6 ounces fat-free plain or flavored yogurt—100 calories or less).

# LUNCH OPTIONS

(400 TO 500 CALORIES)

*Each lunch option is approximately 400 calories. If you'd like to increase to 500 calories, follow the instructions for adding 100 calories.*

## Ham and Cheese Sandwich

Toast 2 slices reduced-calorie whole wheat bread (50 calories or less per slice). On the bottom slice, layer 1 tablespoon reduced-fat mayonnaise, optional spicy mustard, 4 ounces lean ham (or turkey), and 1 slice fat-free or reduced-fat cheese. Top with tomato, onion, and the remaining slice of bread. Enjoy with 1 cup baby carrots.

*To add approximately 100 calories:* Substitute 2 slices regular whole wheat bread for the reduced-calorie bread, or add a side serving of 6 ounces fat-free flavored yogurt or 1 apple.

### Caesar Salad with Grilled Chicken or Shrimp

Top a large bed of romaine lettuce with 4 ounces grilled chicken or cooked shrimp, 3 tablespoons grated Parmesan cheese, and optional anchovies (4 fillets). Toss with 4 tablespoons reduced-calorie Caesar dressing (45 calories or less per tablespoon) or 1 to 2 tablespoons regular Caesar dressing.

*To add approximately 100 calories:* Enjoy with 1 whole wheat pita (70 calories), or add ½ cup croutons to the salad.

### Cottage Cheese with Cantaloupe and Almonds

Fill ½ cantaloupe with 1 cup fat-free or 1% cottage cheese and top with 2 tablespoons slivered almonds (or chopped walnuts or sunflower seeds). For the cottage cheese, you can substitute 1 cup plain or flavored fat-free yogurt.

*To add approximately 100 calories:* Add 2 tablespoons chopped nuts or seeds, for a total of 4 tablespoons.

### Open-Faced Tuna Melt

Mash 3 ounces water-packed light tuna (or canned wild salmon or chicken breast) with 1 to 2 teaspoons reduced-fat mayonnaise, minced onion, and freshly ground black pepper. Spread evenly over 2 slices reduced-calorie whole wheat toast (50 calories or less per slice). Top each slice with tomato and 1 slice fat-free or reduced-fat cheese (any variety, including Cheddar, Swiss, or American). Bake in a 350°F oven until the cheese melts. Enjoy with crunchy celery and red, yellow, and green pepper strips.

*To add approximately 100 calories:* Use the entire 5-ounce can of tuna (or 5 ounces salmon or chicken breast), and add 2 to 4 tablespoons reduced-calorie dressing to your veggies for dipping.

### Turkey Burger with Veggies

Top a 5-ounce lean turkey burger or veggie burger with lettuce, tomato, onion, and optional mustard, ketchup, or salsa. Serve on ½ whole grain bun or in 1 mini (70-calorie) whole wheat pita. Enjoy with 1 cup steamed vegetables (broccoli, cauliflower, or spinach).

*To add approximately 100 calories:* Enjoy the burger on 1 whole bun, and top the steamed vegetables with 1 tablespoon grated Parmesan cheese (or 2 teaspoons reduced-fat, soft tub, trans-fat-free spread).

### Mediterranean Pita and Yogurt

Spread 1 regular-size whole wheat pita (150 calories or less) with ⅓ cup hummus, then stuff with shredded lettuce, tomato, onion, and cucumber. Enjoy with 6 ounces fat-free plain or flavored yogurt (100 calories or less).

*To add approximately 100 calories:* Add 5 sliced olives to the pita sandwich, and enjoy the yogurt with 1 cup fresh berries.

### Broccoli-Cheese Omelet with Salad

Sauté 1 cup broccoli florets in oil spray until soft. Beat 1 whole egg with 3 egg whites and pour around the broccoli. When the bottom is cooked, gently flip. Top with 3 tablespoons shredded fat-free or reduced-fat cheese. Fold the omelet over and cook until the cheese melts and the egg mixture is firm. Season with preferred herbs. Enjoy with a mixed green salad tossed with 1 to 2 teaspoons olive oil and unlimited balsamic vinegar or fresh lemon juice (or 2 to 4 tablespoons reduced-calorie dressing).

*To add approximately 100 calories:* Add 1 slice whole grain bread or 1 mini (70-calorie) whole wheat pita.

### Turkey, Cheese, and Avocado Sandwich

Layer 4 ounces sliced turkey breast (or grilled chicken or lean ham), 1 slice reduced-fat cheese, 2 or 3 thin slices avocado, lettuce, tomato, and onion between 2 slices reduced-calorie whole wheat bread (50 calories or less per slice). Add optional mustard and 2 teaspoons reduced-fat mayonnaise (or hummus). Enjoy with 1 cup crunchy bell pepper strips.

*To add approximately 100 calories:* For the reduced-calorie bread, substitute regular whole wheat bread. Or add 1 apple, 1 pear, or 1 cup berries.

### Edamame with Wild Salmon Dijonnaise

Enjoy 1 cup boiled edamame (green soybeans in the pod), with 5 ounces canned salmon mashed with 1 tablespoon reduced-fat mayonnaise, 1 to 2 teaspoons Dijon mustard, and minced onion and black pepper to taste. Serve on a large bed of leafy greens tossed with fresh lemon juice or 2 tablespoons reduced-calorie dressing.

*To add approximately 100 calories:* Add 2 plain rice cakes or 1 mini (70-calorie) whole wheat pita.

### Spinach Salad with Beets, Goat Cheese, and Walnuts

Top a large bed of baby spinach leaves with ½ cup sliced beets, ½ cup sugar snap peas, 2 ounces soft goat cheese, and 1 tablespoon lightly toasted, chopped walnuts. Toss with 2 teaspoons olive oil and unlimited vinegar or fresh lemon juice (or 2 to 4 tablespoons reduced-calorie dressing).

*To add approximately 100 calories:* Add 2 tablespoons lightly toasted, chopped walnuts (or ½ cantaloupe, 1 cup grapes, 1 cup cherries, 1 apple, 1 pear, or 1 cup berries).

### Baked Potato with Broccoli and Cheese

Top 1 medium baked white potato with unlimited cooked, chopped broccoli and 1 ounce melted fat-free or reduced-fat cheese (or ½ cup fat-free or 1% low-fat cottage cheese). Serve with 2 tablespoons fat-free or reduced-fat sour cream and optional salsa.

*To add approximately 100 calories:* Add 1 cup baby carrots and 2 tablespoons reduced-calorie dressing.

### Grilled Chicken-Pepper Wrap

Sauté unlimited onion and bell peppers in oil spray or 1 teaspoon olive or canola oil. Wrap in a whole grain tortilla (100 calories or less) with 5 ounces grilled chicken. Enjoy with 1 cup crunchy baby carrots and unlimited sliced cucumber.

*To add approximately 100 calories:* Add 1 cup fresh grapes (or 1 cup cherries, 1 small banana, ½ cantaloupe, 1 apple, or 1 pear).

### Salad with the Works

Choose one 4-ounce serving from the following protein options: canned sardines, canned light tuna in water, chicken, turkey, lean ham, lean roast beef, tofu, or a favorite fish or shellfish. Place on top of a large bed of leafy greens and mix with ½ chopped bell pepper (red, yellow, or green), 5 cherry tomatoes, and ¼ cup each sliced mushrooms, chopped cucumbers, sliced beets, chopped red onion, and artichoke hearts. Add 2 tablespoons chickpeas (garbanzo beans) and 5 sliced olives. Toss with 2 teaspoons olive oil and 2 tablespoons vinegar or fresh lemon juice (or 2 to 4 tablespoons reduced-calorie dressing).

*To add approximately 100 calories:* Add ¼ chopped avocado to the salad, or enjoy with 1 slice whole grain bread or 1 small whole grain dinner roll.

### Veggie Tuna Salad with Pita

Enjoy 1 serving of Veggie Tuna Salad (page 271) on a large bed of romaine or spinach leaves with 1 mini (70-calorie) whole wheat pita and 1 cup baby carrots with 2 tablespoons reduced-calorie vinaigrette dressing. (You may substitute chicken breast or wild salmon for the tuna salad.)

*To add approximately 100 calories:* For the 70-calorie mini pita, substitute a regular-size pita.

### Japanese Spread: Miso Soup with California Rolls

Enjoy 1 order miso soup with 1 six-piece California roll; a side order of steamed vegetables; and optional ginger, wasabi, and reduced-sodium soy sauce.

*To add approximately 100 calories:* Add 3 additional pieces California roll (½ order).

## DINNER OPTIONS

### (500 TO 600 CALORIES)

*Each dinner option is approximately 500 calories. If you'd like to increase to 600 calories, follow the instructions for adding 100 calories. For the first week, only select options listed in Week One (these menus do not include starch). During your second week (and weeks that follow), enjoy meal options listed in Week Two, or feel free to repeat the menus from Week One.*

## WEEK ONE

### Rosemary Chicken with Sautéed Spinach and Salad

Enjoy 5 ounces grilled or baked chicken breast with preferred seasonings (or Rosemary Chicken, page 347) with 1 cup sautéed spinach (4 cups raw spinach leaves sautéed in 1 teaspoon olive oil and seasoned with minced garlic and salt and pepper to taste). Serve with a side salad of chopped lettuce, cucumber, carrot, onion, and mushrooms tossed with 1 tablespoon chopped walnuts, 1 teaspoon olive oil, and 1 to 2 tablespoons vinegar or fresh lemon juice (or 2 tablespoons reduced-calorie dressing).

*To add approximately 100 calories:* Add 3 ounces chicken breast (for a total of 8 ounces).

### Pork Tenderloin with Cauliflower Mashed "Potatoes"

Enjoy 5 ounces grilled, baked, or broiled lean pork tenderloin (or grilled chicken breast) with 1 serving Cauliflower Mashed "Potatoes" (page 216). Serve with a side salad of 2 cups chopped lettuce and ¼ cup each chopped pepper, onion, cucumber, mushrooms, and grated or chopped carrots tossed with 1 to 2 teaspoons olive oil and unlimited vinegar or fresh lemon juice (or 2 to 4 tablespoons reduced-calorie salad dressing).

*To add approximately 100 calories:* Add 3 ounces pork tenderloin (for a total of 8 ounces).

### Cheddar-Turkey Burger with Mixed Greens

Top a 5-ounce turkey burger (or lean hamburger or veggie burger) with sliced tomato, onion, 1 ounce reduced-fat Cheddar cheese, and optional 2 tablespoons ketchup or salsa. Serve with unlimited leafy greens tossed with 2 to 4 tablespoons reduced-calorie vinaigrette (or 1 teaspoon olive oil and unlimited vinegar or fresh lemon juice).

*To add approximately 100 calories:* Add ¼ avocado, thinly sliced (or 2 heaping tablespoons guacamole).

### Sirloin Steak with Mozzarella and Tomato Salad

Enjoy 5 ounces grilled sirloin steak (trimmed of fat) with optional 2 tablespoons steak sauce or ketchup and mozzarella and tomato salad (½ sliced red tomato and 1 ounce reduced-fat mozzarella cheese; alternate slices of tomato and cheese on plate and drizzle with 2 tablespoons reduced-calorie balsamic vinaigrette). Serve with unlimited steamed or grilled asparagus spears.

*To add approximately 100 calories:* Add 2 ounces steak (for a total of 7 ounces).

## Sweet Salmon over Arugula with Broccoli

Mix 1 tablespoon reduced-sodium soy sauce and 1 tablespoon honey. Drizzle over 1 wild salmon fillet (6 ounces) and grill or broil 10 to 15 minutes, basting every few minutes. Serve over a large mound of baby arugula leaves tossed with 1 tablespoon lightly toasted, slivered almonds and 2 tablespoons reduced-calorie dressing. Enjoy with unlimited steamed broccoli. For the salmon, you may substitute any preferred grilled or baked fish.

*To add approximately 100 calories:* Add 2 ounces salmon or other fish (for a total of 8 ounces).

## Tofu Salad with Snow Peas, Almonds, and Mandarin Oranges

Toss 6 to 8 ounces extra-firm tofu, cubed and chilled, with 2 to 3 cups baby spinach leaves, 1 cup steamed and chilled snow peas, ½ chopped tomato, and ½ cup mandarin oranges (canned in light syrup or juice). Drizzle with 1 teaspoon sesame oil and 1 tablespoon reduced-sodium soy sauce and top with 1 to 2 tablespoons slivered almonds. For the tofu, you may substitute grilled chicken breast or shrimp.

*To add approximately 100 calories:* Add ½ cup mandarin oranges (for a total of 1 cup) and 1 tablespoon slivered almonds (for a total of 2 to 3 tablespoons).

## Orange Pepper Beef Stir-Fry with Cucumber Slices

Enjoy 1 serving Orange Pepper Beef Stir-Fry (page 97) with 1 sliced cucumber.

*To add approximately 100 calories:* Skip the cucumber and add a mixed vegetable salad of lettuce, tomato, cucumber, onion, pepper, carrots, and mushrooms. Toss with 1 teaspoon olive oil and unlimited vinegar or fresh lemon juice (or 2 tablespoons reduced-calorie dressing).

## WEEK TWO (STARCH ADDED)

### Grilled Fish with Brussels Sprouts and Sweet Potato

Enjoy 1 fish fillet (6 ounces; wild salmon, flounder, sole, tilapia, or trout), grilled with 1 teaspoon olive oil and lemon juice and preferred seasonings, with unlimited steamed Brussels sprouts (or cauliflower, sugar snap peas, or zucchini), topped with 1 tablespoon reduced-fat, soft tub, trans-fat-free spread and ½ plain baked sweet potato.

*To add approximately 100 calories:* Enjoy 1 whole sweet potato.

### Southwestern Meat Loaf with Cauliflower Mashed "Potatoes"

Enjoy 1 serving Southwestern Turkey Meat Loaf (page 59) with 2 servings Cauliflower Mashed "Potatoes" (page 216) or unlimited steamed cauliflower or broccoli topped with 2 to 4 tablespoons grated Parmesan or Romano cheese. Serve with 1 cup crunchy baby carrots.

*To add approximately 100 calories:* Add another ½ serving meat loaf.

### Sweet and Sour Tofu-Veggie Stir-Fry with Brown Rice

Enjoy 1 serving Sweet-and-Sour Tofu-Veggie Stir-Fry (page 245) with ¾ cup cooked brown rice (or ½ medium baked white or sweet potato topped with 1 tablespoon reduced-fat, soft tub, trans-fat-free spread or 2 tablespoons fat-free or reduced-fat sour cream).

*To add approximately 100 calories:* Add ½ cup cooked brown rice (1¼ cups total), or enjoy the whole potato.

### Turkey Tacos with Lettuce, Tomato, and Cheese

Enjoy 3 Turkey Tacos (page 244) with optional salsa and hot sauce.

*To add approximately 100 calories:* Add 1 cup baby carrots dipped in 1 heaping tablespoon guacamole.

### Chinese Takeout

Order 1 seafood, tofu, or chicken entrée with steamed vegetables, and request garlic, black bean, or ginger sauce on the side. Enjoy with 1 cup brown rice and flavor with 1 tablespoon side sauce and unlimited reduced-sodium soy sauce.

*To add approximately 100 calories:* Add 2 steamed vegetable dumplings or an additional ½ cup brown rice.

### Skinny Shepherd's Pie

Enjoy 1 serving Skinny Shepherd's Pie (page 58) with a side salad of chopped lettuce, cucumber, tomato, mushrooms, and onion tossed with 1 teaspoon olive oil and unlimited vinegar or fresh lemon juice (or 2 tablespoons reduced-calorie dressing).

*To add approximately 100 calories:* Add ½ cup chickpeas (garbanzo beans) to the side salad (or 2 tablespoons chickpeas and 1 tablespoon chopped nuts).

### Turkey Chili with Cheese

Top 1 serving (2 cups) Turkey Chili (page 363) with 1 ounce shredded fat-free or reduced-fat Cheddar cheese and 2 tablespoons fat-free or reduced-fat sour cream. Serve with mixed green salad of bell peppers, carrots, onion, and mushrooms tossed with 1 teaspoon olive oil and unlimited vinegar or fresh lemon juice.

*To add approximately 100 calories:* Add ¾ cup chili (for a total of 2¾ cups).

## SNACK OPTIONS

100 CALORIES OR LESS

- ◆ *Best Vegetable Snacks:* up to 2 cups raw or cooked bell peppers (red, green, or yellow), broccoli, cauliflower, tomato, mushrooms, green beans, carrots, asparagus, cauliflower, celery, sugar snap peas
- ◆ *Best Fruit Snacks:* 1 apple, orange, pear, nectarine, tangerine, kiwifruit, or peach; 2 plums or clementines; ½ papaya, ½ mango, ½ banana, or ½ grapefruit; ¼ cantaloupe; 1 cup blueberries, boysenberries, blackberries, raspberries, sliced strawberries, cherries, or grapes; 1 cup cubed watermelon, pineapple, or honeydew; 4 apricots or prunes; 2 dates or figs; 20 whole strawberries; 2 tablespoons raisins

- 10 almonds
- 1 cup fat-free milk
- 1 low-fat hot cocoa (100 calories or less)
- 1 small skim latte or cappuccino
- 1 string cheese (or 1 ounce fat-free or reduced-fat cheese)
- ½ cup fat-free or 1% cottage cheese (with optional cinnamon)
- 1 hard-cooked egg (or 4 cooked egg whites)
- ½ cup natural, unsweetened applesauce
- 4 level tablespoons fat-free cream cheese (or 2 level tablespoons light cream cheese) with celery sticks
- 6 ounces fat-free plain or flavored yogurt (100 calories or less)
- 1 level tablespoon peanut butter with celery sticks

## 100 TO 200 CALORIES

- 10 almonds plus 1 serving fruit (from fruit list)
- 10 almonds plus 1 string cheese (or 1 ounce fat-free or reduced-fat cheese)
- 2 rice cakes, each topped with sliced tomato and half a slice reduced-fat cheese
- 1 cup boiled edamame (green soybeans in the pod)
- Nuts: 1 ounce (about ¼ cup) almonds, cashews, pecans, walnuts, peanuts, or soy nuts
- ½ cup pistachios or sunflower seeds in the shell
- ½ cup 1% cottage cheese topped with ½ cup berries (or 2 tablespoons ground flaxseed or wheat germ)
- 70-calorie whole wheat pita with 1 level tablespoon peanut butter (or 2 tablespoons hummus)
- 1 cup fat-free plain or flavored yogurt (120 calories or less) mixed with 2 tablespoons wheat germ
- 1 cup baby carrots or bell pepper strips with 2 tablespoons hummus or guacamole
- 1 sliced apple with 1 level tablespoon peanut butter
- Frozen banana: Slice one peeled banana into ½-inch wheels, place in a small plastic bag, and freeze before serving.

◆ Berry Yogurt Smoothie: In a blender, mix ½ cup fat-free milk, ½ cup nonfat yogurt, ¾ cup frozen berries, and 3 to 5 ice cubes.

◆ Vanilla Pumpkin Pudding: Mix 1 cup fat-free vanilla yogurt with ½ cup canned 100% pure pumpkin puree and a dash of ground cinnamon.

◆ 1 baked apple with 1 to 2 teaspoons sugar and cinnamon

◆ 1 Banana Almond Muffin (page 412)

## FUN FOODS (150 CALORIES OR LESS)

*In addition to your healthy snack options, here's a list of calorie-controlled fun foods to choose from. Substitute one item from this list for one of your daily snacks, or know that they're available and save them for those occasional cravings. All items are 150 calories or less. If you have a personal favorite that's not on my list, simply portion out 150 calories' worth and enjoy. It's very important that you always remember to count these calories as a snack.*

◆ 1 ounce dark chocolate (preferably at least 70% cacao)

◆ ½ cup fat-free pudding

◆ ½ cup low-fat ice cream, frozen yogurt, or sorbet

◆ 1 low-fat ice cream pop

◆ 4 cups air-popped popcorn

◆ 2 standard cookies

◆ 1 fun-size candy bar

◆ 100-calorie snack pack

◆ 1 ounce baked chips (potato, tortilla, vegetable, or lentil)

◆ 1 ounce pretzels

◆ 1 ounce soy crisps

◆ 10 strawberries with 2 heaping tablespoons reduced-fat whipped topping

◆ 1 glass wine or champagne

◆ 1 bottle beer

◆ 1 serving Warm Dark Chocolate Sauce with Fresh Fruit (page 80)

# SKINNY SHEPHERD'S PIE

*When most people think of shepherd's pie, they imagine splurging on a calorie-heavy meal in an English pub—with a favorite cold ale, of course! Now you can enjoy the delicious taste without any guilt—really. And if you need the cold ale, simply count it as your daily Fun Food.*

**MAKES 4 SERVINGS**

1 tablespoon olive oil

1 cup finely chopped onion

2 cloves garlic, minced

1¼ pounds ground turkey (at least 90 percent lean)

2 tablespoons tomato paste

1 tablespoon Worcestershire sauce

½ teaspoon garlic powder

½ teaspoon dried thyme

¼ teaspoon paprika

1 cup low-sodium beef broth

Kosher salt

Ground black pepper

2 or 3 large sweet potatoes (about 1½ pounds), cubed and boiled (or softened in the microwave)

½ cup buttermilk or reduced-fat sour cream

2 egg whites

2 tablespoons shredded reduced-fat Cheddar or Swiss cheese

1 tablespoon grated Parmesan cheese

Preheat the oven to 350°F. Coat a 6- to 8-cup ceramic or glass gratin dish with oil spray.

Heat the oil in a large skillet over medium-high heat. Add the onion and garlic and cook, stirring, for 4 to 5 minutes, or until softened and translucent. Add the turkey and increase the heat to high. Cook, stirring, for 3 to 4 minutes longer, or until the turkey is browned.

Stir in the tomato paste, Worcestershire sauce, garlic powder, thyme, and paprika. Cook, stirring, for 2 minutes. Add the broth and cook for 2 to 3 minutes, or until the turkey is cooked through and a light sauce forms. Season to taste with salt and pepper. Set aside.

In a large bowl, mash the sweet potatoes with the buttermilk or sour cream until smooth. Season to taste with salt and pepper. In a large metal bowl, beat the egg whites with a pinch of salt on high speed for 4 to 6 minutes, or until stiff but not lumpy. They should cling firmly to the side of the bowl when tilted. With a spatula, gently fold the egg whites, one-third at a time, into the sweet-potato mixture, until all the egg whites are just incorporated and not deflated.

Spread the meat mixture into the prepared casserole dish and top with the sweet-potato mixture. Sprinkle with the Cheddar or Swiss and Parmesan. Bake, uncovered, for 30 to 35 minutes, or until the potato topping is puffed and browned around the edges. Serve immediately.

**Per serving:** 403 calories, 41 g protein, 44 g carbohydrate, 7 g fat (2 g saturated), 61 mg cholesterol, 368 mg sodium, 6 g fiber

# SOUTHWESTERN TURKEY MEAT LOAF

*My recipe has less than half the calories of traditional meat loaf. If you'd like to kick up the heat, add a few hits of hot sauce to the meat mixture or serve with superspicy salsa (like we do in my house). Thanks to the extra bonus of soluble fiber from added oats and corn, your waistline and blood sugar both benefit!*

**MAKES 4 SERVINGS**

1 pound ground turkey (at least 90% lean)

1 cup instant oats

¾ cup fat-free milk

2 egg whites

1 small red onion, minced

½ green bell pepper, minced

½ cup fresh corn kernels or thawed frozen corn kernels

2 cloves garlic, minced

½ teaspoon chili powder

¼ teaspoon ground cumin

Kosher salt

Ground black pepper

5 tablespoons salsa, plus more for serving

Preheat the oven to 350°F. Coat a 1-quart loaf pan with oil spray or line with aluminum foil.

In a large bowl, combine the turkey, oats, milk, egg whites, onion, green pepper, corn, garlic, chili powder, and cumin. Season with salt and pepper. Press into the prepared pan and cover with aluminum foil.

Bake for 40 to 45 minutes. Remove the foil and cover with the salsa. Bake, uncovered, for 5 to 10 minutes longer, or until the center is no longer pink. Serve immediately with additional salsa on the side.

**Per serving:** 254 calories, 34 g protein, 23 g carbohydrate, 3 g fat (1 g saturated), 46 mg cholesterol, 193 mg sodium, 3 g fiber

# PART 3

# LOOKING GREAT

# CHAPTER 4

# BEAUTIFUL SKIN

Everybody wants beautiful, healthy skin—especially women, many of whom are concerned (dare I say obsessed?) with signs of aging. I know, because people approach me all the time with questions about skin health—not just in my office but at cocktail parties, on the street, during interviews, and even backstage during my television appearances.

Their interest is perfectly logical. Skin is, quite literally, the face we show to the world. It is our shell, the most exposed part of us. It is our first line of physiological defense against the external environment, and it reflects our state of health. Skin can turn yellow from liver toxins, red from a rush of blood, blue from a lack of oxygen, or gray from cell death.

But all this versatility and responsibility goes largely unappreciated. Most of us care mainly about the superficial beauty of skin. There's nothing wrong with that. Beautiful skin is healthy skin. If battling acne or wrinkles makes you want to eat healthier . . . if the search for clear, smooth skin leads you to exercise more . . . I can't see anything wrong with that! What's good for your skin is good for the rest of you, too.

## WHAT AFFECTS SKIN HEALTH?

In the search for more beautiful skin, the two most common concerns are acne and wrinkles. Acne happens when hair follicles (sometimes called pores) become blocked with natural oils. If the pore is open to the air, the clog will appear as a blackhead. But if oil is trapped below the surface of the skin, it provides a nice little breeding ground for bacteria, leading to pimples—skin eruptions that can look red and inflamed. Because hormones affect how much oil your skin produces, acne is more likely to flare up during times of hormonal upheaval, including adolescence, pregnancy, and premenstrual weeks, as well as times of stress.

Wrinkles are a fact of life. As we age, collagen and elastin, the substances that keep skin firm and elastic, gradually decrease. Fat pads in the face also thin out. Without this underlying structure, skin sags, creases form, and—ugh!—we have wrinkles.

How quickly your skin shows signs of aging is largely determined by genetics, but the process accelerates if your skin is somehow damaged. Skin damage occurs as a result of oxidation, a chemical process during which unstable molecules called free radicals steal electrons from healthy cells. On the skin, oxidative stress can appear as wrinkling, thickening, discoloration, and decreased elasticity. The most damaging oxidative factors are smoking and sun exposure, and the extent of the damage depends on how long and how much you smoke, how much time you spend in the sun, and how many severe sunburns you've had.

Cigarette smoke fills your body with free radicals. Every lungful sends free radicals coursing through your bloodstream, where they can damage every organ in your body, including your skin. Smoking also impairs bloodflow to your skin, starving the cells of nutrition and oxygen. It also damages underlying collagen and elastin and keeps your skin from its natural renewal process. These problems evolve slowly, so the damage to your skin can take up to ten years to appear. Unfortunately, those effects are irreversible. To prevent skin damage from cigarette smoke, including wrinkles, don't smoke and don't spend extensive amounts of time in smoky rooms.

Sunlight, as pleasant as it is, is a form of radiation. Ultraviolet (UV) radiation, to be more specific. UV radiation not only causes free radical damage, it can also cause cells to mutate and potentially turn cancerous. So excess sun exposure is a triple threat: sunburn in the short run, wrinkles in the long run, and the possibility of skin cancer to boot.

## HOW FOOD AFFECTS SKIN

Skin is built from the inside out. Day to day and year to year, skin draws its healthy glow from good nutrition. Even though acne and wrinkles have different causes and occur at different times in your life, nutrition can help minimize or prevent both of these problems and enhance your skin's natural beauty.

### ANTIOXIDANTS

The best defense against the free radical damage of oxidation is a diet rich in antioxidant vitamins and minerals. Research suggests that certain antioxidants—vitamin C, vitamin E, selenium, and vitamin A (in the form of beta-carotene)—nourish and protect skin to extend its youthful appearance.

Topical preparations of these antioxidants—applied to the skin in a cream or ointment—have been shown to help protect the skin against radiation from the sun and even reverse some of the damage that may already have occurred. They may even help prevent skin tumors. Some—such as the vitamin A prescription medications tretinoin (Retin-A, Renova) and isotretinoin (Accutane)—are common treatments for acne and wrinkles.

Antioxidant-rich foods also can help.

**Vitamin C,** naturally found in the skin, is involved in collagen production and protects cells from free radical damage. Scientific studies found that when lab animals ate vitamin C–fortified food, their skin was better able to fight off oxidative damage. Because vitamin C is destroyed by exposure to sunlight, spending even a short time in the sun can leave skin depleted. It is important to replenish your skin's vitamin C stores by eating plenty of vitamin C–rich fruits and vegetables on a regular basis.

BEST FOODS FOR VITAMIN C: *guava, bell peppers (all colors), oranges and orange juice, grapefruit and grapefruit juice, strawberries, pineapple, kohlrabi, papaya, lemons and lemon juice, broccoli, kale, Brussels sprouts, kidney beans, kiwifruit, cantaloupe, cauliflower, cabbage (all varieties), mangoes, white potatoes, mustard greens, tomatoes, sugar snap peas, snow peas, clementines, rutabagas, turnip greens, raspberries, blackberries, watermelon, tangerines, okra, lychees, summer squash, persimmons*

**Vitamin E** helps protect cell membranes and guard against UV radiation damage. Some research suggests that vitamin E may work in combination with vitamin C to provide an extra boost of antiaging skin protection. However, because some studies have raised questions about the safety of vitamin E supplements, these nutrients should come from your diet, not from potent pills. I recommend you stick with food sources (and the small amount found in a multivitamin).

BEST FOODS FOR VITAMIN E: *almonds and almond butter, sunflower seeds and sunflower butter, wheat germ, hazelnuts, spinach, dandelion greens, Swiss chard, pine nuts, peanuts and peanut butter, turnip greens, beet greens, broccoli, canola oil, flaxseed oil, red bell peppers, collard greens, avocados, olive oil, mangoes*

**Selenium** is an antioxidant mineral that helps safeguard the skin from sun damage and delays aging by protecting skin quality and elasticity. Dietary selenium has been shown to reduce sun damage and even prevent some skin cancers in animals. Be sure to get your selenium from food, though, and not from supplements. The Nutritional Prevention of Cancer Trial found that people with a high risk of nonmelanoma skin cancers who took selenium supplements actually had a 25 percent increased risk of squamous cell carcinomas.

BEST FOODS FOR SELENIUM: *Brazil nuts, tuna (canned light), crab, oysters, tilapia, whole wheat pasta, lean beef, cod, shrimp, whole wheat bread or crackers, wheat germ, brown rice, skinless chicken or turkey, cottage cheese (fat-free, 1%), mushrooms, eggs*

**Beta-carotene,** another nutrient critical for skin health, is converted to vitamin A in the body to aid in the growth and repair of body tissues, including your skin. Beta-carotene also acts as an antioxidant that may protect against sun damage. In extremely high doses, straight vitamin A from supplements can be toxic, so I never recommend taking it this way. However, ample beta-carotene from food is entirely safe.

> BEST FOODS FOR BETA-CAROTENE: *sweet potatoes, carrots, kale, butternut squash, turnip greens, pumpkin, mustard greens, cantaloupe, red bell peppers, apricots, Chinese cabbage, spinach, lettuces (romaine, green leaf, red leaf, butterhead), collard greens, Swiss chard, watercress, grapefruit (pink and red), watermelon, cherries, mangoes, tomatoes, guava, asparagus, red cabbage*

## ZINC

Your skin contains about 6 percent of all the zinc in your body. This mineral is necessary for protecting cell membranes and helping maintain the collagen that keeps skin firm. People with severe zinc deficiencies can develop redness, pustules, scaling, and lesions (there's a pretty picture!). In addition, there are microscopic changes in the structure of skin cells themselves. On top of that, zinc is critically involved in skin renewal—which means that if you want to keep your skin fresh and as youthful as possible, be sure to include zinc-rich foods in your menu.

> BEST FOODS FOR ZINC: *oysters, lobster, lean beef, crab, ostrich, wheat germ, skinless chicken or turkey (especially dark meat), lean lamb, clams, mussels, pumpkin seeds, yogurt (fat-free, low-fat), pork tenderloin, starchy beans (such as black, navy, pinto, garbanzo, kidney), lentils, black-eyed peas, soybeans (edamame), lima beans, pine nuts, cashews, peanuts and peanut butter, sunflower seeds and butter, pecans*

## OMEGA-3 FATTY ACIDS

Healthy fats known as omega-3 fatty acids help maintain cell membranes so that they are effective barriers—allowing water and nutrients in and keeping toxins out. Omega-3s have also been shown to protect skin against sun damage. In a study of skin cancer in sunny, skin-scorching southeastern Arizona, people who ate diets rich in fish oils and other omega-3 fats had a 29 percent lower risk of squamous cell skin cancer than those who got very little omega-3s from food. Not too shabby—grill some fish, prevent some cancer. (My Best Foods list includes only the fatty fish that have been shown to be low in mercury, PCBs, and dioxins.)

> BEST FOODS FOR OMEGA-3 FATTY ACIDS: *wild salmon (fresh, canned), herring, mackerel (not king), sardines, anchovies, rainbow trout, Pacific oysters, chia seeds, ground flaxseed, walnuts, butternuts (white walnuts), seaweed, walnut oil, canola oil, flaxseed oil, soybeans (edamame)*

## WATER

It is so basic, but I can't emphasize enough how important water is for skin's health and beauty. Water helps your body flush away toxins, allows the smooth flow of nutrients into cells, and keeps your organs functioning at their best. Plus, cells that are well hydrated are plump and full, which means that your skin will look firmer and clearer (but not "fat"). Recommendations vary, but according to the Institute of Medicine, the average requirement for women is 9 total cups of fluids from water and other beverages per day. For men, it bumps up to 13 cups.

Although liquids are the main source of water, many foods have such high water content that they contribute to overall hydration. The following foods are at least 75 percent water (by weight) and should regularly be included as part of a healthy skin regimen.

**Fruits:** apples, blackberries, blueberries, cantaloupe, cherries, cranberries, grapefruit, grapes, kiwifruit, lemons, limes, mangoes, nectarines, oranges, papaya, peaches, pears, pineapple, plums, raspberries, strawberries, tangerines, watermelon

**Vegetables:** artichokes, asparagus, beets, broccoli, Brussels sprouts, carrots, cauliflower, celery, cucumbers, kale, lettuce, mushrooms, onions, peas, potatoes, pumpkin, peppers (all types), rhubarb, spinach, squash, tomatoes, turnips

## TEA

Another good option for hydration is tea. Teas contain natural compounds known as polyphenols, which have antioxidant properties. In animal studies, polyphenols helped prevent sun-related skin cancers and improve immune functioning. When

## FAQS

**I've heard that sugary foods can cause breakouts. Is this true?**

Maybe. For decades, health experts have been telling people that food doesn't cause acne, but we're now learning that we may have to eat our words to some extent. A 2007 study by Australian researchers suggests that a "high-glycemic diet" may worsen acne and offers a theoretical explanation for the possible link.

In simplest terms, a high-glycemic diet is rich in poor-quality carbohydrates, including soda, sweetened drinks, candy, sugary breakfast cereals, and baked goods. Refined carbs (found in white bread, white rice, crackers, cookies, pastries, and anything made with white flour) also tend to be high on the glycemic scale because they're rapidly broken down into simple sugars in the gut. High-glycemic foods cause a rapid surge in blood sugar, which triggers the body to start pumping out insulin to clear and store the extra sugar. Here's where the potential acne link comes in: High insulin exposure promotes increased production of male sex hormones called androgens, which may contribute to acne proliferation by boosting oily secretions in the skin. Of course, we'll have to wait and see if future studies corroborate these initial findings.

Eating a better diet won't completely cure your acne, but it may improve your skin, and there's no question that limiting empty calories from sugary foods and drinks will benefit your overall health.

applied to human skin in the form of ointments and creams, topical green and white tea extracts have been shown to help protect skin cells against damage from harsh ultraviolet rays. Although there are no definitive human studies about the effects of drinking tea for skin health, tea—green, white, or black; caffeinated or decaffeinated—is always a better choice than soda, fruit juice, or sugary coffee concoctions.

## BONUS POINTS

- ◆ **Use sunscreen.** Whenever you are going to be spending more than a few minutes outside, protect your skin from some of the sun's damaging rays by applying sunscreen to all exposed areas of your body. Look for formulas designed to filter both UVA and UVB radiation, with a sun protection factor (SPF) of at least 15. The SPF is a general indicator of how long you will be protected, and the higher the number, the more time you can spend outside without burning. Use sunscreen with an SPF of at least 30 if you want longer protection or if you tend to burn easily. Apply moisturizer with SPF every day to guard your skin against even casual sun exposure.

- ◆ **Avoid sweets, sugary drinks, and the "white stuff."** Some researchers have theorized that low-quality carbohydrates raise insulin levels, which, over time, may increase levels of certain acne-causing hormones. These foods also cause inflammation in skin cells and throughout the body, causing premature aging and wrinkles.

- ◆ **Consider a topical antioxidant.** Most drugstore and cosmetic brand serums and creams don't contain enough of these antioxidants to make a difference to your skin's health. The more potent—and potentially irritating—preparations aren't for everybody. Some are available only by prescription, so if you want to try an antioxidant skin cream, talk with your dermatologist.

## SUPPLEMENTS

To improve skin health, I strongly recommend getting all of your nutrients from food sources. However, if you would also like to consider supplements, I recommend:

1. **A multivitamin.** Taking a multivitamin will ensure that you get the minimal amount of vitamins and minerals necessary for good skin health, even on days when you might not eat as well as you should. Choose a brand that contains 100 percent DV for vitamin A (optimally, 100 percent—but at least 50 percent—coming from beta-carotene and/or mixed carotenoids), vitamin C, vitamin E, and zinc. Your multivitamin should also provide 55 to 70 micrograms of selenium.

2. **Fish oil supplement.** People who don't eat fatty fish at least once per week may want to consider taking a fish oil supplement. The two most potent types of

omega-3 fatty acids found in fish oil supplements are DHA (docosahexaenoic acid) and EPA (eicosapentaenoic acid). Aim to take a daily dose of 1,000 milligrams of EPA and DHA combined. Because fish oil supplement companies balance these fatty acids differently, you'll need to read the label carefully and tally up the DHA plus EPA total. You typically have to take more than one pill to reach the 1,000 milligram amount.

To prevent rancidity, store bottles of fish oil supplements in the fridge. To lessen the chance of fishy burps or aftertaste, choose an enteric-coated variety, which is digested in the intestines instead of the stomach, making it less likely to repeat on you. Avoid getting omega-3 fats from cod liver oil because it may contain too much vitamin A. Important note: Because fish oil acts as a blood thinner, it should not be taken by people who have hemophilia or who are already taking blood-thinning medications or aspirin.

## FAQS

### Can dairy foods cause acne breakouts?

Possibly. According to a handful of studies in adolescents, there may in fact be a link between dairy and acne. The current prevailing thought is that the dairy-acne connection may be caused by the hormones in milk. Apparently, dairy cows are allowed to become pregnant while they are lactating, and the pregnancy hormones pass into the milk. (This is an issue with both conventionally and organically raised cows.) If you want to test your personal reaction, I recommend eliminating all dairy foods from your diet for one month. These include milk, yogurt, all cheeses, sour cream, and ice cream. (No matter what your age, be sure to get enough daily calcium from nondairy sources, or take a daily calcium supplement to make up for what you're missing.) If you see no difference in your skin, then dairy is not a problem for you. If your acne improves, add dairy back into your diet—but just two servings a day for a week. If your acne comes back, then dairy is most likely the culprit.

For more information on how food can improve your skin, visit www.joybauer.com/skin

# JOY'S 4-STEP PROGRAM
## FOR BEAUTIFUL SKIN

Follow this program if you want healthier skin, now and in the future.

## Step 1 ... START WITH THE BASICS

◆ See your doctor if you have any unusual skin growths, moles, or freckles that have grown or gotten darker, or a scaly patch or scab that won't heal. These may be early signs of skin cancer that can be treated before they turn deadly.

◆ If you smoke, quit.

◆ Stay out of the sun as much as possible. If you do go outdoors, wear sunscreen to protect your skin.

◆ Drink plenty of water.

## Step 2 ... YOUR ULTIMATE GROCERY LIST

This list contains foods with high levels of nutrients that will help your skin look the best it can, and many are featured in the meal plans and recipes that follow. You don't have to purchase every item, but integrate as many as possible into your diet.

### FRUIT

*All* fruit, but especially:
Apricots
Berries (blackberries, blueberries, raspberries, and strawberries)
Cantaloupe
Cherries
Clementines
Grapefruit
Guava
Kiwifruit
Lemons
Mangoes
Oranges
Papaya
Peaches
Persimmons
Pineapple
Tangerines
Watermelon

## VEGETABLES AND LEGUMES

*All* vegetables, but especially:

Artichokes

Asparagus

Avocados

Beans, starchy (such as black, garbanzo, kidney, navy, and pinto)

Beets

Broccoli

Brussels sprouts

Cabbage

Carrots

Cauliflower

Celery

Cucumbers

Dark leafy greens (such as collard, kale, mustard, Swiss chard, and turnip)

Kohlrabi

Lentils

Lettuce (all varieties)

Lima beans

Mushrooms

Okra

Onions (all varieties)

Peas (black-eyed and green)

Peppers (all varieties)

Potatoes (sweet and white)

Pumpkin

Rhubarb

Rutabagas

Snow peas

Soybeans (edamame)

Spinach

Squash, winter

Squash, summer

Sugar snap peas

Tomatoes

Turnips

## SEAFOOD

*All* fish and shellfish, but especially:

Anchovies

Clams

Cod

Crab

Herring

Mackerel (not king)

Mussels

Oysters (especially Pacific)

Salmon, wild (fresh and canned)

Sardines (fresh and canned)

Shrimp

Tilapia

Trout, rainbow

Tuna (canned light)

## LEAN PROTEINS

Beef, lean

Chicken, ground (at least 90% lean)

Chicken, skinless

Eggs and egg substitutes

Lamb, lean

Pork tenderloin

Tempeh

Tofu

Turkey, ground (at least 90% lean)

Turkey, skinless

Turkey bacon

Turkey burgers, lean

Veggie burgers

## NUTS AND SEEDS (PREFERABLY UNSALTED)

Almonds and almond butter
Butternuts (white walnuts)
Cashews and cashew butter
Flaxseed, ground
Hazelnuts

Macadamia nuts
Peanuts and peanut butter
Pecans
Pine nuts
Pumpkin seeds

Sunflower seeds and
   sunflower butter
Walnuts

## WHOLE GRAINS

Amaranth
Barley
Bread, whole grain (buns,
   crackers, English muffins,
   pitas, tortillas, and wraps)

Bulgur
Cereal, whole grain
Millet
Oats
Pasta, whole grain

Quinoa
Rice (brown and wild)
Waffles, whole grain
Wheat germ

## DAIRY

Cheese (fat-free and
   reduced-fat)
Cottage cheese (fat-free or
   1%)

Cream cheese (fat-free or
   reduced-fat)
Milk (fat-free or 1%)
Milk alternatives (almond,
   rice, and soy)

Sour cream (fat-free or
   reduced-fat)
Yogurt (fat-free or low-fat)

## MISCELLANEOUS

Canola oil
Garlic
Herbs and spices (fresh,
   dried, and ground)
Hot sauce
Hummus
Marinara sauce
Mayonnaise, reduced-fat

Mustard (all varieties)
Olive oil
Salad dressing, reduced-
   calorie
Salsa
Soft tub spread, trans-fat-
   free (reduced-fat or
   regular)

Tea, black, green, and white
   (caffeinated or
   decaffeinated)
Vinegar (all varieties)

# Step 3 . . . GOING ABOVE AND BEYOND

If you want to do everything you can to improve your skin, here are some additional things you might try.

◆ Consider taking a daily multivitamin.
◆ If you don't eat at least one serving of a fatty fish every week, consider taking fish oil supplements.

# Step 4 . . . MEAL PLANS

These sample menus include foods that have been shown to improve skin health—specifically, foods high in vitamins C and E, beta-carotene, selenium, zinc, and omega-3 fatty acids.

Every day, choose one option for each of the three meals—breakfast, lunch, and dinner. Then, one or two times per day, choose from among my suggested snacks. Approximate calories have been provided to help adjust for your personal weight-management goals. If you find yourself hungry (and if weight is not an issue), feel free to increase the portion sizes for meals and snacks. Beverage calories are not included. For the best skin, water and green, white, or black tea are your best bets for beverage selections.

## ACNE AND FRIED FOOD

You'll notice that I didn't warn you to avoid fried, greasy, oily foods in my discussion about acne. That's because eating grease doesn't necessarily cause skin problems. However, if you eat french fries, potato chips, or other oily foods and then scratch your nose or rub your chin, you spread that grease to your skin. That kind of topical oil can block pores and cause acne. In fact, anytime you touch your face, you risk transferring dirt and bacteria that can cloud your complexion. Make a point of washing your hands with soap before laying a finger on your face.

## BREAKFAST OPTIONS

(300 TO 400 CALORIES)

### Yogurt with Almonds and Berries

Mix 8 ounces fat-free plain or flavored yogurt with 1 cup berries, 1 to 2 tablespoons slivered almonds (or pumpkin seeds or chopped walnuts), and 2 tablespoons wheat germ.

### Southwest Omelet with Whole Grain Toast

Coat a small skillet with oil spray or 1 teaspoon canola oil. Sauté ½ cup sliced onion and ½ cup sliced red or yellow pepper until soft. Beat 1 whole egg with two egg whites and pour over the sautéed vegetables. Add ½ cup chopped tomato, season with a pinch of salt and ground black pepper, and cook until the bottom becomes firm. Gently flip and cook until the egg mixture becomes firm. Fold the omelet over and serve. Enjoy with 1 slice toasted whole grain bread (with optional 1 teaspoon soft tub, trans-fat-free spread).

### Oatmeal with Chopped Walnuts and Fruit

Prepare ½ cup dry oats with ½ cup water and ½ cup fat-free milk or soy milk. Sweeten with optional 1 to 2 teaspoons sugar, honey, jam, or sugar substitute. Top with 1 tablespoon chopped walnuts (or almonds or sunflower seeds) and ½ cup berries (or ½ mango or 1 peach).

### Peanut Butter Toast

Spread 2 slices toasted whole grain bread with 1 level tablespoon peanut butter.

### Cottage Cheese with Apricots and Pecans

Top 1 cup fat-free or 1% cottage cheese with 4 diced whole apricots (or 1 cup berries or ½ chopped mango) and 2 tablespoons chopped pecans or slivered almonds. (If you like, sprinkle with ½ teaspoon cinnamon.)

## LUNCH OPTIONS

(400 TO 500 CALORIES)

### Butternut Squash Soup with Salad and Fish

Enjoy 2 servings (3 cups) Butternut Squash Soup (page 79) or 2 cups any prepared low-fat soup without cream, with unlimited leafy greens topped with 3 ounces canned sardines (or wild salmon, light tuna, or grilled chicken) and drizzled with 1 teaspoon olive oil and unlimited fresh lemon juice or vinegar.

### Vegetarian Chili and Sweet Potato

Enjoy 2 cups vegetarian chili or Turkey Chili (page 363) with ½ medium baked sweet or white potato (with optional 1 teaspoon soft tub, trans-fat-free spread or 1 tablespoon fat-free sour cream).

### Open-Faced Tuna Melt

Mash 6 ounces canned, water-packed light tuna (or chicken breast or wild salmon) with 1 tablespoon reduced-fat mayonnaise and minced onion and freshly ground black pepper to taste (or use Veggie Tuna Salad, page 271). Toast 2 slices whole grain bread, spread each slice with the tuna mixture, and top each with tomato and 1 slice reduced-fat cheese. Bake in a 350°F oven until the cheese melts. Enjoy with red, yellow, or green pepper strips.

### Turkey Burger with Sautéed Mushrooms and Broccoli

Top 1 cooked 5-ounce turkey burger (or a 5-ounce lean beef burger or veggie burger) with tomato, sautéed mushrooms, and optional 1 tablespoon ketchup. Serve on a hamburger bun (preferably whole grain). For half of the bun, you may substitute 1 slice reduced-fat cheese. Enjoy with unlimited steamed broccoli.

### Caesar Salad with Grilled Chicken or Shrimp

Top a large bed of romaine lettuce with 4 ounces grilled chicken or cooked shrimp, 1 ounce grated Parmesan cheese (4 to 5 level tablespoons), and optional anchovies (4 fillets). Toss with ¼ cup reduced-calorie Caesar dressing (40 calories or less per tablespoon) or 2 tablespoons regular Caesar dressing.

## DINNER OPTIONS

(500 TO 600 CALORIES)

### Beef Stir-Fry with Brown Rice and Steamed Broccoli

Stir-fry 5 ounces lean beef (round, sirloin, or flank), trimmed, in 2 teaspoons canola oil with ½ cup sliced bell peppers, ½ cup sugar snap peas, and 2 chopped scallions (plus optional minced garlic, reduced-sodium soy sauce, and black pepper to taste). Enjoy with ½ cup cooked brown rice and unlimited steamed broccoli (or spinach, kale, or Swiss chard).

### Lemon-Dill Wild Salmon with Baked Potato

Top 1 poached or baked 5-ounce wild salmon fillet with 1 tablespoon Dijon mustard and ½ teaspoon dried dill, and drizzle with juice from ½ lemon (or enjoy 1 serving Easy! 3-Step Microwave Salmon, page 345). Serve with ½ medium baked sweet or white potato (with optional 1 tablespoon soft tub, trans-fat-free spread) and unlimited steamed asparagus (or spinach, broccoli, kale, Swiss chard, or sugar snap peas).

### Rosemary Chicken with Cauliflower and Butternut Squash Soup

Sauté 5 ounces skinless chicken and minced garlic in 2 teaspoons canola or olive oil, and season with preferred herbs (or enjoy 1 serving Rosemary Chicken, page 347). Enjoy with 2 servings (3 cups) Butternut Squash Soup (page 79) and unlimited steamed cauliflower (or broccoli, spinach, kale, or Swiss chard).

### Whole Wheat Pasta with Turkey Meatballs

Enjoy 1 serving Turkey Meatballs in Red Pepper-Tomato Sauce (page 78) with ½ cup cooked whole grain pasta (or ½ plain medium baked sweet or white potato).

### Grilled Oysters with Cajun Fish and Brussels Sprouts

Enjoy 1 serving Grilled Rockefeller Oysters (page 179) with 6 ounces fish (tilapia, cod, haddock, wild salmon, or trout) rubbed with Cajun spice and baked or grilled, a leafy green salad tossed with 1 teaspoon olive oil and unlimited fresh lemon juice or balsamic vinegar (or 2 tablespoons reduced-calorie dressing), and unlimited steamed or roasted Brussels sprouts (or broccoli, Swiss chard, or spinach).

## SNACK OPTIONS

### 100 CALORIES OR LESS

◆ *Best Vegetable Snacks:* up to 2 cups raw or cooked bell peppers (red, green, or yellow), broccoli, cauliflower, asparagus, carrots, sugar snap peas, mushrooms

◆ *Best Fruit Snacks:* 1 guava, peach, orange, persimmon, kiwifruit, clementine, or tangerine; 4 apricots; 6 lychees; 1 cup blueberries, blackberries, raspberries, or cherries; 1 cup cubed watermelon or pineapple; 20 whole strawberries; ½ mango, cantaloupe, papaya, or grapefruit

◆ 2 level teaspoons peanut butter (or other nut butter) with celery sticks

◆ ½ cup fat-free or 1% cottage cheese with red, green, or yellow bell pepper strips

### 100 TO 200 CALORIES

◆ 1 serving (1½ cups) Butternut Squash Soup (page 79)

◆ 1 serving Warm Dark Chocolate Sauce with Fresh Fruit (page 80)

◆ 1 ounce (about ¼ cup) almonds, cashews, pecans, walnuts, or peanuts

◆ ½ cup pistachios or sunflower seeds in the shell

◆ 1 slice whole grain bread (or 70-calorie pita) topped with 1 level tablespoon peanut butter (or other nut butter)

◆ Red, yellow, and/or green pepper strips and baby carrots dipped in ¼ cup hummus

◆ 1 cup fat-free plain or flavored yogurt mixed with ½ cup berries or cherries plus 1 tablespoon wheat germ

◆ ½ mango or small cantaloupe with ½ cup fat-free or 1% cottage cheese

# TURKEY MEATBALLS IN RED PEPPER–TOMATO SAUCE

*I call these Beautiful Meatballs. By mixing wheat germ, egg whites, and plain yogurt into lean ground turkey meat, I'm able to boost the vitamin E, selenium, and zinc. Together with the red pepper–tomato sauce—rich in vitamin C and beta-carotene—it's a perfect meal for a healthy complexion.*

**MAKES 4 SERVINGS (APPROXIMATELY 5 MEATBALLS EACH)**

½ cup wheat germ

2 egg whites

½ cup fat-free plain yogurt

¼ cup packed fresh basil leaves, chopped

2 small onions, minced

2 cloves garlic, minced

1 pound ground turkey (at least 90% lean)

Kosher salt

Freshly ground black pepper

1 can (28 ounces) whole peeled tomatoes

2 tablespoons olive oil

1 red bell pepper, finely chopped

1 sprig fresh thyme or 1 teaspoon dried

1 teaspoon dried oregano

In a large bowl, combine the wheat germ, egg whites, yogurt, basil, half of the onions, and half of the garlic. Add the turkey. Season with salt and pepper and mix well. (The mixture will be sticky.) Cover and place in the freezer for 20 minutes for easier handling.

Meanwhile, in a blender or food processor, puree the tomatoes with 1 cup water.

Heat 1 tablespoon of the oil in a large nonstick skillet over medium-high heat. Sauté the remaining onion and garlic for 3 to 4 minutes, or until translucent. Add the bell pepper and cook for 5 to 6 minutes longer, or until the pepper softens slightly. Add the thyme, oregano, and pureed tomatoes and bring to a low simmer.

Roll the turkey mixture into about 20 meatballs, each 2 inches in diameter. Coat a nonstick skillet with oil spray. Add the remaining 1 tablespoon oil and heat over high heat. In batches, add the meatballs and sauté until they are browned on all sides, 6 to 7 minutes total.

Carefully transfer the meatballs to the tomato sauce as they finish cooking. Simmer, partially covered, for about 20 minutes longer, or until the meatballs are cooked through. Season with additional salt and pepper if needed. Serve immediately.

**Per serving:** 390 calories, 33 g protein, 25 g carbohydrate, 19 g fat (4 g saturated), 176 mg cholesterol, 536 mg sodium, 6 g fiber; plus 54 mg vitamin C (90% DV), 326 mcg beta-carotene, 3 mg zinc (20% DV)

# BUTTERNUT SQUASH SOUP

*This is, by far, one of my favorite low-calorie comfort soups. It's easy to make, and 1½ cups provide a blast of vitamin C and beta-carotene for radiant skin!*

**MAKES 4 SERVINGS (1½ CUPS EACH)**

1 tablespoon olive oil

2 large leeks, trimmed and chopped

⅛ teaspoon ground cinnamon

⅛ teaspoon nutmeg

1½ pounds butternut squash, peeled and cubed (about 4 cups)

2 large carrots, peeled and grated

3 cups low-sodium chicken or vegetable broth

Kosher salt

Freshly ground black pepper

Coat a large stockpot with oil spray. Add the oil and heat over medium-high heat. Add the leeks and sauté for 6 to 7 minutes, or until translucent and soft. Add the cinnamon and nutmeg and cook an additional minute to release the flavor of the spices. Add the squash, carrots, and broth and bring to a boil.

Reduce to a simmer and cook for 20 to 25 minutes longer, or until the vegetables are tender. Puree the soup with an immersion blender or in a food processor or blender. Season with salt and pepper to taste and serve immediately.

> **Per serving:** 158 calories, 5 g protein, 30 g carbohydrate, 4 g fat (0 g saturated), 0 mg cholesterol, 452 mg sodium, 5 g fiber; plus 43 mg vitamin C (73% DV), 10,160 mcg beta-carotene

# WARM DARK CHOCOLATE SAUCE WITH FRESH FRUIT

*Here's the most wonderful news: Research suggests that consuming flavonol-rich cocoa may improve your skin. If you dip fresh fruit into my guilt-free dark chocolate sauce, you'll get the added benefits of vitamin C. If you're diabetic or would like to lower the calories even further, replace the sugar with your preferred sugar substitute.*

**MAKES 6 SERVINGS (¼ CUP SAUCE EACH WITH FRUIT)**

1 tablespoon cornstarch

1 can (12 ounces) fat-free evaporated milk

½ cup unsweetened cocoa powder

½ cup granulated sugar

½ teaspoon instant coffee

½ teaspoon vanilla extract

⅛ teaspoon kosher salt

1 cup whole strawberries

1 cup fresh pineapple chunks

In a medium saucepan, whisk the cornstarch into the evaporated milk. Place over low heat and stir in the cocoa powder, sugar, coffee, vanilla, and salt. Cook, whisking constantly, for 5 to 6 minutes, or until the ingredients are thoroughly combined and the liquid starts to thicken. Serve immediately with the strawberries and pineapple.

**Per serving:** 153 calories, 6 g protein, 33 g carbohydrate, 1 g fat (0 g saturated), 0 mg cholesterol, 133 mg sodium, 3 g fiber; plus 24 mg vitamin C (40% DV)

# CHAPTER 5

# HEALTHY HAIR

Unless you are balding, chances are good that you take hair for granted. A little shampoo and conditioner, a bit of styling product, and a good hair day is in your future, right? Not necessarily. Like all other body tissues, the state of your hair is related to your overall health and individual physical characteristics.

Hair starts its life span in small, sacklike structures in the skin known as follicles. Each follicle produces a single hair shaft composed of a hard protein called keratin, which is arranged in long, tightly bound strands. New growth begins in the follicle and pushes outward so that the oldest part of the hair is farthest from the scalp.

Each hair has a distinct growth cycle—active growth, maturation, and rest. During the resting phase, the follicle relaxes its hold on the shaft, so hair can easily fall or be pulled out. Every hair on your head goes through the growth cycle, but not all at the same time. At any given moment, about 15 percent of all the hairs on your head are resting and therefore capable of shedding . . . in your hairbrush, in the shower, on the bathroom floor. This is totally normal and not a harbinger of baldness. Between my two daughters and myself, our shower drain needs cleaning about every two weeks—that's about all the "resting" hair it can take before it's thoroughly clogged. Trust me, none of us is even close to bald. But if you have been experiencing unusual hair loss or problems with dryness, splitting, or breakage or you simply want to have more beautiful locks, nutrition can help.

## WHAT AFFECTS HAIR HEALTH?

It is estimated that we each lose about 100 hairs a day. The actual number you'll lose on any given day depends on how abundant and healthy your follicles are, what medications you're taking, and many other factors, some of which are beyond your control. For example, the recommendations in this chapter won't reverse thinning hair due to male pattern baldness or aging—typical male baldness is genetic. As we age, our hair spends more time in the resting phase, which means that we'll shed more hair than usual, and it won't grow back as quickly. For more general hair problems, here are some factors that you should be aware of.

## HORMONAL SHIFTS

Both male and female hormones affect hair growth. Male hormones known as androgens—a category that includes testosterone—stimulate hair growth on the face and body and create fuller, thicker hair on the head. In women, ovaries and adrenal glands naturally produce androgens, but only in very small amounts. If a woman suddenly starts growing facial hair, she should see her doctor—it could be a sign of a hormone-related health problem.

For some men with a genetic susceptibility to baldness, normal testosterone is converted to a more potent form of testosterone (dihydrotestosterone, or DHT), which binds to cells in the follicle. DHT alters the growth/shed cycle and eventually kills the follicle. These men find themselves becoming bald in their twenties, a few years after their testosterone levels peak. Because the follicle itself shrinks and dies, this type of baldness is irreversible. Some prescription medications may short-circuit the balding process if caught early enough, though the medications need to be continued for life.

In both men and women, levels of androgens decrease after about age 40, which leads to thinner, slower-growing, less luxurious hair as we get older.

In contrast to androgens, the female hormone estrogen slows hair growth and creates a finer, thinner shaft of hair, which is why women are, on average, naturally less hairy than men. After menopause, levels of estrogen fall off dramatically, causing some genetically susceptible women to lose significant amounts of hair. Experts believe that female balding follows a process much like male balding—without enough estrogen to offset the tiny amounts of androgens in their bodies, women also can have androgen-related hair loss. But male and female hair loss aren't identical. While men tend to bald in a distinct pattern that includes a receding hairline and hair loss at the crown, women tend to lose hair evenly, leaving them with a sparse head of hair instead of a totally bald scalp.

The "other" female hormone, progesterone, has almost no direct action on hair. However, when levels of estrogen and progesterone are both high, such as during pregnancy, the combination works to synchronize the hair growth cycles, so more hair is in the growth stage at the same time. In the second and third trimester of pregnancy, the percentage of hair in the resting phase falls by one-third, to about 10 percent. For those few months, pregnant women have the fullest, richest heads of hair they'll have in their entire lives. About three months after delivery, the percentage of shedding hairs goes back up to 15. As all those synchronized hairs enter the resting phase together, it can look like you're suddenly losing all your hair. Don't panic! Once the hair starts to regrow, it returns to its usual growth/rest cycle.

## STRESS

Stress is one of the most common causes of unusual hair loss. Accidents, serious illnesses, severe psychological stress, the loss of a loved one, and other traumatic events can send hair follicles into the resting phase prematurely. About three months later, when those resting follicles release the hair shaft, large amounts of hair can seem to fall out simultaneously and for no discernable reason, because several months will have passed since the event that triggered this whole episode. Again, getting through this is simply a matter of waiting it out. Your hair should begin to regrow almost immediately.

## LACK OF PROTEIN

Hair is made of protein. All basic nutrients contribute to keeping us whole and healthy, but protein provides the building blocks that allow us to repair, replace, or grow bones, skin, muscles, and hair. Although we tend to think of dietary protein as coming from steak, fish, chicken, and other meats, it is also found in eggs, legumes (such as beans and lentils), dairy products, soy foods, and—in smaller amounts—some whole grains and vegetables. People who don't get enough protein in their diets, such as those with anorexia nervosa or who follow any extreme weight-loss diet, will slow the rate of new hair growth. As hair is naturally shed, it won't grow back as quickly. With enough hair loss, the scalp will start to show through.

## FAQS

**My doctor tested my iron level in the office, and it came up a little on the low side but still normal. My thyroid, blood sugar, and all other blood tests turned out normal. Is there anything else I should test that might explain my hair loss?**

Since your iron tested low-normal, make sure that you eat lots of iron-rich protein (coupled with foods rich in vitamin C, if you're a vegetarian) for the next several weeks. This will help bring your iron levels back into the mid-normal range. You might also want to go back to your doctor and ask for a more extensive test for iron levels. There are actually three main tests for iron: (1) serum iron, which measures the amount of iron in blood; (2) ferritin, which is a measure of the amount of iron stored in the body; and (3) total iron binding capacity (TIBC), which is a measure of how much iron is available in your blood. Many doctors will test only serum iron, but the ferritin and TIBC tests are more sensitive and can often catch an iron deficiency before it becomes severe. Low ferritin means low iron stores, which means that you may need more iron. High TIBC means that your body has a big gap between how much iron the body has at its disposal and how much it needs. Both of these tests can help diagnose iron-deficiency anemia or pre-anemia. Talk with your doctor about these additional tests. Your iron levels may yet be the problem. You may be a candidate for a supplemental dose, but never take iron pills unless a medical professional confirms that you need them.

## FAQS

**I was losing a lot of hair, had no energy, gained weight, and felt miserable. Finally I was diagnosed with low thyroid hormone (hypothyroid). I've been on Synthroid for a couple of weeks, and I'm feeling better, but my hair still hasn't come back. What's up?**

There's a good chance your hair will come back; you just have to give it more time. Your body needs a chance to recover from illness, and your follicles need a few months to recover from the resting phase. If your hair hasn't started to regrow within six months after your blood levels of thyroid hormone have returned to normal, talk with your doctor to see if there might be another reason for your continuing problem.

Starvation also depletes the body of other nutrients important for hair growth and quality. And over the long term, starvation and extreme weight loss will lead to a reduction in hormone production, which can also lead to thinning hair.

## MEDICATIONS AND SUPPLEMENTS

Most people understand that chemotherapy treatments for cancer can cause widespread balding, but many other commonly prescribed medications may lead to less extensive hair loss. These include anticoagulants (such as warfarin), antidepressants, oral contraceptives, and medications for blood pressure, gout, or arthritis. In addition, very high doses of vitamin A and selenium are toxic and can cause hair loss. This type of toxicity happens only if you take high-dose supplements, so don't take individual supplements for vitamin A or selenium. If you take a multivitamin supplement, it shouldn't contain more than 100 percent DV for vitamin A (5,000 IU) or selenium (70 micrograms). Better yet, make sure your multivitamin provides 50 to 100 percent of its vitamin A in the precursor form of beta-carotene and/or mixed carotenoids. There is no known chance of vitamin A toxicity when you're getting your standard supplemental dose from carotenoids, because beta-carotene in food and supplements is converted to the active form of vitamin A by your body in controlled amounts. Once you stop taking the medication or supplements, hair will usually begin to grow back within a few months.

## THYROID GLAND MALFUNCTION AND OTHER DISORDERS

Thyroid hormones affect the metabolism of all cells, including cells in hair follicles. Too much thyroid hormone (hyperthyroid) or too little thyroid hormone (hypothyroid) can result in thin, brittle hair or hair loss.

With uncontrolled diabetes, body cells (including cells in hair follicles) starve because glucose can't get in; and in systemic lupus erythematosus, the body attacks its own collagen, including the collagen in hair follicles. These disorders and many others—including celiac disease, rheumatoid arthritis, ulcerative colitis, and Crohn's disease—may cause hair loss or damage by altering cell metabolism or structure. Once the underlying disease is treated, hair growth should return to normal. All cases of unexplained hair loss should be investigated by a physician to rule out the possibility of serious disease.

## HOW FOOD AFFECTS HAIR

Hair is a great marker of overall health. Good hair depends on the body's ability to construct a proper hair shaft, as well as the health of the skin and follicles. Good nutrition assures the best possible environment for building strong, lustrous hair. But this is not a quick fix. Changing your diet now will affect only new growth, not the part of the hair that is already visible. You could get a completely fresh start if you shaved your head today and started eating a perfect, hair-improving diet tomorrow. Your new head of hair would positively radiate with health. But there's really no need. Take my word for it: Starting a hair-healthy diet today will mean a more gorgeous head of hair within six months to a year, depending on how fast your hair grows. Hair growth rates vary between about $\frac{1}{4}$ and $1\frac{1}{4}$ inch per month, depending on age, gender, ethnicity, and other genetic and lifestyle factors. On average, a person can expect to have about 6 inches of new growth every year, so it will take about that long to notice the effects of your nutritional changes.

## B VITAMINS: FOLATE, $B_6$, $B_{12}$

These vitamins are involved in the creation of red blood cells, which carry oxygen and nutrients to all body cells, including those of the scalp, follicles, and growing hair. Without enough B vitamins, these cells can starve, causing shedding, slow growth, or weak hair that is prone to breaking.

BEST FOODS FOR VITAMIN $B_6$: *chickpeas (garbanzo beans), wild salmon (fresh, canned), lean beef, pork tenderloin, skinless chicken, potatoes (sweet, white), oats, bananas, pistachios, lentils, tomato paste, barley, rice (brown, wild), peppers, winter squash (acorn, butternut), broccoli, broccoli raab, carrots, Brussels sprouts, peanuts and peanut butter, eggs, shrimp, tofu, apricots, watermelon, avocados, strawberries, whole grain bread*

BEST FOODS FOR VITAMIN $B_{12}$: *shellfish (clams, oysters, crab), wild salmon (fresh, canned), soy milk, trout (rainbow, wild), tuna (canned light), lean beef, veggie burgers, cottage cheese (fat-free, 1%), yogurt (fat-free, low-fat), milk (fat-free, 1%), eggs, cheese (fat-free, reduced-fat)*

BEST FOODS FOR FOLATE: *lentils, black-eyed peas, soybeans, oats, turnip greens, spinach, mustard greens, green peas, artichokes, okra, beets, parsnips, broccoli, broccoli raab, sunflower seeds, wheat germ, oranges and orange juice, Brussels sprouts, papaya, seaweed, berries (boysenberries, blackberries, strawberries), starchy beans (such as black, navy, pinto, garbanzo, kidney), cauliflower, Chinese cabbage, corn, whole grain bread, whole grain pasta*

## BIOTIN

People ask me about biotin for hair health all the time. Usually they've heard about it on a shampoo commercial or read a magazine article that recommended biotin supplements. Biotin is a B vitamin essential for hair growth and overall scalp health. Because our bodies make their own biotin in the intestines and it is plentiful in many common foods, deficiency is very rare. In those few cases where people are very ill and don't have use of their intestines, biotin deficiency causes hair loss. So yes, biotin is important for hair health, but you don't need to take supplements. Just eat a balanced diet that includes some high-biotin foods.

BEST FOODS FOR BIOTIN: *eggs, peanuts and peanut butter, almonds and almond butter, wheat bran, walnuts, Swiss chard, whole wheat bread, wild salmon (fresh, canned), cheese (fat-free, reduced-fat), cauliflower, avocados, raspberries*

## IRON-RICH PROTEIN

Iron helps red blood cells carry oxygen. Iron deficiency can lead to anemia, a condition in which cells don't get enough oxygen to function properly. The result can be devastating to the whole body, causing weakness, fatigue, and possibly hair loss. One large-scale study found that premenopausal women who reported severe hair loss were more likely to have low iron reserves (as measured by a test for an iron storage protein called ferritin) than women who reported little or no hair loss. Women of childbearing age are more likely to experience iron deficiency because they lose a significant amount of iron from the blood shed during menstruation. Women with heavier periods will lose more iron than those with lighter flow.

For most people, foods can provide all the iron necessary for good health and strong hair. I recommend iron-rich protein for two reasons. First, protein is necessary for all cell growth, including hair cells. Hair gets its structure from keratin, and without enough protein for keratin, your strands will weaken and grow more slowly. Second, the iron found in meat (called heme iron) is more easily absorbed by the body than the iron in plant foods (nonheme iron).

Vegetarians can meet their iron requirement by consuming plenty of iron-rich plant foods like beans, lentils, and dark leafy greens. Vitamin C improves the body's ability to absorb nonheme iron, so vegetarians should eat iron-rich foods and foods rich in vitamin C at the same meal. Before menopause, women may want to consider taking a multivitamin that contains iron. (See the following section on supplements for more information.)

BEST FOODS FOR IRON-RICH PROTEIN: *clams, oysters, lean beef and lamb, skinless chicken and turkey (especially dark meat), pork tenderloin, shrimp, egg yolks*

BEST FOODS FOR IRON-RICH PROTEIN (VEGETARIAN SOURCES): *tofu, tempeh, soybeans (edamame), lentils, starchy beans (such as black, navy, pinto, garbanzo, kidney), black-eyed peas*

BEST IRON-RICH VEGETABLES (LOW IN PROTEIN): *spinach, seaweed, Swiss chard, asparagus, Brussels sprouts, mustard greens, kale, broccoli*

## VITAMIN C

Vitamin C is necessary for hair health for many reasons. Vitamin C helps the body use nonheme iron—the type found in vegetables—to assure that there is enough iron in red blood cells to carry oxygen to hair follicles. Vitamin C is also used to form collagen, a structural fiber that helps our bodies—quite literally—hold everything together. Hair follicles, blood vessels, and skin all require collagen to stay healthy for optimal growth. For example, some of the first signs of severe vitamin C deficiency are tiny bumps and red spots around the hair follicles on the arms, back, buttocks, and legs. These bumps are caused when tiny blood vessels leak around the follicles. Hair growth is also affected. On the body, the small hairs on arms and legs can become misshapen, curling in on themselves. On the head, even minor vitamin C deficiencies can lead to dry, brittle hair that breaks easily.

BEST FOODS FOR VITAMIN C: *guava, bell peppers (all colors), oranges and orange juice, grapefruit and grapefruit juice, strawberries, pineapple, kohlrabi, papaya, lemons and lemon juice, broccoli, kale, Brussels sprouts, kidney beans, kiwifruit, cantaloupe, cauliflower, cabbage (all varieties), mangoes, white potatoes, mustard greens, tomatoes, sugar snap peas, snow peas, clementines, rutabagas, turnip greens, raspberries, blackberries, watermelon, tangerines, okra, lychees, summer squash, persimmons*

## BETA-CAROTENE

Beta-carotene in foods is converted to vitamin A in the body, and vitamin A is necessary for all cell growth, including hair cells. A deficiency can lead to dry, dull, lifeless hair and dry skin, which can flake off into dandruff. Note that you can have too much of a good thing when it comes to vitamin A—excessive amounts can cause hair loss. My advice is to add more beta-carotene-rich foods to your meals rather than take vitamin A supplements. If you should choose to take a multivitamin, check the label to make sure that your brand supplies no more than 50 percent DV of vitamin A in the form of retinol. Retinol is listed on supplement labels as palmitate or acetate. The other 50 percent or more should come in the form of beta-carotene or mixed carotenoids, which are converted to vitamin A only as we need it.

## FAQS

**My husband was balding when we met in our twenties. He has tried Rogaine, but it didn't work for him. He's now doing this weird comb-over thing with his remaining hair, and it looks hideous. Are you sure there's nothing that can help him?**

Nutritional cures can't fix male pattern baldness. I always recommend that men who are uncomfortable with their baldness talk with their doctors. They have more options available to them than over-the-counter Rogaine. But I must say that there has never been a better time to be bald! Instead of a comb-over, many men opt to shave their heads entirely for a sleek, modern look. And I wish more men would understand that many women think that confident bald men are sexy. I love my husband's bald head. The measure of a man is not his hair but his loving nature and the strength of his character.

**BEST FOODS FOR BETA-CAROTENE:** *sweet potatoes, carrots, kale, butternut squash, turnip greens, pumpkin, mustard greens, cantaloupe, red peppers, apricots, Chinese cabbage, spinach, lettuces (romaine, green leaf, red leaf, butterhead), collard greens, Swiss chard, watercress, grapefruit, watermelon, cherries, mangoes, tomatoes, guava, asparagus, red cabbage*

## ZINC

The mineral zinc is involved in tissue growth and repair, including hair growth. It also helps keep the oil glands around your hair follicles working properly. Low levels of zinc can cause hair loss, slow growth, and dandruff. The amount you get from eating foods rich in zinc is plenty to keep your tresses gorgeous. Aside from a multivitamin that provides up to 100 percent DV, I don't recommend taking extra zinc supplements because excess zinc can inhibit your body's ability to absorb copper, a minor but necessary mineral.

**BEST FOODS FOR ZINC:** *oysters, lobster, lean beef, crab, ostrich, wheat germ, skinless chicken or turkey (especially dark meat), lean lamb, clams, mussels, pumpkin seeds, yogurt (fat-free, low-fat), pork tenderloin, starchy beans (such as black, navy, pinto, garbanzo, kidney), lentils, black-eyed peas, soybeans (edamame), lima beans, pine nuts, cashews, peanuts and peanut butter, sunflower seeds and butter, pecans*

## BONUS POINTS

◆ **Drink enough water.** Water helps transport vitamins, minerals, and other nutrients throughout the body, including to the scalp and hair follicles. Plus, dehydrated cells in follicles can't build healthy hair. I recommend staying well hydrated throughout each day. On average, women need about nine cups of fluids per day, while men need around thirteen cups per day, and water is always the best hydrator.

## NAILS

Like hair, nails are made mainly of the hardened protein keratin, which means that the foods that create beautiful hair also help nails stay strong. Protein is necessary for nail growth and strength, zinc keeps nails from weakening, and iron keeps nails from distorting into spoon shapes. Just as high doses of selenium can cause hair loss, too much selenium can also lead to nail loss (yikes!).

Although many people believe that calcium supplements help build strong nails, research doesn't support the notion. Researchers from New Zealand examined the effects of calcium on nail health. Nearly 700 postmenopausal women took 1,000 milligrams of calcium every day for a year. At the end of the study, the women reported no change in nail strength. So although I heartily recommend calcium for many different health issues, nail health isn't among them.

Your nails are a good indicator of your overall health and diet quality, so the best prescription for strong, beautiful nails is to eat a well-balanced diet rich in colorful produce, whole grains, lean proteins, and low-fat dairy products.

◆ **See a doctor about unusual hair loss.** Seeing more than the typical number of hairs collecting on your shower floor or pillowcase or noticing more scalp than you're used to could be early indicators of a treatable disorder. Better to be safe than sorry.

◆ **Don't abuse your hair.** Pulling it tight in braids or ponytails, overtreating it with perms or bleach, or manually tugging or twisting on it can cause loss or breakage. Unfortunately, nutrition can't help repair that kind of trauma.

## SUPPLEMENTS

Food is your best bet for gorgeous hair, but if you feel the need to take a supplement, I would recommend a multivitamin that contains 100 percent DV of zinc, copper, vitamin C, the B vitamins (specifically $B_6$, $B_{12}$, and folic acid), and vitamin A (optimally, 50 to 100 percent should come from beta-carotene and/or mixed carotenoids). If you are a woman of childbearing age, look for a multivitamin that contains up to 100 percent DV iron. All men and nonmenstruating women should look for a multi that contains no iron. Unless you've been diagnosed with anemia, you won't need it or want it because too much iron can be toxic. Hint: Look for vitamins labeled "For Men" or "Senior Formula"—those are typically iron free.

For more hair-healthy diet tips, visit www.joybauer.com/hair.

# JOY'S 4-STEP PROGRAM
## FOR HEALTHY HAIR

Follow this program if you have experienced unusual hair loss or if you want healthier, stronger, more beautiful hair.

## Step 1 ... START WITH THE BASICS

♦ If you've been losing more hair than usual, see your doctor to rule out a medical cause.

♦ Stay hydrated. Drink whenever you feel thirsty. On average, men require thirteen cups of fluid per day, and women require nine cups per day. The majority of your fluids should be plain water.

## Step 2 ... YOUR ULTIMATE GROCERY LIST

This list contains foods with high levels of nutrients that help make hair strong and lustrous, plus other overall healthy foods to help round out your grocery list. You don't have to purchase every item, but these foods should make up the bulk of what you eat each week.

### FRUIT

*All* fruit, but especially:
Apricots
Bananas
Berries (blackberries, blueberries, boysenberries, raspberries, and strawberries)
Cantaloupe
Cherries
Clementines
Grapefruit
Guava
Kiwifruit
Lemons
Limes
Lychees
Mangoes
Oranges
Papayas
Persimmons
Pineapple
Tangerines
Watermelon

## VEGETABLES AND LEGUMES

*All* vegetables, but especially:

Artichokes

Asparagus

Avocados

Beans, starchy (such as black, garbanzo, kidney, navy, and pinto)

Beets

Broccoli

Broccoli raab

Brussels sprouts

Cabbage

Carrots

Cauliflower

Celery

Corn

Green beans

Dark leafy greens (such as collard, kale, mustard, Swiss chard, and turnip)

Kohlrabi

Lentils

Lettuce (all varieties)

Lima beans

Okra

Onions (all varieties)

Parsnips

Peas (green, black-eyed)

Peppers (all varieties)

Potatoes (sweet and white)

Pumpkin

Rutabagas

Snow peas

Soybeans (edamame)

Spinach

Squash, summer

Squash, winter (especially acorn and butternut)

Sugar snap peas

Tomatoes

## SEAFOOD

*All* fish and shellfish, but especially:

Clams

Crab

Lobster

Mussels

Salmon, wild (fresh and canned)

Shrimp

Trout (rainbow, wild)

Tuna (canned light)

## LEAN PROTEINS

Beef, lean

Chicken, ground (at least 90% lean)

Chicken, skinless

Eggs and egg substitutes

Lamb, lean

Pork tenderloin

Tempeh

Tofu

Turkey, ground (at least 90% lean)

Turkey, skinless

Turkey bacon

Turkey burgers, lean

Veggie burgers

## NUTS AND SEEDS (PREFERABLY UNSALTED)

Almonds and almond butter

Cashews and cashew butter

Hazelnuts

Macadamia nuts

Peanuts and peanut butter

Pecans

Pine nuts

Pistachios

Pumpkin seeds

Sunflower seeds a͟ sunflower butt͟

Walnuts

## WHOLE GRAINS

| | | |
|---|---|---|
| Amaranth | Bulgur | Quinoa |
| Barley | Cereal, whole grain | Rice (brown and wild) |
| Bread, whole grain (buns, crackers, English muffins, pitas, tortillas, and wraps) | Millet | Waffles, whole grain |
| | Oats | Wheat germ |
| | Pasta, whole grain | |

## DAIRY

| | | |
|---|---|---|
| Cheese (fat-free or reduced-fat) | Cream cheese (fat-free or reduced-fat) | Milk alternatives (almond, rice, and soy) |
| Cottage cheese (fat-free or 1%) | Milk (fat-free or 1%) | Yogurt (fat-free or low-fat) |

## MISCELLANEOUS

| | | |
|---|---|---|
| Canola oil | Mayonnaise, reduced-fat | Salsa |
| Garlic | Mustard (all varieties) | Soft tub spread, trans-fat-free (reduced-fat or regular) |
| Herbs and spices (fresh, dried, and ground) | Olive oil | |
| Hot sauce | Salad dressing, reduced-calorie | Vinegar (all varieties) |

# Step 3 ... GOING ABOVE AND BEYOND

If you want to do absolutely everything you can for hair health, you might try:

◆ Taking a multivitamin. Men and nonmenstruating women should choose a vitamin without iron.

◆ Being extra gentle with your hair—limit pulling, processing, coloring, and even brushing.

## IS A CUT IN YOUR FUTURE?

The next time you go to a hairstylist, ask for an honest assessment of the state of your tresses. If your hair is dry, split, or poorly nourished, those particular strands will never recover. If your hair is fine, too much length can put stress on it and cause breakage and a flat, lifeless appearance. In both cases, you may need to cut several inches off and be patient while your new, glossy, healthy hair grows in.

# Step 4 . . . MEAL PLANS

These sample menus include foods that are full of nutrients that contribute to healthy, strong, shiny hair, including high-quality protein, iron, zinc, beta-carotene, B vitamins, and vitamin C.

Every day, choose one option for each of the three meals—breakfast, lunch, and dinner. Then, once or twice per day, choose from a variety of my suggested snacks. Approximate calories have been provided to help adjust for your personal weight-management goals. If you find yourself hungry (and if weight is not an issue), feel free to increase the portion sizes for meals and snacks. Beverage calories are not included.

## BREAKFAST OPTIONS

(300 TO 400 CALORIES)

### Cantaloupe with Vanilla Yogurt and Sunflower Seeds

Fill ½ cantaloupe with 6 ounces fat-free vanilla yogurt and top with 2 tablespoons sunflower seeds (or slivered almonds or chopped walnuts) and 1 tablespoon wheat germ.

### Broccoli-Cheddar Omelet with Toast

Sauté 1 cup chopped broccoli in oil spray (or 1 teaspoon canola or olive oil) until soft. Beat 1 whole egg and 2 egg whites and add to broccoli; cook until edges brown. Add 1 ounce reduced-fat Cheddar cheese and fold the omelet in half. Continue cooking until the underside is golden brown. Serve with 1 slice toasted whole wheat bread (with optional 1 teaspoon soft tub, trans-fat-free spread).

### Banana-Walnut Oatmeal

Prepare ½ cup dry oats with 1 cup water (and/or optional fat-free milk) and top with 2 tablespoons chopped walnuts and ½ sliced banana. Sweeten with optional 1 teaspoon sugar, honey, maple syrup, or sugar substitute.

### Tropical Cottage Cheese with Almonds

Mix 1 cup fat-free or 1% cottage cheese with 1 cup chopped papaya, pineapple, and/or mango. Top with 1 tablespoon chopped almonds (or walnuts, pecans, or sunflower seeds).

### Whole Grain Cereal with Milk and Fruit

Mix 1 cup whole grain cereal with 1 cup fat-free milk and 1 tablespoon wheat germ. Enjoy with 1 whole grapefruit (or 1 cup berries).

## LUNCH OPTIONS

(400 TO 500 CALORIES)

### Turkey Sandwich with Avocado and Baby Carrots

Layer 4 ounces sliced turkey (or chicken), lettuce, tomato, and 2 thin slices avocado between 2 slices whole grain bread (or in 1 whole wheat pita or wrap) with optional 2 teaspoons reduced-fat mayo and/or mustard. Enjoy with unlimited baby carrots and/or bell pepper strips.

### Japanese Spread: Edamame with California Roll

Enjoy 1 cup boiled edamame (green soybeans in the pod) with 1 six-piece California roll and unlimited steamed vegetables lightly sprinkled with optional reduced-sodium soy sauce.

### Turkey Burger with Salad

Top 1 cooked 5-ounce turkey burger or veggie burger with tomato, onion, and 2 tablespoons ketchup. Serve on a whole grain bun (or toasted whole grain English muffin or pita) with a green salad (baby spinach or dark green lettuce) tossed with 1 teaspoon olive oil and unlimited vinegar or fresh lemon juice (or 2 tablespoons reduced-calorie dressing).

### Spinach Salad with Beets, Goat Cheese, and Walnuts

Top a large bed of baby spinach leaves with ½ cup sliced beets, ½ cup sugar snap peas, 2 ounces soft goat cheese, and 2 tablespoons chopped walnuts. Toss with 2 teaspoons olive oil and unlimited vinegar or fresh lemon juice (or 2 to 4 tablespoons reduced-calorie dressing).

### Lentil Soup with Tomato Cheese Melt

Enjoy 2 cups reduced-sodium lentil or black bean soup with 1 toasted slice of whole grain bread topped with sliced tomato and 1 slice reduced-fat cheese, heated in a 350°F oven until the cheese melts.

## DINNER OPTIONS

(500 TO 600 CALORIES)

### Turkey Chili with Salad

Enjoy 1 serving (2 cups) Turkey Chili (page 363) or any prepared reduced-sodium turkey or vegetarian chili topped with 1 ounce (¼ cup) shredded reduced-fat cheese. Serve with salad (leafy greens and other preferred vegetables) tossed with 1 teaspoon olive oil and unlimited vinegar or fresh lemon juice (or 2 tablespoons reduced-calorie dressing).

### Chicken with Satay Sauce and Brown Rice

Grill 5 ounces chicken breast in 2 teaspoons canola or sesame oil and serve with satay dipping sauce (1 level tablespoon creamy peanut butter mixed with 1 tablespoon reduced-sodium soy sauce and 1 teaspoon minced garlic), unlimited steamed cabbage (or green beans, broccoli, or asparagus), and ½ cup cooked brown rice.

### Spiced Pork Tenderloin with Black-Eyed Peas, Caramelized Onions, and Cauliflower

Enjoy 1 serving (page 98).

### Sautéed Tofu with Peppers and Sugar Snap Peas

Sauté 6 ounces cubed extra-firm tofu, ½ cup sliced bell peppers, ½ cup sugar snap peas, and 2 chopped scallions in 2 teaspoons canola or sesame oil. Sprinkle with 1 tablespoon chopped peanuts and up to 1 tablespoon reduced-sodium soy sauce. Enjoy with ½ cup cooked brown rice (or ½ baked sweet or white potato) and unlimited steamed broccoli or green beans.

### Orange Pepper Beef Stir-Fry with Fresh Fruit

Enjoy 1 serving Orange Pepper Beef Stir-Fry (page 97) with 1 cup fresh berries (or ½ mango, ½ grapefruit, or ¼ cantaloupe).

## SNACK OPTIONS

100 CALORIES OR LESS

- ◆ *Best Vegetable Snacks:* up to 2 cups raw or cooked bell peppers (red, green, yellow), broccoli, sugar snap peas, tomatoes, carrots, asparagus, or cauliflower
- ◆ *Best Fruit Snacks:* 1 orange, tangerine, or kiwifruit; 2 clementines; ½ papaya, mango, grapefruit, or cantaloupe; 1 cup berries, cherries, or sliced strawberries; 1 cup cubed watermelon or pineapple; 4 apricots; 20 whole strawberries
- ◆ 1 hard-cooked egg (or 4 egg whites)
- ◆ ½ cup fat-free or 1% cottage cheese with celery sticks or bell pepper strips
- ◆ 1 string cheese

100 TO 200 CALORIES

- ◆ 1 cup boiled edamame (green soybeans in the pod)
- ◆ 1 slice toasted whole grain bread, topped with 1 level tablespoon nut butter
- ◆ ¼ cup guacamole with bell pepper strips
- ◆ 1 banana with 2 level teaspoons peanut or almond butter
- ◆ 1 ounce (about ¼ cup) almonds, walnuts, pecans, or peanuts
- ◆ ½ cup sunflower seeds or pistachios in the shell
- ◆ 1 cup fat-free plain or flavored yogurt topped with ½ cup berries
- ◆ ½ cup fat-free or 1% cottage cheese mixed with ½ cup berries and topped with optional 1 tablespoon wheat germ

# ORANGE PEPPER BEEF STIR-FRY

*What could be fresher and brighter than orange juice, lime juice, and a rainbow of peppers? Add broccoli, beef, and a few Asian tastes, and you've got a quick and easy dinner that everyone enjoys.*

**MAKES 2 SERVINGS**

½ pound stew beef or top round

½ cup reduced-sodium beef broth

¼ cup reduced-sodium soy sauce

¼ cup orange juice concentrate

2 tablespoons lime juice

1 tablespoon sesame oil

1 tablespoon minced garlic

1 tablespoon minced fresh ginger

1 tablespoon cornstarch

1 tablespoon canola oil

1 red bell pepper, thinly sliced

1 green bell pepper, thinly sliced

1 yellow bell pepper, thinly sliced

1 Vidalia or red onion

1 cup broccoli florets

Kosher salt

3 scallions, thinly sliced

Place the beef in the freezer for 15 to 20 minutes, or until firm but not totally frozen, for easy slicing. Cut into paper-thin slices against the grain.

In a large bowl, whisk the broth, soy sauce, orange juice concentrate, lime juice, sesame oil, garlic, and ginger. Stir in the cornstarch until no lumps remain. Set aside.

Coat a wok or large skillet with oil spray. Add the canola oil and warm over medium heat. Add the peppers, onion, and broccoli and cook, stirring, for 4 to 5 minutes, or until the vegetables begin to soften but are still crisp. Increase the heat to high and add the beef. Cook, stirring, for 3 to 4 minutes, or until the beef begins to take on color.

Reduce the heat to low and add the reserved broth mixture. Cook for 2 to 3 minutes longer, or until the sauce thickens and the beef is no longer pink inside. Season with salt if needed and garnish with the scallions. Serve immediately.

**Per serving:** 485 calories, 43 g protein, 32 g carbohydrate, 21 g fat (4 g saturated), 74 mg cholesterol, 1,284 mg sodium, 5 g fiber; plus 5 mg iron (30% DV), 392 mg vitamin C (653% DV), 3,628 IU vitamin A (73% DV), 7 mg zinc (45% DV), 117 mcg folate (30% DV), 1 mg vitamin B$_6$ (58% DV), 2 mcg vitamin B$_{12}$ (34% DV)

## SPICED PORK TENDERLOIN WITH BLACK-EYED PEAS, CARAMELIZED ONIONS, AND CAULIFLOWER

*Don't let the long list of ingredients put you off—the prep is simple, the taste is sublime. And how many recipes do you know that deliver almost the entire alphabet of vitamins and minerals, from vitamin A to zinc?*

**MAKES 4 SERVINGS**

¼ teaspoon chili powder

¼ teaspoon ground cinnamon

¼ teaspoon ground cumin

¼ teaspoon kosher salt, plus more to taste

¼ teaspoon ground black pepper, plus more to taste

⅛ teaspoon ground red pepper

1 pork tenderloin (1 to 1½ pounds), cut into 4 steaks

2 tablespoons olive oil

1 large red onion, thinly sliced

¼ to ½ cup reduced-sodium chicken broth

1 can (16 ounces) black-eyed peas, drained and rinsed

1 small head cauliflower, cut into florets

1 tablespoon whole wheat bread crumbs

2 tablespoons minced fresh flat-leaf parsley

Zest of 1 lemon

1 tablespoon lemon juice

In a small bowl, combine the chili powder, cinnamon, cumin, salt, black pepper, and red pepper. Coat the pork with oil spray. Rub the spice mixture over the surface of the meat. Wrap in plastic wrap and refrigerate for at least 3 hours, or overnight.

Coat a large skillet with cooking spray. Add 1 tablespoon of the oil and heat over high heat. Add the onion and cook, stirring, for 3 to 4 minutes, or until it begins to brown. Add ¼ cup of the broth and reduce the heat to medium. Cook, stirring occasionally and adding more broth as needed to keep the onion from burning, for 15 to 20 minutes, or until the onion is a deep caramel color. Stir in the black-eyed peas and set aside.

In a steamer or saucepan with a lid, steam the cauliflower over 1 inch of water for 4 to 5 minutes, or until tender. In a bowl, mix the bread crumbs, parsley, and lemon zest and juice. Season with salt and pepper. Sprinkle over the cauliflower.

Coat a large skillet with cooking spray. Heat the remaining 1 tablespoon oil over high heat. Add the steaks and reduce the heat to medium-high. Cook, turning once, for 7 to 8 minutes, or until the steaks are browned and the centers are no longer translucent pink. Serve immediately with the reserved onion mixture and cauliflower.

**Per serving:** 348 calories, 36 g protein, 28 g carbohydrate, 11 g fat (2 g saturated), 90 mg cholesterol, 440 mg sodium, 8 g fiber; plus 4 mg iron (22% DV), 78 mg vitamin C (130% DV), 900 IU vitamin A (18% DV), 2 mg zinc (27% DV), 195 mcg folate (49% DV), 1.5 mg vitamin B$_6$ (75% DV)

# CHAPTER 6

# FEEDING A BEAUTIFUL SMILE

Smile.

Go ahead, try it. Smile . . . right now, wherever you are.

Psychologists have discovered that when people smile, they can activate brain centers that signal happiness, even if they didn't feel particularly happy to begin with. Imagine all the feel-good moments you'll miss out on if you're too self-conscious about your teeth to smile.

Many of us are more concerned with how our smiles look than how healthy our teeth are. Don't believe me? Take a look at these numbers: About 80 percent of adults have some form of periodontal disease, which often goes untreated. Most people don't even floss every day, let alone visit the dentist regularly. On the other hand, tooth whitening is a huge and growing business, a market estimated to be well over $1 billion in the United States alone.

But there's more to dental health than white teeth. To have truly healthy teeth, you'll need to learn some unpleasant truths about the dynamics of food, plaque, decay, tartar, and gum disease. None of it is pretty. Except for your teeth, which can shine with just a few changes to your diet and dental routine.

## WHAT AFFECTS TOOTH HEALTH?

A tooth has a structure similar to a Tootsie Pop. As just about anyone knows, a Tootsie Pop has a hard lollipop outer shell, a soft Tootsie Roll center, and a supporting stick that extends out from the middle of the pop. A tooth has a hard enamel outer shell, a softer dentin center, and a root canal that extends from the middle of the tooth into the jaw. This root canal contains nerves and blood vessels that feed the tooth and keep it alive.

Enamel surrounds the exposed part of the tooth, stopping just inside the gum line. Made primarily of calcium, it is the hardest substance in the body—harder,

## FAQS

**I'm bleaching my teeth to make them whiter. Is there anything I should or should not eat to get the best results?**

During the active phase of bleaching—especially after an in-office bleaching session—the enamel is much more susceptible to stains and demineralization. Be especially careful to avoid eating sugary foods, dried fruits, and other sticky carbohydrates. In addition, avoid foods that can easily stain your teeth, such as coffee, tea, red wine, tomato sauce, and grape juice. If it can stain your clothes, it might stain your newly whitened teeth. Dentists recommend staying away from staining foods for three days after each bleaching procedure. And because all whitening products are not created equal, always ask your dentist about the safest way to brighten your teeth.

even, than bone. But unlike bone, enamel cannot regenerate. If the outer shell is breached, the inner part of the tooth becomes vulnerable and can erode down to the root. That's why any cracks or areas of decay need to be filled by a dentist.

Just under the enamel is the dentin, which contains millions of fluid-filled tubules, tiny canals that lead to the extremely sensitive nerve. When the protective enamel wears away, you've got trouble. Cavities, cracks, gum recession, tooth-grinding, brushing too hard, or even eating too many acidic foods can all provide access to the tubules and, consequently, a tooth's nerve center. Hot foods, cold drinks, sugar, or even sudden puffs of air can ride the tubules into the core of your tooth. Anyone with tooth sensitivity knows that it is both uncomfortable and embarrassing—there's nothing sexy about that pained grimace after a sip of ice water.

So the first key to good tooth health is keeping your enamel shell strong. That can be a challenge all by itself. Consider this: Every minute of every day, our teeth are collecting a film of plaque—a combination of naturally occurring mouth bacteria, food sugars, and other substances. Food sugars come not just from the obvious sources—the sugar in candy, soda, and other sweets—but also from the natural sugars created during the breakdown of fruits, whole grain foods, and other carbohydrates. All these sugars feed the bacteria, which, in turn, produce acid that leeches calcium salts from enamel and weakens it. The process is called demineralization. As long as the bacteria and sugars remain in your mouth, the acid level will remain high—which is why sticky foods like raisins, jam, or gummy bears can wreak havoc on enamel long after you finish eating. Once you stop eating a meal and clear food remnants out of your mouth (by, say, brushing), acid levels remain high for about 30 minutes or so before your saliva slowly returns everything back to normal. If you sip sugary drinks or snack continuously, your teeth may remain bathed in acid all day long, and if you have dry mouth from low saliva flow, the acid remains higher longer.

Plaque remains on the teeth unless you brush or floss it away. After about 24 hours, the soft plaque begins to harden into tartar, which cannot be removed by simple brushing. If tartar forms at or under the gum line, it can cause the gums (also called gingiva) to become inflamed, causing redness, puffiness, and bad breath. This inflammation (or gingivitis) might not sound like a big deal—until you take the long view.

Gingivitis is just the first stage of gum disease. Teeth are embedded in the jaw, held in place by connective tissue and surrounded by your gums. If tartar is not removed, toxins destroy the connective tissue and bacteria can invade the bone around your teeth, creating infection and causing bone loss (a condition known as periodontal disease). If periodontal disease is left untreated, the tooth becomes unanchored, loosens, and eventually falls out.

For healthy teeth, then, start with some basic dental hygiene.

◆ Limit the number of sugary foods (and low-quality carbohydrates) you eat during the day. Dried fruits, crackers, pretzels, cookies, and other foods that get stuck on or between teeth can be particularly devastating to enamel over time. Lollipops and hard candies are also detrimental since they bathe your back teeth in sugars for prolonged periods of time.

◆ Limit your number of "eating episodes" during the day. If you nibble on something every 30 minutes, your mouth will always contain acid, and your enamel will be under constant attack. Of course, eating every few hours is normal and perfectly fine.

◆ Avoid sugary drinks, including sodas, fruit juices, overly sweetened coffee or tea, and sweetened waters. Many dentists also recommend avoiding sugar-free diet beverages because they often contain citric, malic, or phosphoric acids that can be damaging to teeth. If you must drink them, use a straw to bypass your teeth.

◆ Brush your teeth after every meal. If you cannot brush, at least rinse your mouth with water to remove some food debris. Chewing sugarless gum can also help.

**FAQ**

**I kicked my soda habit and have been drinking a lot of seltzer waters instead. They come in natural flavors and contain no sugars or artificial sweeteners. However, I've heard that all carbonated beverages, including seltzers, are bad for your teeth. Is that true?**

No, naturally flavored seltzer water is a smart beverage choice, and it has no negative effects on your teeth. Although it's a touch more acidic than regular, flat drinking water because of the added carbonation, the difference is minimal and nothing to be concerned with. In fact, seltzer water is about 100 times less damaging to your teeth than regular and diet sodas, which contain acids that erode tooth enamel, making them more susceptible to cavities. Just make sure you choose seltzers that list only two ingredients: carbonated water and natural flavors.

◆ Floss at least once a day to remove food particles and plaque between teeth.

◆ Visit the dentist at least once a year for a professional cleaning, or more frequently if your dentist recommends it. Many dentists recommend twice yearly visits to keep on top of tartar, but some people who are more susceptible to tooth decay and/or tartar buildup may need to go even more often.

## HOW FOOD AFFECTS TOOTH HEALTH

Though it may seem like tooth care is all about what not to eat, there are some foods that contribute to a healthy smile.

### CALCIUM AND VITAMIN D

Most people understand that calcium and vitamin D are important for strong bones, but many of us fail to make the connection between our bones and our teeth. Teeth are embedded in the jawbone, so if its bone density falls, your teeth won't have a firm footing. If periodontal disease sets in, a strong jawbone will be your first defense against tooth loss.

In addition, a calcium-poor diet seems to increase the overall risk of developing periodontal disease. Research has shown that women who get less than 500 milligrams of calcium per day from their diets have a 54 percent greater risk of periodontal disease, compared with those who get more than 800 milligrams

## INFLAMMATION AND DISEASE

Many dentists are finding themselves in a position to save lives, thanks to research that has linked periodontal disease with an increased risk of heart disease. What do the two have in common? In a word, inflammation.

You know that if a skunk sprays its scent in your neighbor's yard, the stink will soon be in your yard, too. The same type of thing happens with inflammation. When there is an infection or disease in the gums, the body's immune response increases levels of inflammatory chemicals designed to fight the problem. But these chemicals don't stay just in the mouth—they circulate throughout the body. Inflammatory chemicals can cause collateral damage—and the delicate lining of blood vessels is often in the line of fire. Over time, this can lead to atherosclerosis, blood clots, and heart disease.

Although no one knows exactly which comes first, the mouth inflammation or the heart disease, the link is clear. A 2006 study of middle-aged men in Northern Ireland showed that those with periodontal disease had a risk of heart disease three times higher than that of men with healthy gums. If your dentist tells you that your gums are in trouble, see your primary care physician for a full workup. It just might save your life.

of calcium per day. Calcium cannot be absorbed and used by bone without vitamin D, so it is important to eat foods rich in both nutrients. Women of all ages who don't get enough calcium through diet should consider taking a supplement that contains calcium plus D$_3$ (cholecalciferol, the most potent form of vitamin D). See the Supplements section (page 00) for more information.

BEST FOODS FOR CALCIUM: *yogurt (fat-free, low-fat), milk (fat-free, 1%), soy milk, cheese (fat-free, reduced-fat), tofu with calcium (check nutrition label), soybeans (edamame), frozen yogurt (fat-free, low-fat), low-fat ice cream, bok choy, kale, white beans, collard greens, broccoli, almonds and almond butter*

BEST FOODS FOR VITAMIN D: *wild salmon (fresh, canned), mackerel (not king), sardines, herring, milk (fat-free, 1%), soy milk, fortified yogurt (fat-free, low-fat), egg yolks, vitamin D-enhanced mushrooms\**

*\*These mushrooms are treated with UV light, which dramatically increases their vitamin D content.*

## VITAMIN C

Vitamin C is critical for keeping gums healthy because it strengthens blood vessels and the connective tissue that holds your teeth in your jaw. The antioxidant properties of vitamin C also help reduce inflammation, which may help prevent or slow the progression of gingivitis. In one study, researchers found that people who did not get enough vitamin C in their diets had about a 20 percent greater risk of developing periodontal disease than people who ate plenty of vitamin C–rich produce.

BEST FOODS FOR VITAMIN C: *guava, bell peppers (all colors), oranges and orange juice, grapefruit and grapefruit juice, strawberries, pineapple, kohlrabi, papaya, lemons and lemon juice, broccoli, kale, Brussels sprouts, kidney beans, kiwifruit, cantaloupe, cauliflower, cabbage (all varieties), mangoes, white potatoes, mustard greens, tomatoes, sugar snap peas, snow peas, clementines, rutabagas, turnip greens, raspberries, blackberries, watermelon, tangerines, okra, lychees, summer squash, persimmons*

## WATER AND GREEN TEA

Water not only helps wash away food debris that can get trapped in teeth, it also helps keep saliva levels high. Saliva is your body's best defense against tooth decay because its proteins and minerals counteract enamel-eating acids, keeping your teeth strong. That's why people with dry mouth, no matter what the cause, need to see the dentist more frequently than others. If you have dry mouth, hard candies can be disastrous! Chew sugarless gum instead. Saliva is more than 95 percent water, so stay hydrated throughout the day to keep its flow constant.

If plain water bores you, try unsweetened green tea. Green tea is rich in antioxidants called catechins, which inhibit the growth of bacteria that initiate periodontal disease and break down gum tissue. A 2009 study found that Japanese men who regularly consumed green tea had healthier gums than men who were less frequent tea drinkers. For each additional cup of green tea consumed, markers of gum health improved, suggesting that regularly sipping green tea (unsweetened, of course!) can promote dental health and help ward off gum disease.

## BONUS POINTS

◆ **Talk with your dentist about the importance of fluoride.** Fluoride is one of the most effective measures available for preventing tooth decay: so effective, in fact, that many public water supplies provide safe levels of fluoridation. Studies have consistently found that children who receive fluoride from their water or dental treatments have less than half the number of cavities than children who don't get fluoride. This mineral occurs naturally in some foods, such as tea and seafood, and in foods cooked in fluoridated water. With the popularity of bottled water and water filtration systems, many people are not getting as much fluoride as they might think. (To find out whether your tap water contains fluoride, call your county water department. To check on bottled water or your water filter, call the public information phone number published on the bottle or the filter packaging.) Dentists recommend that everyone brush with a fluoride toothpaste, and they suggest a fluoride rinse for some. Don't take fluoride supplements without a doctor's recommendation, and don't swallow toothpaste—too much fluoride can be toxic.

◆ **If you have heartburn from reflux disease or if you are bulimic, talk with your dentist.** Stomach acids that make their way into the mouth, either from reflux or vomiting, can eat away at tooth enamel. While you are working on solving your medical problem, make sure your dentist knows about it so you can work together to keep your teeth as healthy as possible.

◆ **Stop using tobacco products.** People who smoke cigarettes or cigars or use other tobacco products are more likely to have tartar, periodontal disease, and tooth loss, compared with people who don't. One Swedish study of smokers and nonsmokers found that smokers were more than twice as likely to have periodontal disease—and more severe disease—than nonsmokers. Tobacco also stains your teeth, which is never attractive.

◆ **Go for crunchy.** Raw vegetables and crunchy fruits (like apples) are not only jam-packed with vitamins and minerals, they also help clean your teeth of plaque and bacteria. Think of them as nature's tasty toothbrushes!

◆ **Chew sugarless gum if you can't brush after a meal or snack.** Chewing sugarless gum stimulates saliva to wash away food particles, acts as a natural toothbrush, and buffers acids to protect enamel. In addition, the artificial sweetener xylitol can inhibit tooth decay by actually remineralizing teeth. Many dentists recommend that their patients chew a piece of xylitol-containing gum after every meal. Brands that contain xylitol include most flavors of Trident (except Trident White), Orbit, and Stride sugar-free gum. Because formulations can change, always check the gum's ingredients list for xylitol before purchasing it.

◆ **Drink soda wisely.** I do not recommend drinking soda at all (big surprise!). However, I recognize that some of you may have an ingrained habit. While you are working on breaking the habit, here are some tips for safer (but not totally safe) teeth.

- **Use a straw.** Sipping through a straw will keep the soda farther toward the back of your mouth and prevent it from hitting every tooth.

- **Drink with meals.** If you drink sodas between meals, that sugar and acid combination prolongs the amount of time during which your enamel is being demineralized.

## SUPPLEMENTS

If you want to do everything possible to improve tooth health, you may want to consider these supplements in addition to the food fixes.

1. **A multivitamin.** Tooth health depends on the health of your body. To be assured that you get the vitamins and minerals you need to keep your beautiful smile, consider taking a multivitamin that contains 100 percent DV for vitamin C and at least 800 IU of vitamin D.

2. **Calcium plus vitamin D$_3$.** I always prefer that women get their calcium from food, but if you're not consistently consuming at least three daily servings of calcium-rich foods or beverages, you may want to consider taking a separate supplement. When buying supplements, remember that calcium is worthless without vitamin D, so make sure you're getting a total of at least 800 IU vitamin D$_3$ through your multi and/or calcium supplement. See page 233 in the Osteoporosis chapter for more information on types of calcium supplements and dosing.

Special note for men: I never recommend calcium supplements to men. Some studies have shown a link between high calcium intake and increased risk of prostate cancer. Men's calcium intake should be fine if they stick with food and beverage sources of calcium only.

For more information on how food can improve your smile, visit www.joybauer.com/teeth.

# JOY'S 4-STEP PROGRAM
## FOR FEEDING A BEAUTIFUL SMILE

Follow this program if you want to maintain a gorgeous smile.

## Step 1 ... START WITH THE BASICS

◆ See your dentist. If you haven't been in more than a year, schedule a checkup and cleaning immediately. Some people with extensive gum disease can have no symptoms at all, so let a professional check out your mouth just in case.

◆ If you smoke or use other tobacco products, quit.

◆ Chew sugarless gum if you can't brush after meals.

◆ Limit the number of sugary foods and low-quality carbohydrates in your diet.

## Step 2 ... YOUR ULTIMATE GROCERY LIST

This list contains foods with high levels of nutrients that contribute to tooth health (specifically, foods rich in calcium and vitamins D and C), plus other overall healthy foods to round out your grocery list. Although fruit and whole grain products are incredibly healthy, they are carbohydrates and can increase the level of acid in your mouth. Therefore, make sure to brush, chew sugarless gum, or drink plenty of water and/or unsweetened green tea after meals and snacks.

### FRUIT

*All* fruit, but especially:
Berries (blackberries, blueberries, raspberries, and strawberries)
Cantaloupe
Clementines
Grapefruit

Guava
Kiwifruit
Lychees
Mangoes
Oranges
Papayas

Persimmons
Pineapple
Tangerines
Watermelon

## VEGETABLES AND LEGUMES

*All* vegetables, but especially:

Beans, starchy (especially white and kidney)

Bok choy

Broccoli

Brussels sprouts

Cabbage

Cauliflower

Dark, leafy greens (such as collard, kale, mustard, Swiss chard, and turnip)

Kohlrabi

Okra

Onions (all varieties)

Peppers (all varieties)

Potatoes, white

Rutabagas

Snow peas

Soybeans (edamame)

Squash, summer

Sugar snap peas

Tomatoes

## SEAFOOD

*All* fish and shellfish, but especially:

Herring

Mackerel (not king)

Salmon, wild (fresh and canned)

Sardines (fresh and canned)

## LEAN PROTEINS

Beef, lean

Chicken, ground (at least 90% lean)

Chicken, skinless

Eggs and egg substitutes

Pork tenderloin

Tempeh

Tofu

Turkey, ground (at least 90% lean)

Turkey, skinless

Turkey bacon

Turkey burgers, lean

Veggie burgers

## NUTS AND SEEDS (PREFERABLY UNSALTED)

Almonds and almond butter

Cashews and cashew butter

Hazelnuts

Macadamia nuts

Peanuts and peanut butter

Pecans

Pine nuts

Pistachios

Pumpkin seeds

Sunflower seeds and sunflower butter

Walnuts

## WHOLE GRAINS

Amaranth

Barley

Bread, whole grain (buns, crackers, English muffins, pitas, tortillas, and wraps)

Bulgur

Cereal, whole grain (at least 3 grams fiber; no more than 8 grams sugar per serving)

Millet

Oats

Pasta, whole grain

Quinoa

Rice (brown and wild)

Waffles, whole grain

Wheat germ

## DAIRY

Cheese (fat-free or reduced-fat)

Cottage cheese (fat-free or 1%)

Cream cheese (fat-free or reduced-fat)

Frozen yogurt

Ice cream (low-fat)

Milk (fat-free or 1%)

Milk alternatives (almond, rice, and soy)

Sour cream (fat-free or reduced-fat)

Yogurt (fat-free or low-fat)

## MISCELLANEOUS

Canola oil

Garlic

Herbs and spices (fresh, dried, and ground)

Hot sauce

Hummus

Marinara sauce

Mayonnaise, reduced-fat

Mustard (all varieties)

Olive oil

Salad dressing (reduced-calorie)

Salsa

Soft tub spread, trans-fat-free (reduced-fat or regular)

Sugarless gum

Tea, green

Vinegar (all varieties)

# Step 3 . . . GOING ABOVE AND BEYOND

If you want to do everything you can for tooth health, here are some additional things you might try.

◆ Take a multivitamin for general nutrition. Women should consider a supplement of calcium plus vitamin $D_3$ for strong bones and teeth. Men should consider taking a vitamin $D_3$ supplement.

## HALITOSIS HELP

Worried about bad breath? Your first step should be to visit your dentist to make sure you don't have gum disease. If your mouth is healthy, you might need to alter your diet. Nearly everyone knows that garlic can cause odor problems—it's not called the stinking rose for nothing. But other common foods can also foul your breath. The worst offenders are coffee, cheese, and onions. If you brush your teeth or chew some sugarless gum, you'll take care of most of the problem. But keep in mind that onions and garlic contain smelly compounds that are absorbed into your bloodstream and exhaled from your lungs for hours after you eat them. Extremely low-carb, high-fat diets can also cause "ketone breath" from the metabolism of all the fat, so be sure to enjoy your fair share of high-quality carbs: vegetables, fresh fruit, and whole grains.

◆ If you have heartburn from reflux disease or if you're bulimic, see your
   primary care physician to get treatment.

◆ Add crunchy fruits and vegetables into your daily diet.

# Step 4 . . . MEAL PLANS

These sample menus include foods that have been shown to contribute to good
tooth health.

Every day, choose one option for each of the three meals—breakfast, lunch, and
dinner. Then, once or twice per day, choose from my suggested snacks. Approximate
calories have been provided to help adjust for your personal weight-management
goals. If you find yourself hungry (and if weight is not an issue), feel free to increase
the portion sizes for meals and snacks. Beverage calories are not included.

## BREAKFAST OPTIONS

(300 TO 400 CALORIES)

### Broccoli-Cheese Soufflé

Enjoy 1 serving (page 113).

### Strawberry-Kiwi Smoothie with Cottage Cheese

Enjoy 1 serving (2 cups) Strawberry-Kiwi Smoothie (page 114) with 1 cup fat-
free or 1% cottage cheese.

### Waffles with Maple Yogurt and Fresh Fruit

Toast 2 whole grain waffles (preferably calcium-fortified) and top with maple
yogurt (2 teaspoons pure maple syrup mixed with ½ cup fat-free or low-fat
plain yogurt). Enjoy with 1 orange or ½ grapefruit.

### Egg and Cheese Breakfast Sandwich

Toast 1 whole grain English muffin and layer with sliced tomato, 1 egg
(scrambled or sunny side up), and 1 slice reduced-fat cheese. Enjoy with
½ grapefruit or 1 orange.

### Hard-Cooked Egg with Cereal, Milk, and Berries

Mix 1 cup whole grain cereal with 1 cup fat-free milk and top with ½ cup berries or ½ sliced banana. Enjoy with one hard-cooked egg (or 3 or 4 egg whites).

## LUNCH OPTIONS

(400 TO 500 CALORIES)

### Edamame with Wild Salmon Dijonnaise

Enjoy 1 cup boiled edamame (green soybeans in the pod) with 5 ounces canned wild salmon, drained, mashed, and mixed with 1 tablespoon reduced-fat mayonnaise, 1 to 2 teaspoons Dijon mustard, and minced onion and black pepper to taste. Serve on a large bed of lettuce drizzled with lemon juice and your choice of seasonings (or 1 to 2 tablespoons reduced-calorie dressing).

### Broccoli-Cheese Soufflé with Cottage Cheese and Almonds

Enjoy 1 serving Broccoli-Cheese Soufflé (page 113) with ½ cup fat-free or 1% cottage cheese topped with 1 tablespoon slivered almonds.

### Tomato-Cheese Omelet with Tropical Mango-Citrus Smoothie

Beat 1 whole egg with 2 or 3 egg whites. Cook in a small skillet coated with oil spray. When the bottom is cooked, gently flip and add chopped tomato and 1 ounce (¼ cup shredded) reduced-fat cheese. Fold the omelet in half and continue cooking until the egg mixture firms and the cheese melts. Enjoy with 1 serving (2 cups) Tropical Mango-Citrus Smoothie (page 114).

### Mixed Vegetable Salad with Sardines

Toss 4 ounces (about 8) sardines with unlimited leafy greens, chopped tomatoes, carrots, bell pepper, onion, and ½ cup white or navy beans. Drizzle with 2 to 4 tablespoons reduced-calorie salad dressing (or 1 teaspoon olive oil and unlimited vinegar or fresh lemon juice). Season with ground black pepper to taste.

### Tofu Salad with Snow Peas, Almonds, and Mandarin Oranges

Toss 4 ounces extra-firm tofu, cubed and chilled, with 2 cups leafy greens or lettuce, 1 cup steamed and chilled snow peas, ½ chopped tomato, and ½ cup mandarin oranges (canned in natural juice or light syrup). Drizzle with 1 to 2 teaspoons sesame oil and 1 tablespoon reduced-sodium soy sauce and top with 1 to 2 tablespoons slivered almonds.

## DINNER OPTIONS

(500 TO 600 CALORIES)

### Wild Salmon Salad with Parmesan Baked Potato

Enjoy 1 serving Wild Salmon Salad (page 321) with unlimited leafy greens and ½ plain baked potato topped with 2 tablespoons grated Parmesan cheese.

### Breakfast for Dinner: Almond-Berry Oatmeal

Prepare ¾ cup dry oats with 1½ cups water and top with 2 tablespoons slivered almonds and 1 cup berries. Sweeten with optional 1 teaspoon sugar, honey, pure maple syrup, or sugar substitute. Enjoy with 6 ounces fat-free plain or flavored yogurt on the side.

### Whole Wheat Pita Pizza with the Works

Split and toast 1 whole wheat pita (or use 200 calories' worth of whole wheat pizza crust). Top each pita half with 2 to 3 heaping tablespoons marinara sauce and ¼ cup part-skim ricotta cheese, plus ½ cup sliced bell peppers and unlimited chopped broccoli florets sautéed in oil spray. Sprinkle each pita half with 2 tablespoons shredded reduced-fat mozzarella cheese. Heat in a 350°F oven until the cheese melts and bubbles. Season with crushed red pepper and oregano.

### Healthy Chicken Parmesan and Broccoli

Enjoy 1 serving (page 246).

### Sweet and Sour Tofu-Veggie Stir-Fry

Enjoy 1 serving Sweet and Sour Tofu-Veggie Stir-Fry (page 245) with 1 cup cooked brown rice.

## SNACK OPTIONS

100 CALORIES OR LESS

- ◆ *Best Vegetable Snacks:* up to 2 cups raw or cooked broccoli, bell peppers, cauliflower, tomatoes, sugar snap peas, or snow peas
- ◆ *Best Fruit Snacks:* 1 guava, orange, kiwifruit, or tangerine; 2 clementines; ½ mango, grapefruit, papaya, or cantaloupe; 1 cup cubed watermelon or pineapple; 1 cup raspberries, sliced strawberries, blackberries, or pineapple; 20 whole strawberries
- ◆ 1 hard-cooked egg (or 4 egg whites)
- ◆ 1 cup fat-free milk
- ◆ 1 cup low-fat hot cocoa
- ◆ ½ cup fat-free or 1% cottage cheese
- ◆ 10 almonds

100 TO 200 CALORIES

- ◆ ½ cup frozen yogurt or low-fat ice cream
- ◆ 1 serving (6- to 8-ounce container) fat-free plain or flavored yogurt
- ◆ 1 serving (2 cups) Tropical Mango-Citrus Smoothie (page 114)
- ◆ 1 serving (2 cups) Strawberry-Kiwi Smoothie (page 114)
- ◆ Everyday Fruit Smoothie: In a blender, mix ½ cup fat-free milk (or soy milk), ½ cup fat-free yogurt, ¾ cup fresh or frozen fruit (such as berries, banana, peaches, or mango), and 3 to 5 ice cubes.
- ◆ ¾ cup whole grain cereal with 1 cup fat-free milk
- ◆ 1 cup fat-free milk with 1 cup berries (sliced strawberries, raspberries, or blackberries)
- ◆ 20 almonds

# BROCCOLI-CHEESE SOUFFLÉ

*This guilt-free soufflé provides twice the amount of vitamin C you need every day and more than 40 percent of your daily requirement for calcium. The delicious flavor (and healthy ingredients!) will have you smiling.*

**MAKES 2 SERVINGS**

2 teaspoons grated Parmesan cheese

6 egg whites plus 3 yolks, at room temperature

¼ teaspoon kosher salt, plus more to taste

2 tablespoons reduced-fat, soft tub, trans-fat-free spread

2 tablespoons all-purpose flour

1 cup fat-free milk, heated just to a simmer on stove top or in microwave

½ teaspoon paprika

¼ teaspoon nutmeg

Ground black pepper to taste

1 bunch broccoli, cut into florets (about 3 cups)

¼ cup reduced-sodium chicken broth or water

1 shallot or 1 small onion, minced

¼ cup plus 1 tablespoon finely grated reduced-fat Swiss cheese

Preheat the oven to 375°F. Coat a 6- or 8-cup ceramic gratin dish with oil spray and sprinkle the inside with the Parmesan.

In a large metal bowl, beat the egg whites and ¼ teaspoon salt on high speed for 4 to 6 minutes, or until the whites become stiff but not lumpy. Set aside.

In a medium saucepan over medium-high heat, melt the spread until it begins to foam. Add the flour and mix vigorously for 2 to 3 minutes, or until the flour forms a paste without browning. Remove from the heat, pour in the hot milk, and whisk quickly until the mixture is smooth. Add the paprika, nutmeg, and salt and pepper to taste. Bring the mixture to a slow boil over medium-high heat. Cook, stirring constantly, for 2 to 3 minutes, or until the sauce becomes heavy and thick. Remove from the heat. Add the egg yolks one at a time, mixing well after each addition.

In a blender, puree the broccoli and broth or water. Stir the broccoli mixture, shallot or onion, and ¼ cup of the Swiss into the milk mixture. With a spatula, gently fold in one-third of the egg whites, lifting the milk mixture from the bottom of the pan. Transfer the milk mixture to the bowl with the remaining egg whites and continue to fold, without deflating the egg whites, until just combined.

Pour into the prepared gratin dish and sprinkle with the remaining 1 tablespoon Swiss. Bake, uncovered, for 25 to 30 minutes, or until the soufflé puffs and is golden on the top. Serve immediately.

**Per serving:** 343 calories, 29 g protein, 24 g carbohydrate, 14 g fat (5 g saturated), 317 mg cholesterol, 788 mg sodium, 4 g fiber; plus 77 IU vitamin D (20% DV), 470 mg calcium (48% DV), 120 mg vitamin C (200% DV)

## STRAWBERRY-KIWI SMOOTHIE

*Refreshing and easy to make, one serving of this smoothie provides almost twice the amount of vitamin C you need for an entire day, plus tooth-strengthening calcium and vitamin D—all for only 155 calories.*

**MAKES 2 SERVINGS (2 CUPS EACH)**

1½ cups fat-free milk

1 cup strawberries, hulled and quartered

2 kiwifruit, peeled and quartered (about ½ cup)

2 tablespoon fresh mint, chopped, plus 2 sprigs for garnish (optional)

1 tablespoon granulated sugar or sugar substitute

1 cup crushed ice

In a blender or food processor, combine the milk, strawberries, kiwi, chopped mint, sugar or sugar substitute, and ice. Blend until smooth. Garnish with fresh mint sprigs, if using.

**Per serving:** 155 calories, 8 g protein, 32 g carbohydrate, 0 g fat, 0 mg cholesterol, 81 mg sodium, 4 g fiber; plus 75 IU vitamin D (19% DV), 270 mg calcium (27% DV), 113 mg vitamin C (188% DV)

## TROPICAL MANGO-CITRUS SMOOTHIE

*Here's another fabulous smoothie recipe you can enjoy anytime, for health or just for pleasure.*

**MAKES 2 SERVINGS (2 CUPS EACH)**

1½ cups fat-free milk

1 mango, peeled and chopped (about 1 cup)

1 orange, peeled and chopped (about ½ cup)

1 lime, juiced

1 teaspoon minced fresh ginger

1 cup crushed ice

In a blender or food processor, combine the milk, mango, orange, lime juice, ginger, and ice and blend until smooth.

**Per serving:** 171 calories, 8 g protein, 30 g carbohydrate, 0 g fat, 0 mg cholesterol, 80 mg sodium, 4 g fiber; plus 75 IU vitamin D (19% DV), 277 mg calcium (28% DV), 73 mg vitamin C (122% DV)

# PART 4

# LIVING LONG AND STRONG

# CHAPTER 7

# CARDIOVASCULAR DISEASE

ne spring day, Wendy noticed the world's longest conga line of ants traveling across her driveway, heading into her garage. From there, the ants disappeared into an almost imperceptible crack near an interior wall. She called an exterminator, expecting to get a bill for a hundred dollars or so for spraying around the garage. Instead, she ended up with an estimate of $12,000. It turns out that there was a tiny hole in the floor of their newly installed shower—a hole that dripped water onto the beams holding up the second floor. At first, that small amount of water had no noticeable effect, but over the years it added up to a couple of billion drops. The subflooring and wood studs had rotted—creating the equivalent of ambrosia to carpenter ants, which knew a good thing when they found it and made a nest. So, in addition to the cost of fumigating the whole house, the shower stall had to be removed, tile pried up, subfloor and studs ripped out and replaced, new tile installed, et cetera, et cetera (many thousands of dollars worth of "et cetera").

Cardiovascular disease is a lot like Wendy's house. Many people ignore their doctors' warnings about high cholesterol or blood pressure numbers because they feel perfectly healthy. But those numbers are just the ants on your body's metaphoric driveway, the thing that clues you in to what's going on inside. By the time you get diagnosed with high cholesterol or high blood pressure or high triglycerides, you may already have significant structural damage.

Though I often tell my clients to make nutritional changes at a pace that feels comfortable to them, gradual is not good enough when it comes to cardiovascular disease. The consequences of doing too little are severe—heart attack, stroke, pain, debility, death. Sadly, not everyone gets a second chance. So don't wait until after your next vacation, your daughter's wedding, or that anniversary dinner to start making positive changes. Change your diet, change your habits, and change your lifestyle immediately. I'll show you the how in this chapter. No matter what your risk factors, there is a lot you can start doing now to ensure your cardiovascular health.

## WHAT IS CARDIOVASCULAR DISEASE?

After oxygen enters your bloodstream through your lungs, your heart pumps blood throughout your body to carry oxygen and nutrients to every cell from head to toe. Because blood has to travel to so many areas, the vessels that carry it range in size from the thick arteries and veins that branch off from your heart to the miniature capillaries that feed the tiniest, most distant parts of your body. Cardiovascular disease, also called heart disease, can affect any part of this vast network, from the heart (cardio-) through all the blood vessels (-vascular).

Healthy blood vessels are flexible and strong, capable of containing the pulsing pressure of rushing blood, heartbeat after heartbeat, year after year, for a lifetime. We'd like to think that they are durable, too, but they are in fact relatively fragile. Think about Monarch butterflies. They migrate hundreds of miles in a single season—some more than 1,500 miles—on wings that are so fragile that they can be destroyed with a single touch. That's what blood vessels are like: tough but delicate, sturdy but vulnerable. If anything goes wrong and blood can't flow to all parts of your body, your cells won't receive the nutrition and oxygen they—and you—need to survive. If blood can't get to your heart, the result is a heart attack. If blood can't get to all portions of your brain, the result is a stroke. In other words, the blood must keep flowing.

## HIGH BLOOD PRESSURE (HYPERTENSION)

As your heart contracts to pump blood through your arteries, the force of that rushing blood against the vessel walls is called systolic blood pressure. As your heart relaxes between beats, the blood presses less forcefully against the vessel walls, as reflected by diastolic blood pressure. When you go to the doctor, your blood pressure is given in two numbers: systolic pressure over diastolic pressure, measured in millimeters of mercury (mm Hg).

Physicians recommend that you main-

### FAQS

**I can't tell you how happy I was when I read that chocolate may help improve blood pressure. Is it true?**

Yes, but with limitations. Scientists have discovered that the antioxidant flavonoids in chocolate can lower blood pressure, reduce inflammation, and improve the elasticity of blood vessels and may even increase HDL, or "good," cholesterol. Note that dark chocolate contains more than double the amount of flavonoids as milk chocolate, and the addition of milk may stop the intestines from absorbing the flavonoids. So if you're going to eat chocolate, choose a variety that is at least 70 percent dark chocolate.

Of course, chocolate is also packed with calories and fat that will lead to weight gain if you eat too much of it, so make sure that you stick to 1-ounce portions—and remember to account for the extra 150 calories in your daily calorie allotment.

tain blood pressure at or below 120/80 mm Hg, but high blood pressure (HBP) is medically defined as any reading higher than 140/90 mm Hg. Readings of 121 to 130 systolic or 81 to 89 diastolic are considered prehypertension, a warning that your blood pressure may soon rise into the danger zone. The higher your blood pressure, the more the delicate lining of your blood vessels is battered, increasing the risk of structural damage and inflammation and, consequently, heart attack, stroke, kidney failure, and other blood vessel disorders. In addition, HBP can contribute to a condition called atherosclerosis—the formation of plaque, a fatty substance that builds up on the insides of the vessels, making them narrower and less flexible and choking the blood supply to every part of your body. These narrow vessels must still carry the same amount of blood as they did when they were healthy, which only adds to the pressure the vessel walls must bear. So high blood pressure is a risk factor for even higher blood pressure. That's why blood pressure problems never really go away. Once you have damage from HBP, you'll have to fight forever to control it.

If you've been diagnosed with HBP, your doctor has probably already told you the basics. You can control blood pressure by achieving and maintaining a healthy weight; reducing your bad cholesterol (LDL) if it's high; limiting your salt intake; exercising; and adding calcium, vitamin D, magnesium, and potassium to your diet (see page 131).

For more information on foods to fight high blood pressure, visit www.joybauer.com/blood-pressure.

## BAD CHOLESTEROL NUMBERS

Cholesterol is a natural fatlike substance that exists in all human and animal tissue as a part of cell membranes. Cholesterol is also part of the myelin sheath that surrounds and protects nerves, and it is used to produce vitamin D, bile, and several hormones. Our bodies make all the cholesterol we need for health, but we get extra from eating meat, poultry, and fish. (Incidentally, cholesterol is never found in plant-based foods, so "cholesterol-free!" labels on products like peanut butter are really just stating the obvious.)

Cholesterol comes in two main varieties: low-density lipoprotein (LDL) cholesterol (commonly called bad cholesterol—remember "L for lousy"), and high-density lipoprotein (HDL) cholesterol (good cholesterol—remember "H for hero"). LDL cholesterol is one of the components of vessel-clogging plaque. Over time, plaque can incorporate calcium and other substances and become hard and brittle. If the plaque deposits grow large enough, they can block a blood vessel. In addition, the brittle plaque can break off, travel through your bloodstream, and form a clot anywhere in your body.

The higher your LDL cholesterol, the greater your risk of developing life-threatening plaque, so you want your low-density low. According to the National Institutes of Health (NIH), the optimal level of LDL cholesterol is below 100 mg/dL. High LDL cholesterol is defined as 160 mg/dL and higher—but certainly anything above 130 is worth treating.

HDL cholesterol, on the other hand, is like nature's plaque vacuum cleaner—it picks up the vessel-clogging cholesterol and carries it away to the liver, where it is disposed of in the form of bile. The higher your HDL levels, the cleaner your blood vessels will be, so you want your high-density high. According to the American Heart Association, people with HDL of 60 mg/dL or higher have a lower risk of heart disease, whereas HDL below 40 mg/dL for men and 50 mg/dL for women is considered too low.

Because HDL is so important to the health of blood vessels, some physicians prefer to talk about the cholesterol ratio—your total cholesterol divided by your HDL cholesterol. For example, if your total cholesterol number is 250 and your HDL is 50, your ratio is 250/50, or 5. People are urged to aim for a ratio of 5 or less, but a ratio of 3.5 or lower is considered optimal.

High cholesterol can be caused by factors both in and out of your control. Heredity plays a big part. Some people can lead a perfectly heart-healthy lifestyle and still have skyrocketing cholesterol because their bodies naturally make too much of it. Also, LDL cholesterol increases inevitably with age, so even if you put up all-star numbers when you were younger, you are more likely to have problems with each passing year. Men naturally have higher cholesterol than women, but the female advantage fades when the hormonal changes of menopause lead to a steep rise in LDL.

And as if high LDL cholesterol wasn't dangerous enough on its own, the results of a study published in a 2006 issue of the journal *Hypertension* showed that people who had high LDL cholesterol or a high cholesterol ratio had an increased risk of developing high blood pressure. Really, these results make sense. High LDL cholesterol leads to atherosclerosis, which causes narrowing of the blood vessels—meaning your heart has to pump that much harder to squeeze blood through them—which means increased blood pressure. You can improve your cholesterol profile by losing weight (if you are overweight), increasing physical activity, and following my cholesterol-busting nutrition program.

For more information on a cholesterol-friendly diet, visit www.joybauer.com/cholesterol.

## HIGH TRIGLYCERIDES

*Triglyceride* is just a fancy word for "fat." Triglycerides are found in foods and manufactured and stored in our bodies. As with LDL cholesterol, eating too much unhealthy fat (more about that in the following sections on saturated and trans fats) will raise your blood triglycerides, but some people also have a genetic predisposition that causes them to manufacture excessive triglycerides on their own, no matter how carefully they eat. Triglyceride levels can shoot up after eating foods that are high in saturated fats or carbohydrates or after drinking alcohol. That's why triglyceride tests require an overnight fast. Triglycerides can become elevated because of genetics or in reaction to having diabetes, hypothyroidism, or kidney disease. As with most other heart-related factors, being overweight and inactive also contributes to abnormally high triglycerides.

High triglyceride levels make blood thicker and stickier, which means that it is more likely to form clots. Normal triglyceride levels are defined as less than 150 mg/dL, 150 to 199 is considered borderline high, 200 to 499 is high, and 500 or higher is officially called very high. To me, anything over 150 is a red flag indicating that my client needs to take immediate steps to get the situation under control.

**FAQS**

**I have high cholesterol, and I've heard that red yeast rice works the same as some of the statin drugs. I'll do anything to avoid taking medication. Does red yeast rice work? Is it safe?**

Red yeast rice does work to lower cholesterol, but only because it contains naturally occurring chemicals that are identical to medicinal statins. These chemicals function the same, and they have the same risks and side effects—including possible liver toxicity and muscle pain or weakness. The difference is that prescription medications are standardized, regulated, and produced in a sterile environment. The amount of active ingredient in each dose of red yeast rice can vary from package to package or even from capsule to capsule in the same package. Worse, red yeast rice may contain contaminants, some of which may cause serious illness. This is one of those cases when natural doesn't necessarily mean better. If you want to safely lower your cholesterol level, talk with your doctor about whether you should start taking a statin medication.

Studies have shown that high triglyceride levels are associated with increased risks of cardiovascular disease and stroke—in both men and women—alone or in combination with other risk factors (high triglycerides combined with high LDL cholesterol can be a particularly deadly combination). For example, in one groundbreaking study, triglycerides alone increased the risk of cardiovascular disease by 14 percent in men and by 37 percent in women. But when the test subjects also had low HDL cholesterol and other risk factors, high triglycerides increased the risk of disease by 32 percent in men and 76 percent in women. Fortunately, triglycerides are relatively easily controlled with the diet and lifestyle changes outlined in this chapter. To lower triglycerides, lose weight if you're overweight, avoid foods that are loaded with sugar (soda, sweets, even dried fruit and fruit juice), limit refined carbohydrates (white bread, white rice, regular pasta, and anything made with white flour), reduce saturated and trans fats, cut back substantially on alcohol (when triglycerides are high, alcohol will keep them high), and incorporate omega-3 fats into your diet.

For more information on foods that can lower high triglyceride levels, visit www.joybauer.com/triglycerides.

## METABOLIC SYNDROME

As you might imagine, having one risk factor for heart disease is bad enough, but having more than one amplifies the threat. Metabolic syndrome describes a cluster of risk factors that together create a toxic, inflammatory environment in blood vessels and throughout the body. Metabolic syndrome is like an advanced warning system to put you and your doctor on high alert that unless you make significant changes to your lifestyle, you're at great risk of developing type 2 diabetes or cardiovascular disease. Metabolic syndrome is common in individuals who are overweight (particularly those who carry most of their weight around their waist).

Metabolic syndrome is most commonly diagnosed in people who have at least three of the following issues: elevated blood pressure (130/85 mm Hg or higher), elevated triglycerides (150 mg/dL or higher), low HDL cholesterol (below 50 mg/dL for women; below 40 mg/dL for men), large waist circumference (greater than 35 inches for women; greater than 40 inches for men), and fasting blood sugar levels higher than 100 mg/dL. The combination of three or more of these factors is dangerous, even if the numbers are only slightly out of the normal range. Fortunately, the 4-step plan in this chapter can help improve each of these risk factors, so you can solve all of these issues with one approach.

## HOW FOOD AFFECTS CARDIOVASCULAR DISEASE

Eating well for cardiovascular health means knowing which foods to avoid, which to limit, and which to embrace.

### FOODS TO AVOID OR LIMIT
### Saturated Fats

Saturated fats are found in animal products, including meats, butter, whole-milk dairy (including yogurt, cheese, and ice cream), and poultry skin. We know that saturated fats raise LDL (bad) cholesterol, but whether a diet high in saturated fat directly increases risk of cardiovascular disease is still being hotly debated by researchers and health professionals. A recent meta-analysis of 21 studies failed to find a link between saturated fat intake and risk of developing heart disease. While this study certainly isn't the last word on what has become a very controversial topic, it does illustrate that there's more to a heart-healthy diet than just cutting down on saturated fat. It turns out that how you replace saturated fat with other nutrients is just as important as strictly limiting it.

Exchanging saturated fat for healthier fats, like polyunsaturated fats (found in fatty fish, nuts, seeds, and vegetable oils), lowers LDL cholesterol and definitively reduces the risk of heart attack and cardiac death. A 2010 study found that for every 5 percent increase in calories from polyunsaturated fats (as a replacement for saturated fats), the risk of heart disease drops by 10 percent. That's substantial! Unfortunately, when health organizations started urging Americans to cut back on saturated fat decades ago, most people didn't replace the butter and beef in their diets with nuts and fatty fish . . . they just started eating more sweets, bread, pasta, and white flour products. As it turns out, these refined carbs are just as damaging to your heart and blood vessels as saturated fat (more on this later). Replacing saturated fat with junky carbohydrates definitely doesn't improve heart health—and, though we're still awaiting more definitive research, it's very possible that replacing bad fats with bad carbs actually *increases* your risk of heart disease. Not to worry—my heart-healthy program cuts out both! On my plan you'll be eating plenty of lean proteins; high-quality carbs like vegetables, fruits, and whole grains; and, of course, heart-healthy fats. Before we explore the foods you should be eating, let's focus on getting the saturated fat out of your diet.

◆ Limit or avoid butter, cream cheese, lard, sour cream, doughnuts, cakes, cookies, white and milk chocolate, ice cream, pizza, cream- or cheese-based salad dressings, cheese sauce, cream sauces, animal shortenings, fatty meats (including hamburgers, bologna, pepperoni, sausage, bacon, salami, pastrami, spareribs, and hot dogs), and whole-milk dairy products.

◆ Choose lean meats only (including skinless chicken and turkey, lean beef, and pork tenderloin), fish and shellfish, and reduced-fat or fat-free dairy products. Try substituting soy foods for meat at least some of the time. Although soy itself may not directly reduce your risk of heart disease, it replaces animal fats with healthier proteins. Choose high-quality whole-soy foods, such as tofu, tempeh, soy milk, and edamame.

◆ Always remove skin from poultry.

◆ Prepare foods by baking, roasting, broiling, boiling, poaching, steaming, grilling, or stir-frying in heart-healthy oils, like olive and canola.

## Trans Fats

Trans fats are even more dangerous than the saturated fats I just advised you to limit or avoid. The main source of trans fat is partially hydrogenated oil, which is found in most stick margarines, as well as some packaged baked goods, snack foods, fried foods, and fast-food items (although fortunately, most major fast-food chains have now gone trans-fat-free). By substituting olive oil or vegetable oil for trans fats in just 2 percent of your daily calories, you can reduce your risk of heart disease by 53 percent. There is no safe amount of trans fat, so try to keep it as far from your plate as possible.

Packaged products always list the amount of trans fat on the Nutrition Facts panel, but there's a loophole to be aware of: The FDA allows companies to "round down" and list zero gram of trans fat as long as a product contains less than 0.5 gram of trans fat per serving. Therefore, if a product contains partially hydrogenated oils and you eat *several* servings of that product, you could end up consuming 1 or 2 grams of trans fat—and any amount of trans fat in your diet is detrimental to heart health.

To be a smart consumer, first check a product's nutrition label to ensure that it has zero gram of trans fat. Next, browse the ingredients list to confirm that the product does not contain any "partially hydrogenated oils." If it does, put it back on the shelf. Although a trace amount of partially hydrogenated oil here and there certainly isn't life threatening, there are now so many packaged foods that are completely free of these toxic fats that there's no reason to compromise.

## Cholesterol-Rich Foods

Years ago, doctors used to recommend that people with heart disease avoid all high-cholesterol foods. But dietary cholesterol does not harm health as much as saturated fats and trans fats do. Research into the effects of dietary cholesterol has been mixed, which is not surprising—different people have different susceptibilities. Still, if you want to reduce your risk factors, consider cutting down on all high-cholesterol foods, including egg yolks, shellfish, liver, and other organ meats (like sweetbreads and foie gras). You'll notice whole eggs and shellfish on a couple of my best foods lists because they're high in other heart-healthy nutrients. That said, if your LDL cholesterol is high, limit your intake of egg yolks to no more than three per week (whites are unlimited), and limit shellfish to no more than one portion twice weekly. You may also want to speak with your cardiologist about personal limitations.

## Low-Quality Carbohydrates

Low-quality carbohydrates include sugar, honey, and other sweeteners; soda and other sugary drinks; candy, cakes, cookies, and sugary cereals; anything made with white flour (including white bread, rolls, buns, and regular pasta); and white rice. These unhealthy carbs cause a sudden rise in insulin, which may lead to a spike in triglycerides. Refined carbs can also worsen your cholesterol numbers. A diet high in added sugars has been linked to low HDL (good) cholesterol levels and increased LDL (bad) cholesterol levels. In addition, high blood sugar and insulin levels harm the delicate lining of blood vessels and promote inflammation, which contributes to the buildup of plaque in the arteries. With that in mind, whenever possible, aim for high-quality instead of low-quality carbs. That means cutting back on sweets and embracing whole grain foods such as oatmeal, high-fiber cereals, brown and wild rice, whole wheat pasta, and whole grain breads.

## Salt

For decades, the science has been pretty clear: Salt increases blood pressure in people who are salt sensitive, and the more salt you eat, the greater the potential rise in blood pressure. Sodium in small doses is necessary for the body to function properly, but too much will draw excess fluid into the blood, effectively raising blood pressure. High blood pressure is a major risk factor for stroke and heart disease, so cutting back on salt is a potential lifesaver. A large analysis in the *British Medical Journal* found that reducing people's daily salt intake by 5 grams (about 1 teaspoon) worldwide could prevent 1.25 million deaths from stroke and almost 3 million deaths from cardiovascular disease each year. That's quite a remarkable statistic!

So how much salt should you be eating? In general, healthy people should aim to keep their daily sodium intake below 2,300 milligrams. However, certain populations are advised to further reduce their intake to 1,500 milligrams or less. These populations include people age 51 and older, all African Americans (this ethnic group is at

### FAQ

**I've heard that kosher salt and sea salt are much healthier than regular table salt. Is that true?**

It depends. By weight, all three—kosher, sea, and table salt—contain the same amount of sodium. However, kosher salt has a coarser grain than fine table salt, which means that it contains less sodium by volume. In other words, 1 teaspoon of kosher salt yields less sodium than 1 teaspoon of table salt. (The larger granules of kosher salt can't clump together as closely as the fine ones do.) So, when you're measuring volume amounts for recipes, you'll automatically reduce the sodium content if you make the switch to kosher salt. Sea salt offers the same benefit as kosher salt only if it's a coarse-grained variety. On the other hand, "fine grain" sea salts have the same high sodium content as traditional table salt and therefore don't offer any health advantage.

Nowadays, manufacturers are adding sea salt to potato chips, canned soups, and other packaged foods—probably to make the products seem healthier and more natural. But really it's the amount of salt they're adding, not the type, that's important for health purposes. So don't be swayed by tricky marketing; always check the Nutrition Facts panel to determine the sodium content per serving.

high risk of high blood pressure), and people who already have high blood pressure, diabetes, or chronic kidney disease.

That said, salt consumption is a hard habit to break. Salt actually dulls your sense of taste, which means that, over time, you'll be reaching for that shaker more often to get the flavor you desire from your food. The best thing to do is go cold turkey. Well, almost. First, take the salt shaker off the kitchen table, and try not to add salt to foods you prepare at home. If you miss the flavor, experiment with a variety of salt-free seasonings and perhaps try some of the salt substitutes on the market.

Since up to 80 percent of the sodium in the American diet comes from processed foods (not salt added at the table or during food prep), you'll also want to become a savvy consumer and start reading labels. To get you started, here's a guide to the labeling lingo the FDA uses to regulate sodium claims on food packaging.

◆ "Sodium-free" indicates that a product contains less than 5 milligrams of sodium per serving.

◆ "Very low sodium" indicates that a product contains 35 milligrams of sodium or less per serving.

◆ "Low-sodium" indicates that a product contains 140 milligrams of sodium or less per serving.

◆ "Reduced-sodium" or "less sodium" indicates that a product contains at least 25 percent less sodium than the standard version. Note: Some "reduced-sodium" products are still very high in sodium, so you'll need to check the actual sodium content on the Nutrition Facts panel to see if various foods fit into your low-sodium diet. For example, reduced-sodium canned soups, though considerably lower in salt than regular canned soups, can still contain almost 500 milligrams of sodium per 1-cup serving.

◆ "Light in sodium" indicates that the product contains at least 50 percent less sodium than the standard version. Note: Some "light in sodium" products are still very high in sodium, so as with "reduced" or "less" sodium, check the Nutrition Facts panel. For example, "light" or "lite" soy sauce, though considerably lower in salt than regular soy sauce, still contains 500 to 600 milligrams of sodium per tablespoon.

◆ "Unsalted" or "no salt added" indicates that no sodium (salt) is added to the product during processing, but the product still contains the sodium that naturally occurs in the product's ingredients.

I realize this is a lot of information, and tracking salt intake can be downright confusing, so here are the major points: First and foremost, prepare as many meals as possible at home using whole, unprocessed foods that are naturally low in sodium. When it comes to packaged foods, choose entrées with less than

600 milligrams of sodium; for all other products, aim for less than 200 milligrams of sodium (the lower, the better). For canned foods like soups, tomatoes, vegetables, beans, and broth, go out of your way to purchase only lower-sodium or no-salt-added varieties. If you can find only regular canned beans, be sure to rinse them thoroughly before using. The liquid they are packed in is typically very high in sodium. You'll also want to dramatically limit the saltiest offenders: soy sauce, teriyaki sauce, salad dressings, ketchup, prepared marinades, pickles, sauerkraut, and deli meats.

## GOOD FOODS TO CHOOSE

### Vegetables and Fruits

I know you're probably sick of being told to eat plenty of vegetables and fruits, but it really is important, especially if you are fighting cardiovascular disease. The scientific data all support the same claim: People who eat five or more servings of vegetables and fruits daily have a reduced risk of heart attack and stroke, compared with people who eat fewer than three servings daily. Specifically, heart attack risk is about 15 percent lower, stroke risk is about 30 percent lower, and, on average, the risk of coronary artery disease is reduced by about 5 percent for each additional serving of produce you eat every day.

What's the magic in fruits and vegetables? No one really knows. Sure, they're full of vitamins, minerals, fiber, and antioxidants, but we don't know which ones are most helpful because whenever scientists try to mimic the effects of foods with supplements, their formulations simply don't produce the same protective effects as the real

## FAQ

**I'm watching my sodium intake because I have high blood pressure. Is it safe for me to use salt substitutes instead?**

Yes, probably. However, some salt substitutes are composed of "potassium chloride" (instead of sodium chloride, which is found in regular salt), and extra potassium can be problematic for people who have kidney problems or are taking certain medications (such as potassium-sparing diuretics and other common blood pressure medications). Always speak with your physician before sprinkling this type of salt substitute on your food.

Other salt substitutes (such as Mrs. Dash) do not contain potassium chloride. These products are simply salt-free blends of different herbs and seasonings that add flavor to food. Salt-free seasoning blends that do not contain potassium chloride are safe for everyone to enjoy. (If your physician has instructed you to limit your potassium intake, always double-check the ingredients list to make sure that there is no added potassium chloride, just to be sure.)

You can also experiment with other herbs, spices, and seasonings, such as ground red pepper, garlic powder (not garlic salt), onion powder (not onion salt), cumin, smoked paprika, celery seed (not celery salt), curry powder, wasabi powder, cinnamon, nutmeg, dill, cilantro, thyme, sage, basil, tarragon, chives, lemon and lime juice and zest, wine, flavored vinegars, and extracts (vanilla, almond, etc.).

thing. That means that you have to eat the foods, the whole foods (and nothing but the foods) in order to reap their benefits. Two large caveats: If you're taking any cardiac medication, check with your doctor or pharmacist before eating grapefruit or drinking grapefruit juice. (A compound in grapefruit interferes with the breakdown of many medications, and you'll want to make sure grapefruit are safe for you before incorporating them into your diet.) Also, if you're taking a blood thinner like Coumadin, have your doctor monitor your blood and medication dosage as you increase your intake of dark leafy green vegetables. These vegetables are rich in vitamin K, which plays a key role in blood clotting. (See page 134 for more information on Coumadin and vitamin K.)

## Soluble Fiber

Soluble fiber, especially the viscous type, may help reduce cholesterol by grabbing onto it and escorting it through your digestive system and out of your body. Soluble fiber also may reduce the intestinal absorption of cholesterol and lower blood pressure, and research has shown that eating an additional 5 to 10 grams each day can reduce LDL cholesterol by 3 to 5 percent. If you eat a few foods rich in soluble fiber every day, you'll get at least 5 grams. It is a small improvement, but every percentage point counts!

> BEST FOODS FOR SOLUBLE FIBER: *psyllium seeds (ground), lima beans, starchy beans (such as black, navy, pinto, garbanzo, kidney), Brussels sprouts, oat bran, winter squash, parsnips, turnips, sweet potatoes, lentils, black-eyed peas, split peas, green peas, okra, eggplant, barley, oats, rice bran, guava, oranges, grapefruit, apples, peaches, plums, nectarines, pears, prunes, mangoes, strawberries, blackberries, raspberries, bananas, apricots, raisins, white potatoes, avocados, broccoli, carrots, green beans, spinach, cabbage, kale, wheat germ, ground flaxseed*

## Whole Grains

Whole grains are loaded with many of the same heart-healthy ingredients as vegetables and fruits: fiber, vitamins, minerals, and—surprisingly—high levels of antioxidants. That's because whole grains contain all three parts of the seed: the fiber-rich bran, the micronutrient-dense germ, and the starchy endosperm. In white refined carbs, on the other hand, the most nutritious parts of the grain are stripped away during processing, which explains why they're far less healthy than whole grains.

Plenty of research shows that people who regularly consume whole grains have a lower risk of cardiovascular disease. A 2008 meta-analysis found that individuals who consume an average of 2.5 servings of whole grains per day have a 21 percent lower risk of cardiovascular events (such as heart attack and stroke) than people who eat very few whole grain foods (just 0.2 servings daily). You can easily enjoy 2.5 servings of whole grains by eating a slice of whole wheat bread and ¾ cup of brown rice.

Lately, whole grains have received a lot of attention for their blood pressure perks in particular. Men and women who eat a lot of whole grains are less likely to develop high blood pressure than people who rarely consume them. A 2010 trial made the benefits even clearer. Researchers in the United Kingdom assigned over 200 participants to different groups: One group ate only refined grains, like white bread and refined sugary cereal, while the other groups ate three daily servings of whole grains (whole grain bread, whole grain cereal, or oats). Those in the whole grain groups achieved an average 6 mm Hg drop in their systolic blood pressure, which is a remarkable improvement from just a single dietary change.

To keep your heart healthy and strong, aim to consume at least three servings of whole grains daily (and, of course, dramatically limit those junky, refined grains). If you follow my food plan, you'll automatically meet your daily quota.

## HEALTHY FATS

There was a time when heart researchers slapped the same label—"bad"—on every kind of fat. Now we know that trans fats and saturated fats are dangerous for cardiovascular health, but omega-3 fats and monounsaturated fats are actually good for your heart.

Heart-healthy fish oils are especially rich in omega-3 fatty acids, a type of polyunsaturated fat. Numerous large-scale studies over the past 20 years have found that people who eat diets high in omega-3s have a substantially lower risk of coronary heart disease, as well as sudden death from arrhythmia. Since omega-3s seem to reduce inflammation, lower blood pressure, decrease triglycerides, raise HDL cholesterol, and make blood thinner and less sticky so it is less likely to clot, they are as close to a food prescription for heart health as it gets. I recommend eating omega-3-rich fish at least twice a week. (My Best Foods list includes only the fatty fish that have been shown to be low in mercury, PCBs, and dioxins.) If you cannot manage that, consider taking fish oil capsules. (See the Supplements section, page 138, for more information.)

BEST FOODS FOR OMEGA-3 FATTY ACIDS: *wild salmon (fresh, canned), herring, mackerel (not king), sardines, anchovies, rainbow trout, Pacific oysters, chia seeds, ground flaxseed, walnuts, butternuts (white walnuts), seaweed, walnut oil, canola oil, flaxseed oil, soybeans (edamame)*

Monounsaturated fats, found mainly in olive oil, are thought to protect against heart disease by reducing blood pressure. Scientists discovered the benefits of olive

## FAQS

### I notice you specify wild salmon in your grocery lists and meal plans. Is farmed salmon much less healthy?

I prefer wild salmon over farmed for a number of reasons. From a health perspective, wild salmon is lower in contaminants and has a better nutritional profile. Farmed salmon contains substantially higher levels of toxins—most notably, potential cancer-causing compounds called PCBs. Wild salmon contains significantly more vitamin D—as much as four times the amount found in farmed salmon. And, although wild and farmed salmon contain similar levels of the highly prized omega-3 fats, wild salmon is far leaner overall.

Wild salmon is also better for the environment. Conventional fish farms spread disease and produce large amounts of waste, which pollutes our oceans. Farmed salmon that escape compete with wild species for food and other resources, and they weaken the native gene pool.

In a perfect world, we would all purchase wild seafood caught in a sustainable, eco-friendly manner. Unfortunately, wild salmon is far less plentiful and more costly to harvest, which means it's much more expensive than farmed salmon. I highly encourage you to make room in your food budget for wild salmon, but if that's just not possible (and I realize that for many families, it isn't), you're better off eating some farmed salmon than totally cutting it out of your diet. For the majority of people, the heart-health benefits of eating omega-3–rich farmed salmon outweigh the risks associated with PCBs and other pollutants. However, I strongly advise that young children and pregnant and nursing women consume only wild salmon.

When consuming farmed salmon fillets or steaks, you can reduce your exposure to PCBs by removing the skin. (PCBs are especially concentrated here and in the fat that lies directly beneath.) If you're on a tight budget, canned Alaskan salmon is also a terrific option: It's wild by default, since salmon farming is not permitted in the state of Alaska. Use canned salmon in place of tuna to make a tasty salad, or enjoy a salmon melt with reduced-fat cheese on whole grain bread.

oil by observing Mediterranean populations, which use olive oil more than any other form of fat and typically have low rates of coronary artery disease. Research shows that it doesn't help to just add monounsaturated fats to your diet—you also need to replace some of the unhealthy fats that are already in your diet (all those saturated and trans fats mentioned earlier) with better choices. There is also some evidence that substituting olive oil for some carbohydrates in your diet (particularly those unhealthy, low-quality, refined carbohydrates) can increase HDL.

BEST FOODS FOR MONOUNSATURATED FATS: *olive oil, canola oil, avocados, olives, macadamia nuts, hazelnuts, pecans, almonds, peanuts, cashews, Brazil nuts, pistachios, pine nuts, peanut butter, almond butter, cashew butter, macadamia nut butter, sunflower seed butter*

## CALCIUM AND VITAMIN D

Calcium and vitamin D work as a team—vitamin D helps the body absorb and use calcium. These two nutrients have been shown to help reduce blood pressure by 3 to 10 percent. Although this doesn't sound like much, it could add up to about a 15 percent reduction in risk of cardiovascular disease. Some research suggests that milk proteins may act similarly to antihypertensive (blood pressure–lowering) medications called ACE inhibitors.

BEST FOODS FOR CALCIUM: *yogurt (fat-free, low-fat), milk (fat-free, 1%), soy milk, cheese (fat-free, reduced-fat), tofu with calcium (check nutrition label), soybeans (edamame), frozen yogurt (fat-free, low-fat), low-fat ice cream, bok choy, kale, white beans, collard greens, broccoli, almonds and almond butter*

BEST FOODS FOR VITAMIN D: *wild salmon (fresh, canned), mackerel (not king), sardines, herring, milk (fat-free, 1%), soy milk, fortified yogurt (fat-free, low-fat), egg yolks, vitamin D–enhanced mushrooms\**

*\*These mushrooms are treated with UV light, which dramatically increases their vitamin D content.*

## MAGNESIUM

Although more research is needed, magnesium may turn out to be a potent ally for reducing the risk of cardiovascular disease. In studies done on lab animals, magnesium reduces inflammation and alters the way fats are metabolized. Human studies suggest that eating lots of magnesium-rich foods may reduce triglycerides, lower blood pressure, and increase HDL cholesterol. In a long-term, 15-year study, people who ate plenty of magnesium-rich foods reduced their risk of developing metabolic syndrome by about 30 percent.

## FAQS

**Last year, I found out that I have very high cholesterol. I did everything right—I met with a nutritionist and changed my diet, I started exercising, and I stopped smoking—but my LDL cholesterol is still high. My doctor wants to put me on a statin medication. Why won't my numbers budge?**

Although many people are able to dramatically lower their cholesterol by following a heart-healthy diet and exercising, some people have a genetic predisposition to overproduce cholesterol. No matter how hard they work at their diet and lifestyle, they're just not able to lower their numbers without medication. It sounds like you fall into this category—so definitely take your doctor's advice. At the same time, continue following your new, healthy lifestyle. Although your stellar habits may not be driving your cholesterol numbers into a safe range, the changes you've made are greatly benefiting every part of your body, plus boosting your mood, increasing your energy, and reducing your risk of a whole host of chronic conditions.

BEST FOODS FOR MAGNESIUM: *pumpkin seeds, spinach, Swiss chard, amaranth, sunflower seeds, cashews, almonds, quinoa, tempeh, potatoes (sweet and white), soybeans (edamame), millet, starchy beans (such as black, navy, pinto, garbanzo, kidney), artichoke hearts, peanuts and peanut butter, brown rice, whole grain bread, sesame seeds, wheat germ, flaxseed*

## POTASSIUM

Your blood levels of potassium and sodium are inextricably linked. When potassium is low, your body retains sodium (and, as discussed above, too much sodium raises blood pressure). When potassium is high, your body gets rid of sodium. Eating potassium-rich foods is important for maintaining a healthy balance of both minerals and, by extension, keeping your blood pressure low. Important note: Stick to potassium-rich foods rather than supplements (unless your doctor has prescribed one). High doses of potassium in supplement form will upset the balance and could have serious, even life-threatening, consequences.

BEST FOODS FOR POTASSIUM: *white potatoes, yogurt (fat-free, low-fat), soybeans (edamame), Swiss chard, all fish, sweet potatoes, avocados, cantaloupe, artichokes, bananas, spinach, lettuce, honeydew, pumpkin, milk (fat-free, 1%), carrots, starchy beans (such as black, navy, pinto, garbanzo, kidney), lentils, lima beans, apricots, papaya, split peas, pistachios, winter squash (acorn, butternut), soy milk, watermelon, beets, tomatoes, kale, mushrooms, raisins, peanuts, plums, almonds, sunflower seeds, prunes, oranges, broccoli*

## FAQS

**A friend heard that I'm now taking a statin medication for high cholesterol and recommended that I also take a supplement called CoQ$_{10}$. What exactly is it, and is this something I should consider?**

Coenzyme Q$_{10}$ is an antioxidant necessary for energy production in cells. Without CoQ$_{10}$, cells can't function properly. Our bodies usually make sufficient CoQ$_{10}$ to keep us healthy. Statins work by inhibiting the mechanism that allows the liver to make cholesterol, but they also slow the body's production of CoQ$_{10}$, leading to deficiency. To counteract these effects, I recommend taking 100 to 200 milligrams of CoQ$_{10}$ once a day in a soft gel formulation. Although most people can take CoQ$_{10}$ safely and without side effects, it is always a good idea to talk with your doctor before taking any supplement.

## GARLIC

Studies testing whether garlic is beneficial for heart health have been mixed. Researchers attribute garlic's medicinal capabilities to a naturally occurring compound called allicin, which is released when cloves are minced or crushed. For a long time, garlic's claim to fame was that it improved cholesterol, and many people responded by increasing the garlic in their favorite recipes and popping garlic pills. However, a well-executed 2007 study involving 192 people with moderately elevated LDL cholesterol found that neither raw, fresh garlic nor garlic supplements had any cholesterol-lowering effect. That being said, garlic seems to have other cardiovascular benefits, such as lowering blood pressure. So if you enjoy cooking with garlic, by all means continue to work it into your favorite dishes.

## PLANT STEROLS OR STANOLS

Sterols and stanols are natural substances found in small amounts in the cell membranes of plants, including fruits, vegetables, legumes, nuts, and seeds. Sterols occur in relatively high amounts in pistachios, sunflower seeds, sesame seeds, and wheat germ. In terms of their effects on the human body, plant sterols and stanols are virtually the same.

Sterols and stanols are similar in structure to cholesterol, and they compete with cholesterol for access to receptors in the small intestines. (Imagine 15 people all hoping to get a ride in their friend's Volkswagen Beetle—not everyone is going to be riding in the car.) Research has shown that sterols and stanols can cut the amount of cholesterol absorbed by the small intestines by about 50 percent and, therefore, reduce LDL cholesterol levels by between 5 and 14 percent.

You can reap these cardiovascular benefits with just 2 grams of sterols/stanols per day. Because it's impossible to consume that amount from food alone, you may want to consider using one of the heart-healthy, soft tub spreads that come fortified with plant stanols or sterols. You can spread these on whole grain bread or melt them over heart-healthy vegetables. I recommend trying the light versions of these products to save yourself some calories—and if you're not into spreads, consider taking these compounds in pill form. (See

**FAQS**

**I had blood tests done recently. My LDL cholesterol is normal and my triglycerides are normal, but my HDL cholesterol is abnormally low. Is there anything I can do to boost my HDL?**

Some people have a genetic tendency to have low HDL levels. Although this might seem harmless, it can throw off your cholesterol ratio and may indicate a future risk of heart problems. One of the simplest and most effective ways to boost HDL is through exercise. I recommend you engage in at least 30 minutes of physical activity most, if not all, days of the week. Also, be sure to follow the diet and lifestyle recommendations in this chapter—they will help assure that your blood vessels stay as healthy as possible.

In addition, consider taking a low dosage of omega-3 fatty acids (see the Supplements section, page 138, for more information), and speak with your physician about prescription medications that can specifically raise HDL cholesterol.

**FAQS**

**My doctor just started me on a blood-thinning medication called Coumadin. He told me to avoid all green vegetables rich in vitamin K because it interferes with the medication. I know dark leafy greens are very healthy—do I really have to give them up?**

You may not have to give up green vegetables after all. These days, many doctors understand how important dark leafy greens are in preventing heart disease and for overall health, so they will adjust a patient's dosage of Coumadin (or other blood-thinning medication) according to that person's personal blood test results and typical intake of dark leafy greens. Have another conversation with your physician or cardiologist to see if adjusting your dosage is an option. If it is, you can make dark leafy greens a regular part of your diet, as long as you eat a relatively consistent amount from week to week so there aren't any drastic changes in your vitamin K levels. Top choices include spinach, kale, collard greens, Brussels sprouts, watercress, broccoli, and broccoli raab, since they are particularly heart healthy and loaded with antioxidants.

If for any reason your doctor does decide you should avoid dark leafy greens, here are a few go-to veggies that are low in vitamin K but still highly nutrient dense.

- Carrots
- Bell peppers
- Green beans
- Potatoes (sweet and white)
- Pumpkin
- Tomatoes
- Beets
- Winter squash

the Supplements section, page 138, for more information about nonfood sources of plant sterols/stanols.)

## ALCOHOL

The benefits of alcohol depend, in part, on what your cardiovascular risk factors are. If your problem is high triglycerides, alcohol should be considered a rare treat, if you indulge at all. Even small amounts of alcohol can increase triglyceride levels dramatically.

For other risk factors, research suggests that one or two servings of alcohol per day may be good for your heart—that's no more than one serving per day for women and no more than two servings per day for men. Studies have shown that drinking moderate amounts of alcohol reduces the risk of coronary artery disease by about 25 percent and reduces the risk of death from heart disease by about 12 percent. Alcohol seems to increase the good HDL cholesterol and prevent clots.

There are right ways and wrong ways to use alcohol for heart health. The right way is to drink moderately and with a meal. The optimal amount is one or two drinks per day (one serving is 12 ounces of beer, 5 ounces of wine, or one shot of hard alcohol). Although all alcohol has heart-healthy benefits, red wine also contains antioxidants such as resveratrol that provide an extra boost of nutrition. Studies show that people who drink these moderate amounts of alcohol have a lower risk of disease than abstainers—though I can't recommend starting to drink if you're a teetotaler.

The wrong way to use alcohol is to drink heavily. People who regularly drink five or more servings of alcohol per day have a higher risk of disease than people who drink moderately or abstain completely. Even three or more drinks per day raises blood pressure and increases triglycerides. The worst risks are for binge drinkers—people who occasionally consume large amounts of alcohol. Women who have five or more drinks and men who have nine or more drinks in a single drinking episode put themselves at risk of what scientists call major coronary events—heart attacks, strokes, and death.

If you are currently taking medication for lowering blood pressure or cholesterol or if you have diabetes, always talk with your doctor about whether drinking alcohol makes sense for you. There are some questions about whether alcohol might interact with medications or complicate potential liver problems.

## MULTIPLE CHANGES, MEGA BENEFITS

I saved my client story for this point in the chapter because I'm guessing you're probably feeling a little overwhelmed right about now. Take heart . . . as Sean did.

Sean was 36 years old and about 35 pounds overweight. He had high blood pressure, LDL cholesterol of 170, HDL cholesterol of 48, and triglycerides of about 300. His internist was also a cardiologist, and he wanted to put Sean on medication before he developed serious heart disease. Sean

### FAQS

**I have high blood pressure. Is it okay to drink regular caffeinated coffee?**

Despite the extensive amount of research that has gone into answering this question, we still don't have a definitive answer. What we do know is that the caffeine in regular coffee causes a temporary boost in blood pressure. For healthy people without blood pressure issues, this is perfectly safe and nothing to worry about. In fact, the rise in blood pressure is typically far less substantial in regular coffee drinkers because they develop a tolerance to caffeine.

If you already have high blood pressure and you're reluctant to switch to decaf, you'll need to speak with your physician or cardiologist. That's because caffeine sensitivity varies dramatically from person to person, and this decision should be made on a case-by-case basis. If you're taking all of the necessary steps to manage your blood pressure (exercising regularly, limiting sodium, eating plenty of produce, and keeping your weight in check), your physician may not have a problem with you enjoying one to two 8-ounce cups of regular coffee per day.

couldn't stand the thought of going on medication, so he made a deal with his doctor: If he didn't get his numbers down within two months, he would fill his prescription.

When Sean came to see me, his diet was a mess. He ate, partied, and smoked cigarettes like he was still in college. Weekends were orgies of buffalo wings, beer, pizza, and ice cream—all things he was loath to give up, but he did. We made up a game called Beat the Medication. Sean stopped smoking. He started walking every evening with his wife and baby. He took fish oil capsules and plant stanol supplements. And he started eating only heart-healthy foods, including those with plenty of potassium, calcium, and magnesium. He cut out salt and fruit juice and even stopped drinking beer. That was the hardest part, and it was a real struggle for Sean, but he was playing for keeps.

After two months, Sean had lost 17 pounds. His LDL cholesterol dropped 30 points to 140, his HDLs stayed the same, and his triglycerides—slashed by more than half—were down to 120. His doctor was thrilled and gave him another two months to get his LDLs closer to 100.

Sean continued the program and ultimately dropped another 16 pounds. He got all his risk factors under control. His blood pressure was normal, his HDL remained around 50, his LDL dipped right under 100, and his triglycerides fell to 105. He did it! He beat the medication. Even better, he felt energetic and empowered.

Do you want to be like Sean? You can be. It is never too late to make healthy changes. Study after study has shown that the more heart-healthy living you do, the greater the benefits.

## BONUS POINTS

- ◆ **Know all your numbers.** Don't rely on your doctor to keep track of your blood pressure, triglycerides, and cholesterol levels—those numbers don't do you much good sitting in a medical file drawer. Every time you have your blood tested, write down your numbers and track your progress. Most doctors recommend follow-up blood work every year or every six months, depending on your individual health concerns. There's nothing more motivating than results—in this case, seeing your numbers drop steadily lower and lower. Work with your doctor to set goals for each of the following tests: blood pressure, LDL cholesterol, HDL cholesterol, cholesterol ratio (total cholesterol divided by HDL cholesterol), and triglycerides.

- ◆ **Ask about testing your iron and thyroid.** Heart disease risk can be affected by elevated ferritin (a measure of iron), and high cholesterol can be a side effect of low levels of thyroid hormones. Talk with your doctor about whether you need additional blood work done.

- ◆ **If you smoke, quit.** Smoking causes inflammation in your lungs and throughout your entire body, which can contribute to atherosclerosis, blood clots, and risk of heart attack. Smoking makes all heart health indicators worse. If you have high cholesterol, high triglycerides, or high blood pressure, smoking magnifies the danger.

♦ **If you are overweight, focus on dropping some pounds.** Body fat produces and secretes hormones, including inflammatory chemicals that play a key role in the development of atherosclerosis. In addition, being overweight increases blood pressure and LDL cholesterol and decreases HDL cholesterol. Even if your cholesterol levels, blood pressure, and other cardiovascular indicators are in the normal range, obesity is recognized as an independent risk factor for heart disease. And every little bit of weight loss helps. Research has shown that losing just 10 pounds can reduce LDL cholesterol by 5 to 8 percent. (See Weight Loss on page 17 for more information on how to lose weight while following this heart-healthy program.)

♦ **Become more physically active.** Even moderate exercise can help improve cholesterol, triglycerides, and blood pressure. Aerobic activity seems to be able to stop the sharp rise in triglycerides after eating, perhaps because of a decrease in the amount of triglycerides released by the liver or because active muscle clears triglycerides out of the bloodstream more quickly than inactive muscle does. If you haven't exercised regularly (or at all) for years, I recommend starting slowly by walking at an easy pace for 15 minutes a day five days a week. Then, as you get more comfortable, increase the amount of time by 5 minutes each day. Strive to work up to at least 30 minutes each day—but of course, the more the better. (Always get clearance from your doctor before beginning an exercise program.)

♦ **If you have diabetes, control your blood sugar.** Uncontrolled blood sugar can increase your risk of coronary artery disease, heart attack, and stroke. Part of your heart care is diabetes care. (For more information about diabetes, see Type 2 Diabetes on page 183.)

♦ **Manage stress.** High blood pressure has been linked to emotional stress and anxiety. It is so common that the phrase "white-coat hypertension" has been used to describe the spike in blood pressure some people experience in the stressful setting of the doctor's office. Some of the best stress reducers include meditation, yoga, biofeedback, guided relaxation, and cognitive-behavioral therapy. Taking time to play with pets also seems to help. (In case you're wondering, watching TV does not work as a stress reliever—scientists have checked.) Research has shown that reducing stress can reduce blood pressure by as much as 10 percent—not bad for a few minutes of meditation or quiet relaxation every day.

♦ **If you have hypertension, avoid soaking in hot tubs.** You should also avoid saunas, steam rooms, and hot baths or otherwise trying to relax your body with heat. This can raise your heart rate and blood pressure and cause dizziness.

◆ **Get enough sleep.** Research shows that people who get six to eight hours of sleep per night have less risk of developing hypertension than people who get five hours or less per night. It could be that sleeping too little increases stress and that lack of rest leads to less follow-through on healthy diet and exercise plans. When you make time for sleep, you may also find that it's easier to make time for healthy habits, too.

## SUPPLEMENTS

If you are trying to get your cholesterol under control and want to consider supplements in addition to the food fixes, I recommend the following. (If you are taking a prescription cholesterol-lowering medication, talk with your doctor before taking supplements.)

1.  **A multivitamin.** To ensure you're getting all the nutrients necessary for good health, consider taking a daily multivitamin. There is no need to take megadoses—about 100 percent DV of most vitamins and minerals is sufficient. Men and postmenopausal women should take a formulation without iron.

2.  **Soluble fiber.** I recommend getting as much soluble fiber from the foods in your diet as possible. However, if you don't regularly eat five to eight servings of fruits and veggies a day, consider adding a psyllium fiber supplement. Respected brands include Metamucil and Konsyl. Start by taking one dose (typically, 1 teaspoon to 1 tablespoon of powder) mixed with at least 8 ounces of water. You can gradually increase to two or three doses per day, if desired. Because fiber supplements can interfere with some medications, talk with your doctor before taking them. Common side effects include bloating and flatulence.

3.  **Omega-3s from fish oil.** People who don't eat fatty fish at least twice per week may want to consider taking a fish oil supplement. The two most potent types of omega-3 fatty acids found in fish oil supplements are DHA (docosahexaenoic acid) and EPA (eicosapentaenoic acid). Aim to take a daily dose of 1,000 milligrams of EPA and DHA combined. Because fish oil supplement companies balance these fatty acids differently, you'll need to read the label carefully and tally up the DHA plus EPA total. You typically have to take more than one pill to reach the 1,000 milligram dosage.

    Fish oil supplements also have been shown to lower triglycerides by 20 to 50 percent, but this effect requires a higher dosage of 2 to 4 grams (that's 2,000 to 4,000 mg) of DHA and EPA combined. Important note: Dosages this high should be taken only under a doctor's supervision. (It is possible to get a prescription for these higher doses, so you may want to check to see if your medical prescription plan will cover it.)

Store capsules in the fridge to prevent rancidity. To prevent fishy burps or aftertaste, buy enteric-coated varieties, take them with food, and divide up your doses throughout the day. Because fish oil acts as a blood thinner, do not take it if you have hemophilia, are already taking blood-thinning medications, or are on aspirin therapy (unless it's been approved by your doctor). If you have diabetes, talk with your doctor before trying fish oil supplements, because they may affect blood sugar.

4. **Sterols/stanols.** If you don't use soft tub spreads and want to get the benefits of plant sterols and stanols without extra calories, you might consider taking supplements. Follow usage directions carefully; most brands advise taking pills two or three times daily, with or just prior to meals.

For more information on foods that promote heart health, visit www.joybauer.com/heart.

# JOY'S 4-STEP PROGRAM
## FOR CARDIOVASCULAR DISEASE

Follow this program if you have high cholesterol, high blood pressure, or a history of cardiovascular disease, including heart attack and stroke. If heart disease runs in your family, you may want to follow this program to help prevent future health problems.

## Step 1 ... START WITH THE BASICS

These are the first things you should do to get control over your cardiovascular risk factors.

◆ If it has been more than a year since your last doctor visit, consider going in for a heart disease checkup. Blood levels of cholesterol, triglycerides, and other risk factors can change dramatically in one year. Get your most recent numbers. Ask about whether you should also be checked for blood ferritin, thyroid, and blood sugar levels.

◆ If you smoke, quit.

◆ If you are overweight, lose weight.

◆ Begin a program of regular exercise. Always talk with your doctor before starting, and consult her immediately if you experience unusual chest pain, left arm pain or tingling, or general weakness during or after exercise.

## Step 2 ... YOUR ULTIMATE GROCERY LIST

The foods you choose are critical for good cardiovascular health. This list contains foods with high levels of nutrients that can help you get your risk factors under control, including potassium, fiber, omega-3 fatty acids, magnesium, calcium, and vitamin D. You don't have to purchase every item, but these foods should make up the bulk of what you eat during the week. If you find yourself getting bored, try some unfamiliar foods from these groups—they may become new favorites. Skip dried fruit, fruit juice, and alcohol if you have high triglycerides. If you're on medication, check with your physician or pharmacist before putting grapefruit or grapefruit juice in your shopping cart, because a compound in grapefruit interacts with many medications. When choosing canned and packaged products, look for low-salt alternatives.

For a printable version of this list, visit www.joybauer.com/cholesterol.

## FRUIT

*All* fruit, but especially:

Apples

Apricots

Bananas

Berries (blackberries, blueberries, boysenberries, raspberries, and strawberries)

Cantaloupe

Dates

Figs

Grapefruit (skip if you're taking an incompatible medication)

Honeydew

Oranges

Papayas

Peaches

Pears

Plums

Prunes

Raisins

Watermelon

## VEGETABLES AND LEGUMES

*All* vegetables, but especially:

Artichokes

Asparagus

Avocados

Beans, starchy (such as black, garbanzo, kidney, navy, and pinto)

Beets

Bok choy

Broccoli

Broccoli raab

Brussels sprouts

Cabbage

Carrots

Cauliflower

Corn

Dark leafy greens (such as beet, collard, dandelion, kale, mustard, Swiss chard, and turnip)

Lentils

Lettuce (all varieties)

Mushrooms

Okra

Olives

Onions

Parsnips

Peas (black-eyed, green, and split)

Peppers (all varieties)

Potatoes (sweet and white)

Pumpkin (fresh and canned 100% pure pumpkin puree)

Soybeans (edamame)

Spinach

Squash, summer

Squash, winter (acorn and butternut)

Sugar snap peas

Tomatoes

Zucchini

## SEAFOOD

*All* fish and shellfish, but especially:

Anchovies

Herring

Mackerel (not king)

Salmon, wild

Sardines

Rainbow trout

## LEAN PROTEINS

Beef, lean

Chicken, ground (at least 90% lean)

Chicken, skinless

Eggs and egg substitutes

Pork tenderloin

Tempeh

Tofu

Turkey, ground (at least 90% lean)

Turkey, skinless

Turkey bacon

Turkey burgers, lean

Veggie burgers

## NUTS AND SEEDS (PREFERABLY UNSALTED)

Almonds and almond butter

Butternuts (white walnuts)

Cashews and cashew butter

Chia seeds

Flaxseed, ground

Hazelnuts

Macadamia nuts

Peanuts and peanut butter

Pecans

Pine nuts

Pistachios

Pumpkin seeds

Sunflower seeds and sunflower butter

Walnuts

## WHOLE GRAINS

Amaranth

Barley

Bread, whole grain (buns, crackers, English muffins, pitas, tortillas, and wraps)

Bulgur

Cereals, whole grain (at least 3 grams fiber; no more than 8 grams sugar per serving)

Millet

Oat bran

Oats

Pasta, whole grain

Quinoa

Rice (brown and wild)

Waffles, whole grain

Wheat berries

Wheat germ

## DAIRY

Cheese (fat-free or reduced-fat)

Cottage cheese (fat-free or 1%)

Cream cheese (fat-free or reduced-fat)

Frozen yogurt

Ice cream, low-fat

Milk (fat-free or 1%)

Milk alternatives (almond, rice, and soy)

Sour cream (fat-free or reduced-fat)

Yogurt (fat-free or low-fat)

## MISCELLANEOUS

Canola oil

Garlic

Herbs and spices (fresh, dried, and ground)

Hot sauce

Hummus

Marinara sauce

Mayonnaise, reduced-fat

Mustard (all varieties)

Olive oil

Salad dressing, reduced-calorie

Salsa

Salt substitute

Soft tub spread, trans-fat-free (reduced-fat or regular)

Stanol/sterol spread, soft tub (reduced-fat or regular)

Vinegar (all varieties)

# Step 3 . . . GOING ABOVE AND BEYOND

If you want to do everything you can to reduce your risk factors, here are some additional things you might try.

◆ Consider taking a standard multivitamin.

◆ Avoid eating foods high in saturated fats, trans fats, cholesterol, salt, and refined carbohydrates.

◆ Talk with your doctor about whether omega-3 fish oil, sterol/stanol, or soluble fiber supplements might be right for you.

◆ Try to get at least seven hours of sleep a night.

# Step 4 . . . MEAL PLANS

These sample menus include foods that have been shown to protect against cardiovascular disease.

Every day, choose one option for each of the three meals—breakfast, lunch, and dinner. Then, once or twice per day, choose from my suggested snacks. Approximate calories have been provided to help adjust for your personal weight-management goals. If you find yourself hungry (and if weight is not an issue), feel free to increase the portion sizes for meals and snacks. Beverage calories are not included.

## BREAKFAST OPTIONS

(300 TO 400 CALORIES)

### Oatmeal with Milk and Fresh Berries

Prepare ½ cup dry oats with 1 cup water or milk (fat-free, 1%, or soy) and top with 2 tablespoons ground flaxseed (or wheat germ) and ½ cup berries. Sweeten with optional 1 teaspoon sugar, honey, or sugar substitute.

### Hearty Eggs with Vegetables and Toast

Beat 1 whole egg plus 2 egg whites. Cook in a hot skillet coated with oil spray, adding 2 tablespoons chopped tomato and unlimited spinach, mushrooms, peppers, and onion. Serve with toasted whole grain English muffin (or 2 slices whole wheat toast), dry or with 2 teaspoons soft tub spread (with or without stanols/sterols). Instead of half of the English muffin or 1 slice toast, you may substitute 1 serving fruit (1 orange, 1 plum, 1 apple, 1 small banana, $\frac{1}{2}$ grapefruit, or $\frac{1}{4}$ cantaloupe).

### Apple Slices with Peanut Butter

Spread $2\frac{1}{2}$ level tablespoons peanut butter (or other nut butter) on 1 sliced apple (or banana).

### Cereal with Milk, Nuts, and Wheat Germ

Mix 1 cup whole grain fortified cereal with 1 cup milk (fat-free, 1%, or soy) and top with 1 tablespoon chopped walnuts and 1 tablespoon wheat germ (or ground flaxseed). Enjoy with 1 orange (or $\frac{1}{2}$ banana or $\frac{1}{2}$ grapefruit).

### Breakfast Burrito

Beat 1 whole egg with 2 egg whites. Cook on a griddle coated with oil spray. Mix the cooked eggs with $\frac{1}{4}$ cup black beans and 2 tablespoons shredded fat-free or reduced-fat cheese. Wrap in a whole grain tortilla (150 calories or less). Serve with optional onions, peppers, salsa, and hot sauce.

### Strawberry-Banana Cottage Cheese with Almonds

Mix 1 cup 1% or fat-free cottage cheese (or 8 ounces fat-free plain or flavored yogurt) with $\frac{1}{2}$ sliced banana, $\frac{1}{2}$ cup chopped strawberries, and 1 tablespoon slivered almonds.

### Broccoli-Cheese Egg White Omelet with Turkey Bacon

Sauté 1 cup broccoli florets in a skillet coated with oil spray until soft. Beat 1 whole egg with 3 egg whites and add to the broccoli. When the bottom is cooked, gently flip and cook the other side. Top with 2 tablespoons shredded fat-free or reduced-fat cheese. Fold the omelet over and cook until the cheese melts. Season with optional salt substitute and ground black pepper. Enjoy with 2 strips turkey bacon and $\frac{1}{2}$ grapefruit (or $\frac{1}{4}$ cantaloupe or 1 orange).

## LUNCH OPTIONS

(400 TO 500 CALORIES)

### Turkey-Avocado Sandwich

Layer 4 ounces sliced turkey breast (or grilled chicken breast), 2 or 3 thin slices avocado, romaine lettuce or spinach leaves, tomato, and onion between 2 slices whole grain bread or in a pita. Spread with optional mustard, 2 teaspoons reduced-fat mayonnaise, or hummus. Enjoy with a large handful of baby carrots or bell pepper strips (red, green, or yellow).

### Hearty Grilled Chicken Salad

Serve 4 ounces grilled skinless chicken breast on a large bed of mixed leafy greens (romaine, spinach, etc.) with cherry tomatoes, chopped bell pepper, mushrooms, artichoke hearts, ¼ cup chickpeas (garbanzo beans), and ¼ chopped avocado. Toss with 2 teaspoons olive oil and unlimited vinegar or fresh lemon juice (or 2 to 4 tablespoons reduced-calorie dressing).

### Edamame with Wild Salmon Dijonnaise

Enjoy 1 cup boiled edamame (green soybeans in the pod), with 5 ounces canned wild salmon, drained, mashed, and mixed with 1 tablespoon reduced-fat mayonnaise, 1 to 2 teaspoons Dijon mustard, and minced onion and black pepper to taste. Serve on large bed of leafy greens (spinach, romaine, etc.) tossed with unlimited fresh lemon juice or vinegar (or 2 tablespoons reduced-calorie dressing).

### Vegetable-Cheese Omelet with Baked Potato

Beat 1 whole egg with 2 or 3 egg whites. Cook in a skillet coated with oil spray. Add 3 tablespoons chopped tomato, ½ cup sliced mushrooms, and optional dried basil. When the bottom is cooked, gently flip and cook some more. Top with 1 ounce (¼ cup) shredded reduced-fat or fat-free cheese. Fold the omelet and continue cooking until the egg mixture firms and the cheese melts. Enjoy with 1 plain medium baked white or sweet potato.

### Heart-Smart Turkey Burger with Veggies

Top a 5-ounce lean turkey burger (or any store-bought turkey or veggie burger) with optional 2 tablespoons guacamole, lettuce, tomato, onion, and salsa. Enjoy on ½ whole grain bun (or in 70-calorie pita). Serve with unlimited raw or cooked vegetables (broccoli, cauliflower, carrots, kale, Brussels sprouts, green beans, mushrooms, Swiss chard, beets, artichokes, spinach, collard greens, or asparagus).

### Mixed Vegetable Salad with Sardines

Toss 4 ounces (about 8) sardines (canned in oil or tomato sauce) with unlimited leafy greens, tomatoes, carrots, mushrooms, peppers, and onions and ½ cup starchy beans. Drizzle with 2 to 4 tablespoons reduced-calorie salad dressing (or 1 teaspoon olive oil and unlimited vinegar or fresh lemon juice) and season with optional freshly ground pepper.

### Hearty Yogurt Fruit Fiesta

Mix 1 cup fat-free vanilla yogurt (or 1% or fat-free cottage cheese) with 1 chopped apple and ½ cup berries (may substitute favorite fruits). Top with 2 tablespoons sunflower seeds or chopped walnuts.

## DINNER OPTIONS

(500 TO 600 CALORIES)

### Heart-Smart Surf and Turf

Enjoy 1 serving Tuscan Bean Dip (page 152) with unlimited carrots, celery, and pepper strips and 5 ounces grilled or baked tilapia (or wild salmon, cod, halibut, trout, or red snapper) seasoned with 1 teaspoon olive oil and preferred herbs, pepper, and fresh lemon juice.

### Pork Tenderloin with Roasted Balsamic Carrots and Potato

Enjoy 5 ounces grilled, baked, or broiled pork tenderloin with 2 servings Roasted Balsamic Carrots (page 151) and ½ plain medium baked potato (or ½ cup brown or wild rice).

### Whole Wheat Penne with Sea Bass and Pea Sauce

Enjoy 1 serving Whole Wheat Penne with Sea Bass and Pea Sauce (page 323; feel free to substitute fish of your choice) with a side salad of leafy greens, mushrooms, carrots, and 1 tablespoon chopped walnuts tossed with 2 teaspoons olive oil and vinegar or fresh lemon juice (or 2 to 4 tablespoons reduced-calorie dressing).

### Hearty Turkey Meat Loaf with Salad

Enjoy 1 serving Hearty Turkey Meat Loaf (page 149) with a large salad of leafy greens and optional sliced peppers, mushrooms, carrots, tomatoes, beets, and artichokes tossed with ½ cup starchy beans and 2 teaspoons olive oil and unlimited vinegar or fresh lemon juice (or 2 to 4 tablespoons reduced-calorie salad dressing).

### Pesto Salmon with Roasted Artichoke Hearts

Enjoy 1 serving Pesto Salmon with Roasted Artichoke Hearts (page 150) with ½ plain medium baked white or sweet potato topped with optional 2 teaspoons soft tub spread (with or without stanols/sterols).

### Chopped Chicken Salad with Apples and Walnuts

Enjoy 1 serving (page 321).

### Turkey Chili with Salad

Enjoy 1 serving (2 cups) Turkey Chili (page 363) topped with 1 ounce (¼ cup) shredded fat-free or reduced-fat Cheddar cheese and a mixed salad of leafy greens (optional peppers, carrots, beets, and artichokes) tossed with 1 teaspoon olive oil and unlimited balsamic vinegar or fresh lemon juice (or 2 to 4 tablespoons reduced-calorie dressing).

## SNACK OPTIONS

100 CALORIES OR LESS

◆ *Best Vegetable Snacks:* up to 2 cups raw or cooked bell peppers (red, green, or yellow), broccoli, tomatoes, mushrooms, green beans, carrots, asparagus, sugar snap peas, or cauliflower

◆ *Best Fruit Snacks:* 1 apple, banana, orange, pear, or peach; 2 plums; ½ papaya, grapefruit, or cantaloupe; 1 cup berries (boysenberries, blackberries, blueberries, raspberries, or sliced strawberries); 1 cup cubed watermelon or honeydew; 4 apricots or prunes; 2 dates or figs; 20 whole strawberries; 2 tablespoons raisins

◆ 1 level tablespoon peanut butter with celery sticks

◆ 6 ounces fat-free flavored or plain yogurt

◆ 10 almonds, unsalted

◆ 25 pistachios (in shell)

◆ 1 cup Vegetable Oatmeal Bisque (page 322)

◆ 1 cup fat-free milk

## 100 TO 200 CALORIES

◆ 10 almonds (or 25 pistachios in shell) plus 1 serving fruit (see Best Fruit Snacks above)

◆ 1 cup boiled edamame (green soybeans in the pod)

◆ Unsalted whole nuts: 1 ounce (about ¼ cup) of your choice of almonds, cashews, pecans, walnuts, or peanuts

◆ ½ cup pistachios or sunflower seeds in the shell

◆ ½ cup fat-free or 1% cottage cheese mixed with 2 tablespoons ground flaxseed (or wheat germ)

◆ 1 slice whole grain toast (or 70-calorie pita) with 1 level tablespoon peanut butter

◆ 1 cup fat-free plain yogurt mixed with ¾ cup berries

◆ 1 cup baby carrots or pepper strips with ¼ cup hummus or guacamole

◆ 1 sliced apple with 1 level tablespoon peanut butter

◆ Frozen banana: Peel one banana, slice into ½-inch wheels, place in a small plastic bag, and freeze before serving.

◆ Strawberry-Banana Fruit Smoothie: In blender, mix 1 cup fat-free milk, 1 cup frozen strawberries, ½ frozen banana, and 3 to 5 ice cubes

◆ 1 serving Warm Dark Chocolate Sauce with Fresh Fruit (page 80)

◆ Vanilla Pumpkin Yogurt Pudding: 1 cup vanilla fat-free flavored yogurt mixed with ½ cup canned 100% pure pumpkin puree, sprinkled with ground cinnamon

# HEARTY TURKEY MEAT LOAF

*You won't miss the high-fat beef in my heart-smart version of meat loaf. It's got great flavor and health-boosting ingredients—even oats (instead of white bread crumbs), which add soluble fiber and create the perfect consistency.*

**MAKES 4 SERVINGS**

1 pound ground turkey (at least 90% lean)

1 small zucchini, grated

1 cup instant oats

½ cup mushrooms, chopped

¼ cup fat-free milk

¼ cup fresh basil, thinly sliced

2 tablespoons reduced-sodium soy sauce

2 egg whites

4 cloves garlic, minced

½ teaspoon dried thyme

½ teaspoon dried oregano

Ground black pepper to taste

Preheat the oven to 350°F. Coat a 1-quart loaf pan with oil spray or line with aluminum foil.

In a large bowl, mix the turkey, zucchini, oats, mushrooms, milk, basil, soy sauce, egg whites, garlic, thyme, and oregano and season with pepper.

Press into the loaf pan and cover with aluminum foil. Bake for 40 minutes. Remove the foil and bake for 5 to 10 minutes longer, or until the top begins to brown and the center is no longer pink. Serve immediately.

**Per serving:** 239 calories, 33 g protein, 20 g carbohydrate, 3 g fat (0 g saturated), 45 mg cholesterol, 380 mg sodium, 3 g fiber; plus 46 mg magnesium (12% DV)

# PESTO SALMON WITH ROASTED ARTICHOKE HEARTS

*Swimming with omega-3 fats, salmon is one of the world's most heart-healthy foods. You'll up the ante with my pesto variation, which incorporates walnuts, garlic, olive oil, and artichokes—ingredients that will satisfy your ticker as well as your tastebuds.*

**MAKES 2 SERVINGS**

2 cups fresh basil leaves

1 tablespoon walnuts, chopped

3 cloves garlic, minced

¼ teaspoon kosher salt (optional)

1 can (16 ounces) artichoke hearts, rinsed and drained, or 1 package (9 ounces) frozen artichoke hearts, rinsed and thawed

1 large tomato, diced

1 teaspoon fresh thyme, chopped

Ground black pepper

2 fillets (6 ounces each) wild salmon, skin removed

1 tablespoon olive oil

Preheat the oven to 350°F. Line an 8" x 11" baking pan with parchment paper or aluminum foil.

In a blender or food processor, combine the basil, walnuts, half of the garlic, and optional salt. Blend until the mixture resembles a coarse meal.

Arrange the artichoke hearts in 2 separate mounds in the prepared pan. Top with the tomato and sprinkle with the remaining thyme and pepper to taste. Place one salmon fillet on top of each artichoke mound and season with pepper. Spread the basil mixture on the fillets. Drizzle each fillet with ½ tablespoon of the oil.

Bake for 20 to 25 minutes, or until the fillets are no longer translucent in the center and the fish flakes when pressed with a fork. Serve immediately.

**Per serving:** 430 calories, 41 g protein, 22 g carbohydrate, 20 g fat (3 g saturated), 93 mg cholesterol, 440 mg sodium, 5 g fiber

# ROASTED BALSAMIC CARROTS

*Carrots deliver two all-star nutrients for heart health: soluble fiber and potassium. In this recipe, the addition of olive oil and garlic makes the carrots that much more tasty and beneficial. Just another way to enjoy an all-time favorite vegetable!*

**MAKES 4 SERVINGS**

1 pound carrots, peeled and cut into wedges

¼ cup balsamic vinegar

2 tablespoons minced fresh rosemary

2 cloves garlic, minced

¼ teaspoon paprika

¼ teaspoon kosher salt (optional)

Ground black pepper

1 tablespoons olive oil

Preheat the oven to 400°F.

Tear a large piece of aluminum foil, about 24" long. Spread the carrots out evenly over one half. Sprinkle with the vinegar, rosemary, garlic, and paprika. Season with optional salt and pepper. Drizzle with the oil and fold the opposite end over, folding around the edges to make a neat package with no openings. Place the package on a baking sheet and bake for 20 to 25 minutes, or until the carrots are tender when pierced with a knife. Serve immediately.

**Per serving:** 90 calories, 1 g protein, 15 g carbohydrate, 4 g fat (0 g saturated), 0 mg cholesterol, 145 mg sodium, 4 g fiber; plus 540 mg potassium (15% DV)

# Tuscan Bean Dip

*Vegetables go down easy when you have something delicious to dip them in. A friend once watched in shock as her vegetable-hating daughter cleared a plate of crudités with this dip. Give it a try—it's loaded with taste and, thanks to the beans, provides lots of protein, magnesium, and fiber.*

**MAKES 3 SERVINGS (½ CUP EACH)**

1 can (16 ounces) cannellini or navy beans, rinsed and drained (preferably no salt added)

2 tablespoons balsamic vinegar

2 teaspoons olive oil

2 tablespoons thinly sliced basil

½ teaspoon chopped fresh sage or rosemary

2 cloves garlic, minced

⅛ teaspoon red-pepper flakes

¼ teaspoon kosher salt (optional)

Ground black pepper

In a large bowl, mash the beans with the back of a fork or a handheld potato masher. Stir in the vinegar, oil, basil, sage or rosemary, garlic, and pepper flakes. Season to taste with optional salt and black pepper. Serve immediately with vegetable sticks.

**Per serving:** 210 calories, 12 g protein, 33 g carbohydrate, 3.5 g fat (0 g saturated), 0 mg cholesterol, 110 mg sodium, 8 g fiber; plus 75 mg magnesium (20% DV) and 462 mg potassium (13% DV)

# CHAPTER 8

# ARTHRITIS

s anyone with arthritis can tell you, arthritis sufferers truly suffer. Osteoarthritis can wear down the knees. Rheumatoid arthritis can twist and deform the fingers. And gout can make walking an exercise in masochism.

Arthritis is not a single disease but a category that includes about 100 joint-related disorders. According to the National Institutes of Health, arthritis affects about one in every five people in the United States—most of whom don't realize how much nutrition can improve the way they feel. In some cases, such as with gout, a change in diet can dramatically reduce symptoms. Because arthritis can have such debilitating effects, stumbling on even a single piece of helpful information can feel like unearthing buried treasure. I remember that the first time I talked about arthritis on the *Today* show, I got an overwhelming number of phone calls—hundreds of them!—asking for more details. This chapter is all about helpful details that could bring your pain level down a few critical notches.

## WHAT AFFECTS ARTHRITIS?

In medical lingo, the suffix *itis* means "inflammation." Arthritis, then, means any disease that involves inflammation of the joints. But let's start at the very beginning and talk about what joints are made of.

Joints are places where bones come together. Some, such as those that connect the bones of the skull, are stable and immovable. Other joints have minimal mobility, such as those connecting the vertebrae of the spine. But most joints of the body are synovial joints, which allow for varying degrees of movement, depending on their structure. For example, shoulders and hips are able to move freely in every direction because of their ball-and-socket design, while elbows and knees bend in a single direction, like a hinge.

All synovial joints share certain features.

1. The ends of the bones are coated with a soft, smooth substance called cartilage, which helps to cushion the bones and reduce friction.

2. The joint is encased by a ligament that holds the bones together. This ligament forms a capsule around the entire joint.

3. The inside of the capsule is covered by a special lining called the synovial membrane.

4. The synovial membrane secretes a lubricating fluid called synovial fluid.

Of all the different types of arthritis, the two most common are osteoarthritis and rheumatoid arthritis.

## OSTEOARTHRITIS

Osteoarthritis (OA) occurs when the cartilage covering the ends of the bones deteriorates, causing pain and swelling when the bones rub against each other. Over time, the bones can become misshapen from wear, and small bone spurs can grow at the bone ends, causing even more pain. If pieces of bone or cartilage break off, they can remain in the joint, causing still greater pain. In some people, the damage can be so extensive that the joint may have to be replaced.

Although we tend to think of OA as the logical outcome of wear and tear on the joints, scientists aren't so sure. Yes, wear and tear can affect some people's joints, but not everyone's. OA is the result of a combination of factors, including genetics, past injury, joint use and overuse, and the aging process in general. We can't help our genetics, past injuries, or the aging process. And I'm certainly not going to recommend that you stop participating in your favorite sport just to preserve your joints. In fact, exercise can help keep joints mobile (more about that later!). However, there is something you can do to protect your joints from overuse. The word *overuse* implies that it's a problem for serious athletes—and it is—but it also happens when excess body weight places too much stress on a joint.

Being overweight can compress joints. Imagine that you are balancing a book on your head, and someone comes along and places another book on top—and then another and then another. With each book, the vertebrae in your neck will become jammed closer and closer together. When you carry too much weight, that same kind of compression affects your knees and hips. Weight loss can help in a big way. Every 1 pound of weight you lose equates to 4 pounds less stress and pressure on your knees.

The benefits of weight loss go beyond knees. For example, one study followed 48 men and women who had gastric bypass surgery for extreme weight loss. Before surgery, all 48 had musculoskeletal pain, including joint pain, usually in more than one part of their bodies. After surgery, only 11 of them (23 percent) reported musculoskeletal pain, and there was improvement in pain in their spines, necks, arms, hands, legs, and feet. Osteoarthritis stiffness and joint function improved significantly, and the participants reported better quality of life. Surgery for weight loss is a drastic step, and it isn't necessary for most people. The vast majority of overweight people can lose enough weight to reduce their osteoarthritis symptoms through dietary changes alone. (See Weight Loss on page 17 for more information about the best ways to lose weight.)

## RHEUMATOID ARTHRITIS

Rheumatoid arthritis (RA) is a disease that causes inflammation of the lining of the joint capsule—the synovial membrane. Early in the disease process, affected joints can feel swollen, painful, hot, and tender to the touch. As the disease progresses, the synovial membrane thickens and begins to release enzymes that can dissolve bone and cartilage inside the joint. If these enzymes eat away at enough tissue, the joint can become deformed—and the pain can be excruciating. Although some people have constant active disease, others have periods of rest or remission when symptoms may ease up or disappear.

RA is an autoimmune disease, which means that the immune system, which typically defends the body against foreign invaders (such as bacteria or viruses), suddenly turns on itself. In this case, the immune system attacks synovial membranes. Scientists don't know what triggers the process, why it goes into remission, or why it flares up periodically. Genetics plays at least some role. Hormones may also play a part, as RA affects women more often than it affects men and because flares often occur after pregnancy. Some researchers believe that a bacterial or viral infection may set the wheels in motion, but that has not been proven. What we do know is that although RA cannot be cured, it can be managed with medication and lifestyle changes.

## HOW FOOD AFFECTS ARTHRITIS

Because arthritis is a disease of inflammation, the most effective—and logical—treatment is anything that fights inflammation. Medical management of arthritis usually starts with ibuprofen and other anti-inflammatory medications, and nutritional care starts with anti-inflammatory foods.

Inflammation is a complex physiological reaction that begins whenever there is some assault on the body, such as injury, viral or bacterial infection, or exposure to allergens or chemicals. Whenever the body senses danger, it goes on high alert and bursts into action—it begins manufacturing and pumping out interleukins, cytokines, and other substances that rush to the site of the problem. The purpose of those substances is to protect tissue from the assault of foreign invaders.

Most of the time, this defensive system works marvelously well, but not always. Imagine that your house has an infestation of houseflies. If you wanted to be certain to eliminate the problem, you could buy a flyswatter, set glue traps, fumigate with a powerful insecticide, and bring in a thousand spiders to spin webs to trap the flies. But that response would be overkill. Once the flies were gone, you would have a new set of problems—namely, a house full of airborne toxins and way, way too

## FAQS

### I keep hearing about different herbal remedies for my arthritis. How do I know which ones are worth trying?

Herbs have been used as medical treatments for thousands of years by many cultures around the world. Research, however, is limited, and the results are inconsistent. Depending on which herbs you choose, they can help or hurt your health, sometimes in ways we can't predict. I recommend that you talk with your doctor if you have specific questions or health concerns. Among the dozens of potential herbal treatments for arthritis, the most promising are boswellia, devil's claw, and cat's claw.

Boswellia comes from the *Boswellia serrata* tree, which grows in some parts of India. Its anti-inflammatory properties may help relieve some of the pain and stiffness of osteoarthritis. If you want to try boswellia, look for extracts standardized to 60 percent boswellic acids. The typical dosage is 300 to 400 milligrams of boswellic acids three times daily.

Devil's claw is an African plant used to treat arthritis pain. The typical dosage is 750 milligrams three times per day. Look for an extract standardized to contain 50 to 100 milligrams of the active ingredient harpagoside. Long-term safety hasn't been tested, and short-term side effects can include diarrhea, headache, and loss of taste. Because devil's claw can lower blood sugar, it may not be safe if you have diabetes or hypoglycemia.

Cat's claw is a vine that grows in rain forests in South America and Asia. Limited studies have shown that it may be helpful for relieving the pain of osteoarthritis and rheumatoid arthritis. It's available in various forms, including capsules, tablets, liquids, and tea bags. Dosage varies. The public is advised to buy only products that contain *Uncaria tomentosa*. Another plant (*Acacia greggii*), also called cat's claw, is highly toxic. For osteoarthritis, 100 milligrams daily of a specific freeze-dried aqueous cat's claw extract has been used. For rheumatoid arthritis, 60 milligrams daily in three divided doses of a specific cat's claw extract (free of tetracyclic oxindole alkaloids) has been used. Cat's claw can cause allergic reactions and gastrointestinal upset and can also lower blood pressure, so you should not take this supplement if you are on antihypertensive medications or blood thinners. There has been at least one report of kidney failure possibly triggered by cat's claw. For all these reasons, I recommend talking with your doctor before trying it.

many spiders. The immune system often opts for overkill, and we're left with hot, red, swollen, painful joints. The inflammation comes and stays, and there's no way to just turn it off. That's why the best way to fight the pain of nearly any kind of arthritis is to fight inflammation with medication and/or nutrition.

An anti-inflammatory diet excludes foods that fan the flames of inflammation and embraces plenty of foods that reduce it. To get the most out of nutritional changes, you should adopt both sets of recommendations.

## FOODS TO AVOID

I already mentioned that being overweight puts extra stress on your joints, which increases the risk of wear and tear. But there is another reason being overweight is a problem. Body fat is not an inert substance—it is metabolically active, capable of producing hormones and chemicals that actually increase levels of inflammation. By losing weight—and avoiding excess calories that can cause weight gain—you'll automatically reduce the level of inflammation in your body.

Specific food groups that increase inflammation include:

### Saturated Fats

This category includes fats in and from animal products, such as fatty beef or pork, poultry skin, ice cream, butter, whole or 2% milk, regular cheese, bacon, bologna, salami, pepperoni, and beef sausage. Saturated fats are also found in palm oil and palm kernel oil. My guess is that you won't find bottles of any of those oils in your pantry, but chances are you will find them in the ingredients lists of any number of items on your shelves, including crackers, cookies, nondairy creamers, and other packaged baked goods. Try to dramatically limit your intake. In addition to carefully reading labels, choose reduced-fat or fat-free dairy products, lean cuts of beef and pork, and skinless chicken and turkey.

### Trans Fats

In an effort to give baked goods a longer shelf life, scientists took common vegetable oil and added hydrogen molecules in the right places. The result was that the liquid oil turned solid—and dangerous. This man-made substance is called partially hydrogenated oil, and it is the main source of trans fats in packaged foods. Trans fats are thought to be at least as damaging as saturated fats in terms of inflammation and other health problems. They may even be worse. You won't have to go to great lengths to determine whether a food contains trans fats or not. Manufacturers are now required to list the amount of trans fats right after listing the saturated fats on the nutrition label. Also check the ingredients list for partially hydrogenated oils—even products that list zero gram trans fats can have trace amounts.

### Simple and Refined Carbohydrates

Sugary foods, white flour baked goods, white rice, bread, crackers, and other refined carbohydrates set up a state of inflammation in the body, causing increases in cytokines and other pro-inflammatory compounds. Limit these foods if you want the best chance of reducing arthritis pain and progression.

## FOODS TO ADD

These foods all help to reduce some aspect of inflammation and, in turn, may help prevent and manage arthritis as part of an overall healthy lifestyle.

### Omega-3 Fatty Acids

The healthiest of fats for people with arthritis or other inflammatory disorders are omega-3 fatty acids, one of the polyunsaturated fats. Omega-3s work to decrease inflammation by suppressing the production of cytokines and enzymes that erode cartilage.

More than a dozen studies have demonstrated that omega-3 fish oils can reduce symptoms of RA. Study participants reported greater strength and reduced fatigue, joint swelling and tenderness, stiffness, and pain.

Although the evidence is less clear about how fish oil affects OA, the anti-inflammatory effects of omega-3s are so potent that I recommend an omega-3-rich diet and fish oil supplements to my clients with either RA or OA. (My Best Foods list includes only the fatty fish that have been shown to be low in mercury, PCBs, and dioxins.) I've seen some amazing results. Take Colleen: She was in her mid-forties, was about 10 pounds overweight, and had a problem with high cholesterol. I put her on a cholesterol-lowering program that included fish oil capsules. After a month, she returned for a follow-up appointment, and I was pleased to see that she had lost a couple of pounds and her cholesterol had begun to return to healthy levels. But Colleen was ecstatic! She explained that her joint pain—which she'd never mentioned—had almost entirely disappeared. The fish oil supplements made Colleen feel like a new person.

Emma was in her early seventies and had diagnosed OA. She needed to lose about 45 pounds, which contributed to her problem, but the extraordinary level of pain she felt in her knees and hands couldn't be explained by weight alone. I put her on a healthy, calorie-controlled food plan and recommended that she take fish oil capsules, and she also began seeing an acupuncturist. Today, Emma swims and walks on a treadmill without pain, and she is more active than she has been in years. She still has pain flare-ups, but she feels much, much better. We don't know which of the treatments was most effective, and Emma doesn't really care. She feels healthy, and she is unwilling to stop taking any of her supplements, which she sees as her lifeline. (For more information about fish oil and other supplements, see the Supplements section, page 166.)

BEST FOODS FOR OMEGA-3 FATTY ACIDS: *wild salmon (fresh, canned), herring, mackerel (not king), sardines, anchovies, rainbow trout, Pacific oysters, chia seeds, ground flaxseed, walnuts, butternuts (white walnuts), seaweed, walnut oil, canola oil, flaxseed oil, soybeans (edamame)*

## Antioxidants: Vitamin C, Carotenes, Flavonoids

Inflammation produces free radicals, those cell-damaging molecules that are formed in response to toxins or natural body processes. The synovium in your joint cells is just as prone to free radical damage as your skin, eye, and any other body tissue cells are. Antioxidants protect the body from the effects of free radicals and are a critical part of an anti-inflammation diet. Research has demonstrated that certain antioxidants may help prevent arthritis, slow its progression, and relieve pain. The most powerful antioxidants are vitamin C, carotenes, and flavonoids.

Vitamin C is one of the nutrients most responsible for the health of collagen, a major component of cartilage. In addition, research suggests that people who eat a diet low in vitamin C may have a greater risk of developing some kinds of arthritis. For those reasons, it is important to make vitamin C–rich foods a major part of your daily diet. However, researchers at Duke University found that long-term, high-dose vitamin C supplements may make OA worse. (I say *may* because the research was conducted on guinea pigs. The researchers' assumption is that it will have the same effect in people.) If you have OA, I recommend you get vitamin C from food sources or a standard multivitamin only—not from a high-dose individual supplement.

BEST FOODS FOR VITAMIN C: *guava, bell peppers (all colors), oranges and orange juice, grapefruit and grapefruit juice, strawberries, pineapple, kohlrabi, papayas, lemons and lemon juice, broccoli, kale, Brussels sprouts, kidney beans, kiwifruit, cantaloupe, cauliflower, cabbage (all varieties), mangoes, white potatoes, mustard greens, tomatoes, sugar snap peas, snow peas, clementines, rutabagas, turnip greens, raspberries, blackberries, watermelon, tangerines, okra, lychees, summer squash, persimmons*

Carotenes are a group of powerful antioxidant nutrients found in many fruits and vegetables. The best known is beta-carotene, but there are many others. The carotene called beta-cryptoxanthin may reduce the risk of developing inflammation-related disorders, including rheumatoid arthritis. Researchers from the United Kingdom found that people who ate diets high in beta-cryptoxanthin were half as likely to develop a form of inflammatory arthritis as those who ate very few beta-cryptoxanthin foods. They found that adding just one additional serving each day of a food high in beta-cryptoxanthin helped reduce arthritis risk.

BEST FOODS FOR BETA-CRYPTOXANTHIN: *winter squash (acorn, butternut), pumpkin, persimmons, papayas, tangerines, red bell peppers, corn, oranges, apricots, carrots, nectarines, watermelon, peaches, red chile peppers*

BEST FOODS FOR BETA-CAROTENE: *sweet potatoes, carrots, kale, butternut squash, turnip greens, pumpkin, mustard greens, cantaloupe, red bell peppers, apricots, Chinese cabbage, spinach, lettuces (romaine, green leaf, red leaf, butterhead), collard greens, Swiss chard, watercress, grapefruit (pink, red), watermelon, cherries, mangoes, tomatoes, guava, asparagus, red cabbage*

The flavonoids quercetin and anthocyanins are both forms of antioxidants.

The anti-inflammatory effects of quercetin seem to be similar to those of non-steroidal anti-inflammatory medications (such as aspirin and ibuprofen). The synovial fluid in the joints of people with rheumatoid arthritis contains a highly inflammatory chemical called tumor necrosis factor (TNF), and, in research, quercetin was able to limit its inflammatory effects.

BEST FOODS FOR QUERCETIN: *onions, kale, leeks, cherry tomatoes, broccoli, blueberries, black currants, elderberries, lingonberries, cocoa powder (unsweetened), apricots, apples with skin, grapes (red, purple, black), tomatoes, tea, green beans, lettuces (butterhead, Boston, iceberg, Bibb), hot chile peppers, celery, chives, red cabbage, lemons, grapefruit*

Anthocyanins and proanthocyanins are powerful antioxidants known to reduce inflammation. They seem to inhibit production of certain inflammatory chemicals, including cytokines and prostaglandins. They contribute to the health of connective tissue and are more powerful than vitamin C for defusing dangerous free radicals that can irritate body tissues and cause inflammation.

BEST FOODS FOR ANTHOCYANINS: *blackberries, black currants, blueberries, eggplant, elderberries, raspberries, cherries, boysenberries, grapes (red, black, purple), strawberries, plums, cranberries, rhubarb, red onions, red apples, peaches, cabbage (red, purple), red beets, blood oranges*

## Olive Oil

Olive oil contains the "good" monounsaturated fat, along with antioxidants called polyphenols that protect the body against inflammation. In animal studies, rats with arthritis were fed diets high in various kinds of oils. The researchers found that both fish oil and olive oil prevented arthritis-related inflammation. I recommend using olive oil instead of vegetable oil or butter in cooking. Don't pour it on—just substitute one for the other in equal or lesser amounts. Extra-virgin olive oil has the highest concentration of polyphenols, but it's also more expensive than standard olive oil. If you can't afford to use extra-virgin regularly, save it for recipes that really showcase its delicate flavor, such as salad dressings, dips, and cold marinades.

## Vitamin D

Although vitamin D is associated primarily with bone strength, it is also critical for a number of other bodily functions, including joint health. Studies have shown that

# FAQS

**There are so many different kinds of foods to avoid. I think I can figure this out for meals I cook at home, but are there guidelines for what to eat in restaurants?**

You're right—meal planning can be difficult at first, but after a few weeks, making smart food choices will become second nature. When you are eating out, I recommend:

### American Fare

- Grilled fish or skinless chicken breast in olive oil and seasonings, with brown rice or a baked potato (sweet or white) and lots of grilled, roasted, or steamed vegetables

- Salad entrées: a variety of vegetables (request extra red peppers) with grilled chicken, shrimp, turkey breast, or salmon; for dressing, use vinaigrette or request olive oil and vinegar on the side

- Sandwiches: turkey breast, grilled chicken breast, or grilled vegetables on whole grain bread or in a whole wheat pita or whole grain wrap; optional avocado, roasted peppers, lettuce, onion, tomato, and any other preferred vegetables

- Soups: gazpacho, black bean, lentil, vegetable, and butternut squash (without cream)

### Japanese Food

- Edamame, seaweed salad, California rolls (take advantage of sliced ginger!), and steamed or sautéed vegetables

- Chicken or salmon teriyaki with steamed or sautéed vegetables and brown rice

### Chinese Food

- Steamed whole fish with ginger, plus brown rice and sautéed or steamed vegetables

- Steamed entrée of chicken, shrimp, or tofu with any vegetable combination (request ginger and black bean or garlic sauce on the side). Use 1 to 2 tablespoons of the sauce on your entrée and enjoy with steamed brown rice.

### Indian Food

- Chicken, fish, or tofu tikka (no masala), tandoori, or vindaloo with curried vegetables

- Dal (made with lentils) with a side of curried vegetables

getting adequate amounts of vitamin D reduces the risk of both rheumatoid arthritis and osteoarthritis. Among people who already have OA, those who have a vitamin D deficiency are more likely to develop worsening disability over time. Getting even the basic daily requirements of vitamin D leads to greater muscle strength, improvement in physical functioning, and preservation of cartilage. That's at least 600 IU daily until age 70 and at least 800 IU daily for folks 70 and older.

> BEST FOODS FOR VITAMIN D: *wild salmon (fresh, canned), mackerel (not king), sardines, herring, milk (fat-free, 1%), soy milk, fortified yogurt (fat-free, low-fat), egg yolks, vitamin D-enhanced mushrooms\**
>
> *\*These mushrooms are treated with UV light, which dramatically increases their vitamin D content.*

### Spices: Ginger and Turmeric

Most people don't realize that spices are for more than, well, spicing things up. They're an important source of essential nutrients. Like fruits and vegetables, spices come from plant sources, and they can have powerful effects on health. Certain spices seem to have anti-inflammatory effects and therefore should be considered for arthritis treatment. Among the most promising are ginger and turmeric.

Ginger has been shown to lessen the pain of knee osteoarthritis when taken in highly purified, standardized supplement form. Ginger contains chemicals that work similarly to some anti-inflammatory medications, so its effects on arthritis pain are not surprising. However, ginger can also act as a blood thinner, so if you're adding ginger and taking a blood-thinning medication, work with your physician to monitor and possibly adjust your medication if needed.

Turmeric is a mustard yellow spice from Asia and the main ingredient in yellow curry powder. Scientific studies have shown that a compound in turmeric called curcumin may help arthritis by suppressing inflammatory body chemicals. Because of its effects on enzymes related to inflammation, turmeric may work the same was as Celebrex and similar medications do. Note: Turmeric is also used as a dye, so be cautious when handling it—it can discolor clothing and some surfaces. Be sure to try my Chicken Curry and Vegetables recipe on page 178!

## BONUS POINTS

- ◆ **See a doctor about symptoms.** Don't be complacent about joint pain, stiffness, swelling, or weakness, and don't assume that joint pain is a normal part of growing older. Early treatment of OA, RA, or other arthritis can help slow the disease's progression and provide a lot of pain relief.

- ◆ **Work to reduce cholesterol.** Although no one knows what triggers RA, an interesting European study may provide at least one clue. Researchers analyzed 10-year-old blood samples of people who later developed RA and compared them with the blood of a random sample of healthy individuals. They discovered that people who developed RA had higher than normal levels of low-density lipoprotein (LDL) cholesterol, triglycerides, and apolipoprotein B; and lower than normal levels of high-density lipoprotein (HDL) cholesterol. The theory is that these blood results indicate the start of atherosclerosis, which means more inflammation in the body. Could it be that a higher level of inflammation could turn into inflammatory joint disease? More research is needed, but it certainly gives you an added reason to treat your cholesterol problem as early as possible.

◆ **Drink plenty of water.** Cartilage is 65 to 80 percent water, so staying hydrated is important for the health and lubrication of joints. My recommendation is to drink throughout the day and choose water, seltzer, and unsweetened tea or coffee instead of soda or sugary drinks.

◆ **Exercise.** Many people stop exercising at the first twinge of pain in a joint, but this can be a big mistake. Exercise can help you lose or maintain weight, which reduces the overall stress on joints. Strong muscles can absorb shock from daily movements, keep joints stable, and protect against additional joint injury. Stretching and yoga can improve flexibility and range of motion. Exercise of all sorts can also help you sleep better. Talk with your doctor about the best kind of exercise for you, because the best choices will depend on your particular medical situation and pain levels. Swimming and water aerobics are usually good for everyone because they allow free movement without added stress on the joints. No matter which exercise you choose, don't overdo it when you are just starting out, and don't do anything that threatens your balance. And by all means, stop if the pain worsens.

◆ **Try acupuncture.** Among people with osteoarthritis, studies suggest that traditional Chinese acupuncture can help reduce joint pain and improve function. People who had about one treatment per week felt better after just four weeks, and the positive effects grew week after week. It is important to choose a qualified, skilled acupuncturist who knows how to treat osteoarthritis. I prefer that my clients go to an acupuncturist who also has a traditional medical degree to be sure that they are receiving the best combination of Western medicine and Eastern acupuncture. (Ask your rheumatologist or primary care physician for a referral. You can also find certified acupuncturists at the Web site for the National Certification Commission for Acupuncture and Oriental Medicine at www.NCCAOM.org.) Also, watch out for those who are more concerned with business than with health care—the most reputable will treat you only when you have pain and will not pressure you to come in for a set number of treatments.

## GOUT

Imagine needle-sharp shards of glass inserted between the bones of your joints, grating and grinding with every move. That not-so-happy image is the pain of gout, one of the more common forms of arthritis. In some people with a genetic susceptibility—men more often than women—the body converts excess uric acid into crystals that can accumulate in joints.

In most cases, the extreme pain of gout starts in the big toe. I've known clients who have had so much swelling and agony that they can't wear shoes. At the very least, the discomfort is enough to make walking difficult (and, according to one of my clients, "ruin an otherwise great vacation"). Gout can also settle into other joints of the feet, ankles, knees, fingers, wrists, and elbows.

Most cases of gout are controllable. Treatment involves medication and avoiding any food, drink, or medicine that raises levels of uric acid. Because uric acid is a by-product of the metabolism of purine, a substance naturally found in body tissues, you'll never get rid of it entirely. However, if you have gout or have been told you're at high risk, there are several ways to keep uric acid levels as low as possible.

- **Maintain a healthy weight.** Extra body tissue means extra uric acid production from normal processes of breakdown and turnover.

- **Avoid purine-rich meats and seafood.** Studies have shown that eating a diet heavy in high-purine meats and seafood increases the risk of gout by raising uric acid levels in your blood. (The latest research suggests that high-purine vegetables don't seem to increase the risk of gout and therefore don't need to be avoided.) I advise limiting your total intake of animal protein (meat, poultry, and seafood combined) to no more than 6 ounces per day. You should also avoid or dramatically limit your intake of proteins that are highest in purines: organ meats (such as kidney and liver); fatty cuts of beef, lamb, and pork; and certain fish and shellfish (anchovies, herring, sardines, and mackerel).

- **Avoid sugary beverages and foods.** Fructose, a type of sugar found in soda and other sweetened beverages, as well as candy, cookies, and other baked goods, appears to increase gout risk by raising uric acids levels in the blood. A 2008 study found that men with the highest

◆ **Stop smoking.** There are many good reasons to stop smoking, but now we can add healthy joints to the list. Smoking delivers toxins throughout the body, causing inflammation and increasing the risks of rheumatoid arthritis and osteoarthritis. In one study, smokers were more than twice as likely as non-smokers to develop RA. Smokers who also had a genetic susceptibility for RA were more than seven times more likely to develop the disease than the average intake of fructose were twice as likely to develop gout as men with the lowest fructose intake. That's reason enough to cut out all sugary beverages, including soda, fruit drinks, sweetened waters, sugary coffee drinks, sweet tea, and even 100 percent fruit juice. You'll also want to dramatically reduce your intake of sugar and other sweeteners, especially agave, which is about 90 percent fructose.

- **Reduce alcohol intake.** Alcoholic beverages interfere with the body's ability to clear uric acid, increasing your risk of gout. In 2004, Harvard researchers reported that beer was the greatest offender—men who drank two or more beers per day had more than twice the risk of gout, compared with men who didn't drink beer. Spirits also caused an increase in gout but to a lesser degree. Wine did not seem to increase the risk of gout, but I still recommend limiting your consumption.

- **Eat more reduced-fat or fat-free dairy foods.** A 2004 study found that people who eat two or three servings daily—especially of milk and yogurt—can cut their risk of gout by about half, compared with those who eat few dairy foods. Add reduced-fat or fat-free milk or yogurt to your diet.

- **Drink plenty of water.** I recommend that my clients with gout drink at least eight glasses of water daily to help flush uric acid out of the body.

- **Coffee may be protective.** Recent studies in men and women have shown that regularly drinking coffee (both regular and decaf) reduces the risk of developing gout. If you're a coffee lover, by all means continue to enjoy your daily brew.

- **Take aspirin sparingly.** Salicylates—the active ingredients in aspirin—can raise uric acid levels.

- **Get a checkup.** About 75 percent of people diagnosed with gout also have metabolic syndrome, a serious condition that increases the risk of heart disease. If you receive a diagnosis of gout, insist on getting tested for metabolic syndrome. (More information about metabolic syndrome is on page 122.)

person. The effects of smoking on osteoarthritis are less clear, but researchers from a multicenter study reported in 2005 that smokers had a greater risk of osteoarthritis of the knee, possibly because smoking interferes with the body's ability to repair its own cartilage. If you quit smoking, you'll immediately reduce your inflammation load and improve blood flow to all parts of your body, including your aching joints.

◆ **De-stress.** Some experts believe that autoimmune disorders, including rheumatoid arthritis, can flare up in response to stress. Plus, people who feel stressed are more sensitive to pain. Stress reduction can be as important to your health as medication, so make it a priority. Carve out time in your schedule to relax, and, if necessary, downsize your to-do list by asking others to help out. Chances are friends and family will offer to help when they learn of your condition—take them up on it. Check with your local hospital to see if it offers classes in stress-reduction techniques, such as guided imagery, meditation, and progressive relaxation.

◆ **Control your pain.** When it comes to the pain of arthritis, don't try to be a hero. You have nothing to gain by toughing it out. If you hurt, see your doctor. If your doctor prescribes medication, take it. If you still hurt, make another appointment. People in constant pain may stop doing the things they love, and before long their quality of life takes a real turn for the worse. Some arthritis patients become depressed as a result of their constant pain. If you don't have the pain under control and your current doctor seems to have exhausted the options, research pain specialists in your area through organizations such as the American Academy of Pain Management (www.aapainmanage.org).

## SUPPLEMENTS

If you have arthritis and want to consider supplements in addition to the food fixes, I recommend:

## FOR BOTH OSTEOARTHRITIS AND RHEUMATOID ARTHRITIS

1. **A multivitamin.** If you would like to consider a multivitamin to supplement your healthy diet, I recommend brands that provide at least 800 IU vitamin D (in the form of $D_3$, the most potent form of vitamin D) and no more than 100 percent DV of vitamin C and vitamin A (with at least half of the vitamin A coming from beta-carotene and/or mixed carotenoids). Definitely do not choose megadose varieties, because some vitamins may make certain cases of arthritis worse.

2. **Omega-3 fatty acids from fish oil.** Of course you should eat foods rich in omega-3s, but for serious arthritis relief, you'll want to try fish oil supplements. I recommend you start with a daily dose of 2 grams of DHA and EPA combined. If there's no relief after four weeks, speak with your physician about increasing to 3 to 4 grams. Store the supplements in the fridge to prevent rancidity. To prevent fishy burps or aftertaste, buy enteric-coated varieties, take with food, and divide up your doses throughout day. Because fish oil acts as a blood thinner, it should not be taken by people who have hemophilia or who are already taking blood-thinning medications or aspirin (always consult your physician).

## FOR OSTEOARTHRITIS

**SAMe.** Some studies have shown that SAMe (S-adenosylmethionine) may be as effective as certain arthritis medications. One study conducted by researchers from the University of California, Irvine, compared the effects of SAMe with the anti-inflammatory medication Celebrex in 56 people with osteoarthritis. After one month, people who took Celebrex had greater pain relief, but after two months, Celebrex and SAMe reduced pain to the same degree. Joint function also improved. So although SAMe took longer, it ended up working just as well as a prescription pain reliever. The recommended dose of SAMe for arthritis is 1,200 milligrams per day. Though SAMe is generally thought to be safe, it can have side effects, including gastrointestinal problems and mild insomnia. To be safe, talk with your doctor before starting treatment with SAMe.

## FOR RHEUMATOID ARTHRITIS

**GLA (gamma-linolenic acid).** This fatty acid is found in evening primrose oil, borage oil, and black current oil. Studies show that GLA seems to reduce pain, joint tenderness, and morning stiffness of rheumatoid arthritis by suppressing certain inflammatory substances. The recommended dosage is between 1.5 and 3 grams per day. Because the action of this supplement may interfere with certain medications, always talk with your doctor before taking GLA.

## FAQS

**I have arthritis in both of my knees and heard I should take a supplement called glucosamine chondroitin. What is your opinion?**

Unfortunately, recent studies of glucosamine chondroitin haven't been encouraging. Glucosamine and chondroitin sulfate are two compounds that are naturally found in human cartilage, and they're often sold in combination as supplements to strengthen cartilage and slow the progression of arthritis. A large-scale trial funded by the National Institutes of Health tested glucosamine and chondroitin sulfate supplements in a group of people suffering from osteoarthritis in their knees. After taking the pills for two years, participants experienced no reduction in knee pain. An accompanying study conducted in the same group of participants found that glucosamine chondroitin did not reduce the amount of cartilage lost in the knee joint over the two-year period. Based on these results, I no longer recommend glucosamine, chondroitin, or combination supplements, but it doesn't hurt to speak with your physician and see what he or she advises, based on your specific medical history. If your doctor thinks it's worth a shot, take the supplement for three months and see if you notice any difference in symptoms. (Make sure to get a quality brand recommendation from your physician.) If you don't feel an improvement, it's not worth taking.

For more information about foods that promote joint health, visit www.joybauer.com/arthritis.

# JOY'S 4-STEP PROGRAM
## FOR ARTHRITIS

Follow this program if you have osteoarthritis, rheumatoid arthritis, or other arthritis (except gout—see page 164 for more information).

## Step 1 ... START WITH THE BASICS

These are the first things you should do to take control of inflammation, which feeds your arthritis pain.

- ◆ See a doctor if you have new or uncontrolled joint pain. It is important to get early and effective treatment for arthritis.
- ◆ Ask your doctor if taking omega-3 fish oil supplements makes sense for you.
- ◆ If you smoke, quit.
- ◆ Begin a program of gentle, low-stress exercise.
- ◆ Drink plenty of water.
- ◆ Avoid foods high in saturated and trans fats.
- ◆ Avoid foods high in sugar and refined carbohydrates.

## Step 2 ... YOUR ULTIMATE GROCERY LIST

This list contains foods with high levels of nutrients that help reduce inflammation and control arthritis pain. You don't have to purchase every item, but these foods should make up the bulk of what you eat each week.

For a printable version of this list, visit www.joybauer.com/arthritis.

## Special Note to Gout Sufferers:

Because animal proteins are generally high in purines, you'll want to moderate portions of beef, pork, lamb, seafood, and poultry. Consume no more than 6 ounces total of these animal proteins each day. Some animal proteins are especially high in purines and should therefore be completely avoided or eaten only occasionally if you suffer from gout. These include organ meats (such as kidney and liver) and certain fish and shellfish (anchovies, herring, sardines, and mackerel).

## FRUIT

*All* fruit, but especially:

Apples with skin

Apricots

Berries (blackberries, blueberries, boysenberries, elderberries, lingonberries, raspberries, and strawberries)

Cantaloupe

Cherries

Clementines

Grapefruit

Grapes (black, purple, and red)

Guava

Kiwifruit

Lemons

Limes

Lychees

Mangoes

Nectarines

Oranges (especially blood oranges)

Papayas

Peaches

Persimmons

Pineapple

Plums

Tangerines

Watermelon

## VEGETABLES AND LEGUMES

*All* vegetables, but especially:

Asparagus

Beans, green

Beans, starchy (such as black, garbanzo, kidney, navy, and pinto)

Beets, red

Broccoli

Brussels sprouts

Cabbage (Chinese, purple, and red)

Carrots

Cauliflower

Celery

Chives

Corn

Eggplant

Dark leafy greens (such as beet, collard, dandelion, kale, mustard, Swiss chard, and turnip)

Kohlrabi

Leeks

Lettuce

Mushrooms

Okra

Onions (all varieties)

Peas, sugar snap

Peppers (all varieties)

Potatoes (sweet and white)

Pumpkin (fresh and 100% pure canned pumpkin)

Rhubarb

Rutabagas

Seaweed

Snow peas

Soybeans (edamame)

Spinach

Squash, summer

Squash, winter (acorn and butternut)

Tomatoes

Watercress

Zucchini

## SEAFOOD

*All* fish and shellfish, but especially:

Anchovies

Herring

Mackerel (not king)

Pacific oysters

Rainbow trout

Salmon, wild (canned and fresh)

Sardines

## LEAN PROTEINS

Beef, lean

Chicken, ground (at least 90% lean)

Chicken, skinless

Eggs and egg substitutes

Pork tenderloin

Tempeh

Tofu

Turkey, ground (at least 90% lean)

Turkey, skinless

Turkey bacon

Turkey burgers, lean

Veggie burgers

## NUTS AND SEEDS (PREFERABLY UNSALTED)

Almonds and almond butter

Butternuts (white walnuts)

Cashews and cashew butter

Chia seeds

Flaxseed, ground

Hazelnuts

Macadamia nuts

Peanuts and peanut butter

Pecans

Pine

Pistachios

Pumpkin seeds

Sesame seeds

Sunflower seeds and sunflower butter

Walnuts

## WHOLE GRAINS

Bread, whole wheat (buns, crackers, English muffins, pitas, tortillas, and wraps)

Bulgur

Cereal, whole grain (at least 3 grams fiber; no more

than 8 grams sugar per serving)

Millet

Oats

Pasta, whole grain

Quinoa

Rice (brown and wild)

Waffles, whole grain

Wheat germ

## DAIRY

Cheese (fat-free or reduced-fat)

Cottage cheese (fat-free or 1%)

Frozen yogurt

Ice cream, low-fat

Milk (fat-free or 1%)

Milk substitutes (almond, rice, and soy)

Yogurt (fat-free or low-fat)

## MISCELLANEOUS

Canola oil

Cocoa powder, unsweetened

Garlic

Ginger, fresh and ground

Herbs and spices (fresh, dried, and ground)

Hot sauce

Hummus

Marinara sauce

Mayonnaise, reduced-fat

Mustard (all varieties)

Olive oil

Salad dressing, reduced-calorie

Salsa

Soft tub spread, trans-fat-free (reduced-fat or regular)

Turmeric/yellow curry powder

Vinegar (all varieties)

# Step 3 ... GOING ABOVE AND BEYOND

If you want to do everything you can for arthritis pain and stiffness, here are some additional things you might try.

◆ If you have osteoarthritis, ask your doctor about what supplements you might take. The ones with the best track records are omega-3s and SAMe. (See the Supplements section, page 166, for cautions and more information.)

◆ If you have rheumatoid arthritis, ask your doctor about what supplements you might take. The ones with the best track records are GLA and omega-3s.

◆ Incorporate ginger and turmeric into your recipes and meals.

◆ Consult a qualified acupuncturist about pain relief.

◆ Try to find ways to reduce stress, which can amplify pain and even trigger flareups of rheumatoid arthritis.

## A GINGER PRIMER

Ginger is a versatile spice that has anti-inflammatory properties. It can be used in any course, from appetizers to dessert. Look for fresh ginger in the produce section of most grocery stores—it is a tan root about the size of very fat fingers. Powdered ginger, found in the spice aisle, is used most often in baking and gives a stronger taste to foods than fresh ginger does, so do not automatically substitute the same amount of powdered ginger for fresh. A common accompaniment to sushi, pickled ginger (also called gari) is made by soaking thin slices of fresh ginger in rice vinegar and sugar for a week or longer. Candied or crystallized ginger is sweet and can be eaten as an occasional treat or baked into cakes and muffins.

# Step4 ... MEAL PLANS

These sample menus include foods that have been shown to help ease inflammation and arthritis pain. Specifically, they include antioxidants, omega-3 fats, vitamin D, and inflammation-reducing spices.

Every day, choose one option for each of the three meals—breakfast, lunch, and dinner. Then, one or two times per day, choose from a variety of my suggested snacks. Approximate calories have been provided to help adjust for your personal weight-management goals. If you find yourself hungry (and if weight is not an issue), feel free to increase the portion sizes for meals and snacks. Beverage calories are not included, and I encourage you to drink plenty of water throughout the day.

## BREAKFAST OPTIONS

(300 TO 400 CALORIES)

### Vanilla Pumpkin Breakfast Pudding

Mix 1 cup fat-free vanilla yogurt with ½ cup canned 100% pure pumpkin puree and top with 2 tablespoons chopped walnuts and 1 tablespoon wheat germ.

### Scrambled Eggs with Tomatoes, Mushrooms, and Onion

Beat 1 whole egg with 2 or 3 egg whites. Cook in a hot skillet coated with oil spray. Add 2 tablespoons each chopped tomato, sliced mushrooms, and sliced onion. Serve with toasted whole grain English muffin, dry or with 1 to 2 teaspoons soft tub, trans-fat-free spread.

### Grapefruit with Cottage Cheese

Mix 1 pink or red grapefruit (or blood orange), sectioned, with 1 cup fat-free or 1% cottage cheese. Top with 1 to 2 tablespoons wheat germ.

### Fiery Breakfast Burrito

Sauté ½ cup chopped onion, ½ cup sliced bell pepper, and 1 sliced jalapeño chile pepper (with flesh and seeds) in oil spray until soft. Beat 1 whole egg with 2 egg whites and scramble with the sautéed vegetables until the eggs are cooked through. Wrap in a whole grain tortilla (150 calories or less) and add optional salsa and/or hot sauce.

### Tropical Mango-Citrus Smoothie with Toast

Enjoy 1 serving (2 cups) Tropical Mango-Citrus Smoothie (page 114) with 1 slice whole wheat bread, toasted and topped with 2 heaping tablespoons fat-free or 1% cottage cheese and sprinkled with 1 tablespoon wheat germ.

### Cereal with Milk, Nuts, and Berries

Mix 1 cup whole grain cereal with 1 cup fat-free milk (or soy milk) and top with 1 tablespoon chopped walnuts and ½ cup fresh berries (any variety).

### Pumpkin Oatmeal

Prepare ½ cup dry oats with 1 cup fat-free milk (or soy milk) and mix with 2 teaspoons vanilla extract, ½ cup canned 100% pure pumpkin puree, a pinch of salt, and 2 teaspoons sugar (or 1 packet sugar substitute). Top with optional 1 tablespoon wheat germ.

## LUNCH OPTIONS

(400 TO 500 CALORIES)

### The Ache-Less Salad

Top 3 cups leafy greens with 4 ounces (total) of any of the following high-protein options: wild salmon, sardines, mackerel, turkey breast, grilled chicken, or tofu. Mix with ½ chopped tomato, ¼ chopped red onion, ¼ cup sliced mushrooms, 1 sliced red bell pepper, 2 chopped beets, ½ cup chopped carrots, and ¼ cup corn. If desired, add optional red cabbage and chopped celery. Toss with 1 to 2 teaspoons olive oil and unlimited balsamic vinegar or fresh lemon juice (or 2 to 4 tablespoons reduced-calorie dressing).

### Greek Chicken Pita Pocket

Lightly toast 1 whole wheat pita and fill with romaine lettuce, 3 to 4 ounces cooked chicken breast, 1 ounce crumbled feta cheese (preferably reduced-fat), and thin slices of tomato and red onion. Drizzle with plain balsamic vinegar or fresh lemon juice. Season with salt and pepper to taste. Enjoy with crunchy celery sticks and red pepper strips.

### Turkey and Roasted Pepper Sandwich

Layer 4 ounces sliced turkey breast (or chicken breast), unlimited lettuce, sliced tomato, onion, and roasted red peppers between 2 slices whole grain bread. Add optional mustard and 1 to 2 teaspoons reduced-fat mayonnaise. Enjoy with a large handful of baby carrots.

### Butternut Squash Soup with Fish

Enjoy 2 to 3 cups Butternut Squash Soup (page 79) or any prepared low-fat soup without cream with a salad of unlimited leafy greens topped with 3 ounces canned sardines, wild salmon, light tuna packed in water, or grilled chicken. Drizzle the salad with fresh lemon juice or plain vinegar and season with salt and pepper to taste.

### Vegetable Omelet and Baked Potato

Beat 1 whole egg with 2 or 3 egg whites. Cook in a heated skillet coated with oil spray. When the bottom is cooked, gently flip over. Top with any of the following vegetables: mushrooms, onion, peppers (bell and hot), broccoli, kale, spinach, or tomato. Fold the omelet over and cook until the egg mixture is firm. Enjoy with 1 medium plain baked white or sweet potato (or 2 cups hearty vegetable soup).

### Wild Salmon Salad

Enjoy 1 serving Wild Salmon Salad (page 321), or drain and mash 5 to 6 ounces canned Alaskan salmon and mix with 2 teaspoons reduced-fat mayonnaise and minced onion and mustard to taste. Serve over a bed of leafy greens with 1 mini whole grain pita, split and toasted (or 100 calories' worth of whole grain crackers).

### Turkey Burger with Veggies

Top a 5-ounce lean turkey burger (or vegetarian burger) with optional sliced tomato, onion, and roasted peppers and serve on ½ whole grain bun (or in a mini pita pocket). Enjoy with unlimited vegetables (broccoli, cauliflower, kale, Brussels sprouts, sugar snap peas, Swiss chard, beets, spinach, or asparagus), steamed, grilled, roasted, or lightly sautéed in 1 teaspoon olive oil or oil spray.

## DINNER OPTIONS

(500 TO 600 CALORIES)

### Baked Tilapia with Vegetables and Sweet Potato

Season 6 ounces tilapia fillet (or other fish) with 1 teaspoon olive oil, freshly ground pepper, a pinch of kosher salt, and fresh lemon juice. Bake, uncovered, in a 400°F oven for 10 to 12 minutes. Serve with unlimited steamed broccoli (or cauliflower, kale, Brussels sprouts, sugar snap peas, Swiss chard, beets, spinach, or asparagus) and 1 medium baked sweet potato topped with optional ground cinnamon.

### Sweet and Sour Tofu-Veggie Stir-Fry with Brown Rice

Enjoy 1 serving Sweet and Sour Tofu-Veggie Stir-Fry (page 245) with 1 cup cooked brown rice. (Chicken or shrimp may be substituted for the tofu.) Add ½ cup sliced red onion and, if your tastebuds can handle it, double up on the jalapeño chile peppers.

### Oysters Rockefeller with Grilled Salmon over Greens

Enjoy 1 serving Grilled Rockefeller Oysters (page 179) with 5 ounces grilled wild salmon or other fish seasoned with 1 teaspoon olive oil, a pinch of kosher salt, ground black pepper, and preferred seasonings. Serve over a large mound of leafy greens mixed with optional sliced red onion, pepper, mushrooms, and tomato. Drizzle with 2 tablespoons reduced-calorie dressing (or plain balsamic vinegar or fresh lemon juice).

### Sirloin Steak with Gingered Carrots and Baked Potato

Enjoy 5 ounces lean sirloin steak with optional horseradish dip (2 teaspoons horseradish mixed with 1 tablespoon reduced-fat mayonnaise), ½ medium baked potato topped with 1 to 2 tablespoons warm marinara sauce, and 1 serving Gingered Carrots (page 181).

### Chicken Curry and Vegetables with Brown Rice

Enjoy 1 serving Chicken Curry and Vegetables (page 178) over ½ cup cooked brown basmati rice (or regular brown rice).

### Angel Hair Pasta with Roasted Pumpkin, Sage, and Walnuts

Enjoy 1 serving Angel Hair Pasta with Roasted Pumpkin, Sage, and Walnuts (page 381) or 2 cups cooked whole wheat pasta mixed with ½ cup marinara sauce and 1 cup of any vegetable from the grocery list (page 168). Serve with a leafy green salad tossed with 1 teaspoon olive oil and unlimited vinegar or fresh lemon juice (or 2 tablespoons reduced-calorie dressing).

### Rosemary Chicken with Sautéed Swiss Chard

Enjoy 5 ounces grilled Rosemary Chicken (page 347) with 2 cups Sautéed Swiss Chard (page 346) and 1 cup baby carrots.

## SNACK OPTIONS

100 CALORIES OR LESS

- ◆ *Best Vegetable Snacks:* up to 2 cups raw or cooked bell peppers (red, green, yellow), broccoli, sugar snap peas, snow peas, tomatoes, mushrooms, green beans, carrots, asparagus, or cauliflower
- ◆ *Best Fruit Snacks:* 1 apple, orange, blood orange, tangerine, peach, persimmon, or guava; 2 kiwifruit, clementines, tangerines, or plums; ½ papaya, mango, grapefruit, or cantaloupe; 1 cup cubed watermelon, honeydew, or pineapple; 1 cup cherries, grapes (red, black, purple), or berries (blackberries, blueberries, boysenberries, elderberries, lingonberries, raspberries, sliced strawberries); ½ cup lychees; 4 apricots or prunes; 20 whole strawberries; 2 tablespoons raisins
- ◆ ½ cup fat-free or 1% cottage cheese (optional: mix with 1 minced jalapeño chile pepper)
- ◆ ¼ cup Fiery Nectarine Chutney (page 182) with celery sticks and red pepper strips

100 TO 200 CALORIES

- ◆ 1 baked apple with cinnamon and 1 teaspoon sugar or honey
- ◆ 1 ounce (about ¼ cup) whole nuts
- ◆ ½ cup fat-free or 1% cottage cheese with 1 serving fruit (see Best Fruit Snacks above)
- ◆ 1 serving (2 cups) Tropical Mango-Citrus Smoothie (page 114)
- ◆ 1 Ginger-Spiced Pumpkin Muffin (page 180)

◆ 1 serving Warm Dark Chocolate Sauce with Fresh Fruit (page 80)

◆ 1 serving Butternut Squash Soup (page 79)

◆ 1 cup fat-free plain or flavored yogurt mixed with ½ cup berries and 1 table-spoon wheat germ

◆ 1 cup fat-free vanilla yogurt mixed with ½ cup canned 100% pure pumpkin puree and sprinkled with ground cinnamon

# CHICKEN CURRY AND VEGETABLES

*Curry, turmeric, and ginger make this the ultimate anti-inflammatory meal. The traditional version incorporates whole-milk yogurt, but I use fat-free to reduce the saturated fat in the recipe.*

**MAKES 4 SERVINGS (1½ CUPS PER SERVING)**

3 tablespoons curry powder

1 tablespoon olive oil

2 cloves garlic, minced

1 teaspoon turmeric

1 teaspoon minced fresh ginger

1½ pounds boneless, skinless chicken breasts, cut into 2" chunks

Kosher salt

1 head cauliflower (about 1½ pounds), cut into 1" florets, stem discarded

1 large onion, chopped

1 can (15 ounces) chickpeas, rinsed and drained

3 large tomatoes (about 1 pound), chopped

1 cup fat-free plain yogurt

2 tablespoons chopped cilantro, for garnish

**To make in a slow cooker:** Combine the curry powder, oil, garlic, turmeric, and ginger in a zip-top bag. Sprinkle the chicken with salt and place it in the bag. Shake until the curry mixture evenly coats the chicken.

Place the cauliflower and onion in the bottom of a 4- to 5-quart slow cooker. Add the chickpeas and arrange the chicken evenly on top. Add the tomatoes. Cover and cook on high for 3 to 3½ hours, stirring once during cooking time, until the chicken is no longer pink in the center and the vegetables are tender.

Transfer the chicken curry to a large bowl and stir in the yogurt. Season with additional salt, if needed, and garnish with the cilantro. Serve immediately with brown basmati rice.

**To make on the stove top:** Season the chicken with salt. In a large skillet, heat the oil over high heat. Add the chicken and cook, stirring, for 3 to 4 minutes, or until the chicken begins to brown. Transfer the chicken to a plate. Add the onion and cook for 3 to 4 minutes, or until it begins to soften and become translucent. Add the garlic, turmeric, ginger, and curry powder and cook, stirring, for 1 to 2 minutes, or until the mixture becomes fragrant.

Add ¼ cup water and the cauliflower, chickpeas, and tomatoes. Lower the heat to a simmer, and add more water if the mixture becomes dry. Cover and cook for 8 to 10 minutes, or until the cauliflower is tender. Uncover, return the chicken to the pan, and cook, stirring occasionally, for 10 to 15 minutes longer, or until the chicken is cooked through but still tender and the liquid thickens.

Remove from the heat. Stir in the yogurt. Season with salt, if needed, and garnish with the cilantro. Serve immediately with brown basmati rice.

**Per serving:** 437 calories, 52 g protein, 39 g carbohydrate, 8 g fat (1 g saturated), 99 mg cholesterol, 447 mg sodium, 11 g fiber; plus 537 mcg beta-carotene

# GRILLED ROCKEFELLER OYSTERS

*When it comes to oysters, people either love them or hate them. My own household is divided. If you're a lover, you're in luck. Pacific oysters provide omega-3 fats, which have been shown to reduce inflammation in people who suffer from swollen joints.*

**MAKES 4 SERVINGS (6 OYSTERS EACH)**

2 tablespoons olive oil

2 tablespoons all-purpose flour

Zest and juice of 1 lemon

2 cups spinach, wilted and chopped

½ cup fresh basil, chopped

3 cloves garlic, minced

⅛ teaspoon hot sauce

Kosher salt

Ground pepper

2 dozen large, tightly closed fresh Pacific oysters in the shell

2 tablespoons grated Parmesan cheese

Heat the oil in a small skillet over medium heat. Add the flour and cook for 3 to 4 minutes, stirring continuously until a thick, smooth paste forms. Remove from the heat and add ¼ cup water, lemon zest and juice, spinach, basil, garlic, and hot sauce. Whisk quickly until a thick sauce forms. Season with salt and pepper to taste.

Preheat a grill or an oven to 400°F. Shuck the oysters, reserving the shells. Arrange the oysters in the deepest reserved half-shells, one oyster per shell. Top with a spoonful of the spinach mixture and sprinkle with the cheese.

If grilling, set the half-shells on the grill, filling side up. Cover loosely with a sheet of aluminum foil and grill for 8 to 10 minutes, or until the oysters are no longer translucent but are still tender. If baking, place the half-shells on a baking sheet covered with aluminum foil and bake for 8 to 10 minutes, or until the oysters are cooked inside and the filling begins to brown and the oysters are no longer translucent but are still tender. Serve immediately.

**Per serving:** 183 calories, 13 g protein, 9 g carbohydrate, 10 g fat (2 g saturated), 58 mg cholesterol, 178 mg sodium, 2 g fiber

# GINGER-SPICED PUMPKIN MUFFINS

*I call these Muffins with a Mission! Enjoy one as a midday snack, or couple with an egg, fat-free yogurt, or glass of fat-free milk for a balanced breakfast. Either way, it's win/win—just 131 calories and created to help ease the aches and pains of arthritis.*

**MAKES 12**

½ cup packed brown sugar

1½ cups whole wheat flour

2 teaspoons baking powder

1 teaspoon ground cinnamon

1 teaspoon ground ginger

½ teaspoon kosher salt

1 egg

1 cup fat-free milk

½ cup canned 100% pure pumpkin puree

¼ cup canola oil

½ teaspoon grated orange zest

Preheat the oven to 375°F. Lightly coat 12 muffin cups with oil spray.

In a large mixing bowl, stir together the brown sugar, flour, baking powder, cinnamon, ginger, and salt.

In a small bowl, beat the egg for 30 seconds, or until foamy. Add the milk, pumpkin, oil, and orange zest. Beat well. Add the egg mixture to the flour mixture and stir until the flour mixture is moistened.

Fill the muffin cups three-quarters full with batter. Bake for 15 minutes, or until the tops spring back when you touch them with a finger. Turn out the muffins onto a wire rack to cool. Once cool, you can freeze the muffins, tightly wrapped, for up to 2 months.

**Per muffin:** 131 calories, 3 g protein, 19 g carbohydrate, 5 g fat (0 g saturated), 18 mg cholesterol, 20 mg sodium, 2 g fiber; plus 463 mcg beta-carotene, 75 mcg beta-cryptoxanthin

# GINGERED CARROTS

*I'm always looking for creative ways to prepare one of my favorite veggies: carrots. This chapter gave me a reason to experiment with ginger, and I'm thrilled with the finished product. I hope your joints—and tastebuds—agree!*

**MAKES 4 SERVINGS**

1 pound carrots, peeled and cut into 1" wedges

2 tablespoons reduced-fat, soft tub, trans-fat-free spread

¼ cup grated fresh ginger

2 teaspoons ground ginger

Kosher salt

Ground black pepper

Preheat the oven to 400°F. Tear a large piece of aluminum foil, about 24" long. Spread the carrots evenly over one half. Rub the carrots with the soft tub spread, fresh ginger, and ground ginger. Season with salt and pepper.

Fold the opposite end of the foil over, folding around the edges to make a neat package with no openings. Place the package on a baking sheet and bake for 20 to 25 minutes, or until the carrots are tender when pierced with a knife. Serve immediately.

> **Per serving:** 77 calories, 1 g protein, 12 g carbohydrate, 3 g fat (0 g saturated), 0 mg cholesterol, 129 mg sodium, 3 g fiber; plus 470 mcg beta-carotene, 142 mcg beta-cryptoxanthin

# FIERY NECTARINE CHUTNEY

*My sweet and spicy chutney made its debut years ago on the* Today *show. Since then, I've discovered that it goes great with just about anything! Jalapeño chile peppers and ginger possess anti-inflammatory properties, which may assist in alleviating the aches and pains associated with arthritis. What's more, chopped onions supply quercetin, and the nectarines, red pepper, and orange juice provide disease-fighting antioxidants like beta-cryptoxanthin and vitamin C. Serve as a dip with crudités and baked tortilla chips, or spoon a few tablespoons on top of grilled fish, poultry, lean turkey sausages, or veggie burgers.*

**MAKES 12 SERVINGS (¼ CUP EACH)**

2 large, ripened nectarines (about 1 pound), finely chopped with skin

1 large red bell pepper, chopped

½ cup finely chopped red onion

4 teaspoons minced jalapeño chile pepper, or more if you can take the heat (wear plastic gloves when handling)

2 tablespoons fresh lime juice

2 tablespoons orange juice

2 to 3 teaspoons sugar (optional)

¼ teaspoon ground ginger

¼ teaspoon ground allspice

¼ teaspoon kosher salt

In a medium bowl, stir together the nectarines, bell pepper, onion, chile pepper, lime juice, orange juice, sugar (if using), ginger, allspice, and salt. Refrigerate until serving time.

**Per serving:** 19 calories, 0 g protein, 5 g carbohydrate, 0 g fat, 0 mg cholesterol, 49 mg sodium, 1 g fiber; plus 23 mg vitamin C (38% DV)

# CHAPTER 9

# TYPE 2 DIABETES

Of all the disorders I treat, diabetes is among the sneakiest and most destructive.

Sneaky because unless you know you're at risk and are checking for signs, symptoms might not appear until your body is damaged in some way. Over one-quarter of people who have diabetes don't know it. If you suspect there's a problem but wait until you feel sick to get help, you may be well on your way to developing complications.

Destructive because if it goes untreated, it can lead to one (or several) serious complications, including heart attack or stroke, continuous pain from degenerated nerves, the need for foot or leg amputations from gangrene, kidney failure, or vision loss from retinopathy.

It's not a pretty picture. This condition is serious and deserves your undivided attention if you've been diagnosed or know—or even suspect—you're at risk!

On a positive note, if you work with your doctor to closely monitor and control your blood sugar and commit to eating right and exercising regularly, there's great reason to believe you'll live a long, healthy life without serious complications. New medications, clever blood-testing devices, and breakthrough information about foods and supplements mean that successful glucose control is within everyone's reach.

## WHAT IS DIABETES?

Your body's primary source of energy is glucose, a simple sugar created when carbohydrates are broken down during digestion. If everything is working properly, glucose enters the bloodstream and triggers the pancreas to release insulin, which allows glucose to leave the blood and enter every cell in your body. That's how cells get their nourishment. This energy transfer at the cellular level fuels all your bodily functions, from thinking to digestion to all the fantastic physical feats the human body is capable of. Think of glucose as the electricity in a house—you have one main line that branches off into each room and branches again to supply power to the outlets within them. Skimp on the glucose and your power goes out.

If you have diabetes, there is a problem with the way your body produces or uses insulin. If glucose can't move into the cells, it stays in the bloodstream, leading to the high blood sugar levels characteristic of the disease.

There are three main types of diabetes. With type 1 diabetes, the insulin-producing cells of the pancreas are destroyed, so there is no insulin available to let glucose enter body cells. It is as if a circuit breaker tripped, and the power is simply cut off. No insulin means no energy getting to the cells. Type 1 diabetes is an auto-immune disorder for which there is no known prevention. It requires treatment with insulin and carefully planned meals.

With type 2 diabetes, there are two potential insulin problems: Either the pancreas can't make enough insulin, or the cells have become resistant to the insulin your body produces. Either or both of these conditions may be present. Going back to the electricity analogy, insulin resistance is like having a dimmer switch on your body's power supply stuck on low—some energy gets through to the cells, but much of the glucose is blocked from entering cells and stays in the bloodstream. Treatment options vary from person to person, depending on the severity of the condition. Some people with type 2 diabetes can manage their disease with dietary changes alone. Others require medications or insulin replacement.

There is also a third type of diabetes called gestational diabetes, which affects about 4 percent of pregnant women. Although this type of diabetes usually disappears after the baby is born, research suggests that women who develop gestational diabetes have an increased risk of developing type 2 diabetes later in life.

The information in the rest of this chapter pertains only to type 2 diabetes. People with type 1 or gestational diabetes should consult a private nutritionist or trained diabetes educator for one-on-one dietary counseling.

## WHAT AFFECTS TYPE 2 DIABETES?

Type 2 diabetes was once called adult-onset diabetes, but now we know that even young children can develop it. The number one risk factor—by far—is being overweight. Genetics, age, and lack of exercise also contribute to your personal risk, but body weight is the biggest contributor. The American Diabetes Association recommends that anyone who is overweight talk with his or her physician to see if testing is appropriate. If your doctor believes you're at significant risk, she'll order blood tests to rule out a thyroid disorder and determine if you have diabetes or prediabetes. There are three tests used to check for diabetes.

A fasting plasma glucose test (FPG) measures blood glucose after an overnight fast. It is quick, convenient, and inexpensive. Normal fasting blood sugar is below 100 mg/dL. If your blood glucose is 126 mg/dL or higher, the test will be repeated. Two readings of 126 mg/dL or higher means a diagnosis of diabetes. If your blood glucose is 100 to 125 mg/dL, your diagnosis is prediabetes. (Prediabetes used to be called impaired glucose tolerance or impaired fasting glucose.)

An oral glucose tolerance test (OGTT) measures blood glucose after an overnight fast and again 2 hours after you drink a high-glucose liquid. This test is more sensitive than FPG, but it is inconvenient because of the 2-hour wait between blood draws. Normal 2-hour blood glucose is below 140 mg/dL. If your 2-hour blood glucose is 200 mg/dL or higher, the test will be repeated. Two readings of 200 mg/dL or higher means a diagnosis of diabetes. If your 2-hour blood glucose is 140 to 199 mg/dL, your diagnosis is prediabetes.

The glycated hemoglobin test (more commonly called A1C) was recently approved as a third method of diagnosing diabetes. The A1C test is a simple blood test that measures your average blood sugar level over a two- to three-month period. An A1C reading above 6.5 percent indicates a diabetes diagnosis. This test has many advantages over older tests, and many experts now consider it the gold standard.

## WHAT ARE THE DANGERS OF PREDIABETES?

It's probably obvious, but the greatest danger of prediabetes is that it can lead to diabetes. In fact, research shows that most people with prediabetes will develop diabetes within 10 years unless they make significant lifestyle changes. By losing weight (at least 5 percent of body weight), becoming more active, and making broad changes to their eating habits (like embracing the eating plan I'll tell you about later in this chapter), people with prediabetes can stop the progression and avoid a full-fledged diagnosis.

Prediabetes is also one of the hallmarks of another disorder called metabolic syndrome. "Metabolic syndrome" describes a cluster of risk factors that, when taken together, create a toxic environment in your blood vessels. Doctors typically diagnose metabolic syndrome in patients who have at least three of the following conditions: high blood pressure (130/85 mmHg or higher), high triglycerides (150 mg/dL or higher), low HDL cholesterol (below 50 mg/dL for women, below 40 mg/dL for men), large waist circumference (greater than 35 inches for women, greater than 40 inches for men), or fasting blood sugar higher than 100 mg/dL. The combination of any three is dangerous, even if the numbers are only slightly out of the normal range. People with metabolic syndrome have an increased risk of heart attack and stroke. If you have been diagnosed with metabolic syndrome but have a normal fasting glucose level (below 100 mg/dL), follow the 4-step plan outlined in my cardiovascular disease chapter (page 140). If you have been diagnosed with metabolic syndrome and your fasting glucose level is elevated (higher than 100 mg/dL), follow the 4-step program outlined at the end of this chapter. You should also read the cardiovascular disease chapter to learn about which foods you

## FAQS

### Is it safe for people with diabetes to drink coffee?

Many studies have linked moderate coffee drinking with a lower risk of developing type 2 diabetes. A large review published in the *Journal of the American Medical Association* found that people who drank four to six cups of coffee per day were 28 percent less likely to develop diabetes than individuals who drank zero to two cups. Caffeinated or decaffeinated, filtered or instant, all types seem to be protective.

However, for people who already have diabetes, the picture gets cloudier. That's because some studies show that the caffeine in coffee reduces insulin sensitivity, which means insulin and blood sugar levels may in fact increase. If you have diabetes and you're having a tough time keeping your blood sugar down, I recommend switching to decaf for a week or two to see if your blood sugar readings improve. If they do, decaf is clearly the way to go.

should and should not eat in order to bring down all other elevated numbers, such as blood pressure, LDL cholesterol, and triglycerides.

As I mentioned, the good news is that prediabetes doesn't necessarily progress to diabetes. The Diabetes Prevention Program, which studied more than 3,000 people with prediabetes, showed that participants who changed their diets, lost weight, and started exercising reduced their risk of developing diabetes by an astounding 58 percent. That's slashing your risk of diabetes by more than half, without drugs! Treatment with the medication metformin reduced the risk of diabetes by 31 percent—still significant but less than the combined effects of diet and exercise. Every step you take—and I mean that both literally and figuratively—can help prevent or delay the onset of disease. Every year you don't have to deal with the complications of diabetes is a blessing for your future health.

One of my clients is counting those blessings. Dina, 49, went to her doctor for a routine checkup and blood work before her second marriage, and that's when she discovered that she had metabolic syndrome. Her fasting blood sugar was 125—just shy of full-fledged diabetes. In addition, she had triglycerides of about 200, high blood pressure, and total cholesterol of 340—her "bad" LDL cholesterol alone was over 200! (Although LDL cholesterol is not a diagnostic marker for metabolic syndrome, optimal levels are less than 100.). At 5 foot 5 and 163 pounds, Dina was also overweight and carried a significant amount of fat around her middle. She also had a family history of heart disease—her brother had died of a heart attack in his late thirties. Before her test results came back, Dina ate whatever she wanted and didn't care about exercise. Her doctor set her straight: "Those days are over. You're getting married and have a whole new adventure ahead of you. You have a lot to live for." He wrote her a prescription for a cholesterol-lowering medication and sent her to me.

After just 2 months of following every point of my 4-Step Program for Diabetes, Dina lost 16 pounds and trimmed 4 inches off her waist. Her fasting blood sugar was down to 105—still too high but a significant improvement. Her blood pressure was now in the normal range, and her blood lipids were lower, too, thanks to medication and nutrition changes. Her triglycerides had fallen to 130 (now considered normal), and her total cholesterol had fallen to about 210 (the bad LDL cholesterol dropped below 130!). She drew her motivation from both fear and hope—fear of meeting the same early death as her brother and hope for the years of love and happiness that she dreamed of sharing with her new husband. Hope, for many of us, blooms as we see the powerful effects making just a few changes can have on our overall health.

## WHAT ARE THE DANGERS OF TYPE 2 DIABETES?

If you have diabetes, it is important to understand that it's a chronic condition. You can control the disease, but it will never go away. The best you can hope for is that your disease will go into a form of remission—contained but subject to return. You'll need to monitor your blood sugars daily, and your doctor will want to periodically check your progress, too. The A1C test I mentioned earlier as a diagnostic tool is also incredibly useful for tracking how well you're controlling your sugars. This test provides a status report on your average blood glucose level over a two- to three-month period. So A1C captures more than your blood sugar reading at the moment your doctor draws blood for the test—it is also a measure of whether you're controlling your diabetes or your diabetes is controlling you.

High A1C levels mean a high risk of complications from diabetes. To put it bluntly, uncontrolled blood sugar is a poison. Because all cells need and use glucose, many different body systems are affected. People with diabetes face a common set of problems.

### CARDIOVASCULAR

Although a little extra blood sugar doesn't sound dangerous, it is toxic to your blood vessels. High levels of glucose form free radicals, which are unstable molecules that damage cellular membranes, including the delicate cell membranes of your blood vessels. Over the long term, the damage may trigger the immune system to secrete inflammatory chemicals that further assault the blood vessels. The process can lead to serious cardiovascular problems, which in turn may cause a heart attack or stroke. (For more information about the cardiovascular system, see page 117.)

### VISION

Diabetes increases your risk of cataracts, which cloud the lens of your eye, and glaucoma, which can lead to blindness from damage to the optic nerve. In addition, uncontrolled blood glucose damages the delicate blood vessels in the retina, leading to a condition called diabetic retinopathy. Diabetic retinopathy is the leading cause of blindness in America, but that doesn't mean it's in your future. Studies show that people can prevent retinopathy by keeping their blood sugar levels as close to normal as possible. Once retinopathy develops, careful blood sugar control can keep the disease from progressing.

## NEUROPATHY (NERVE DAMAGE)

Uncontrolled diabetes exposes your nerves to something like a sugar bath, which leads to degeneration of nerve axons—the bodies of the nerve cells. In addition, the protective coating around the nerves—the myelin—may be stripped, slowing the speed at which nerves can transmit sensory messages. If the blood vessels that feed the nerves are damaged by diabetes, then those nerves can die.

Early nerve damage may not cause any discomfort. Mild symptoms can include tingling or numbness, particularly in the feet. Over time, neuropathy progresses and may cause pain or large areas of numbness. Scientists estimate that about 26 percent of people with type 2 diabetes have painful neuropathy. If nerves die, muscles in the feet or hands can whither. As the nerve damage becomes more extensive, it can cause impotence, dizziness, gastrointestinal problems, and general weakness.

Because the feet are usually affected first, good foot care is critically important. You may overlook a blister, sore, or cut if that part of your foot is numb. If your foot becomes infected, it could eventually spread internally to the bone. In some cases, an infection can become so severe that it becomes necessary to amputate the limb. The longer you have uncontrolled diabetes, the greater your risk of neuropathy and the greater the potential damage. But, as with eye diseases and other complications, studies have shown that neuropathy can be delayed and even prevented if you control your blood glucose.

## HOW FOOD AFFECTS DIABETES

Let's talk about food on a grand scale for a minute. Regardless of whether you have prediabetes or diabetes, the best thing you can do for your health is to lose weight. But you don't have to slim down to swimsuit shape to reap the benefits. Research has shown that losing even small amounts of weight—as little as 10 pounds over two years—can reduce your risk of developing diabetes by up to 30 percent. That's a small amount of weight to lose for such a large return on the quality of your life! Among people with diabetes, weight loss improves insulin sensitivity and glycemic control, reduces triglycerides and LDL cholesterol, and lowers blood pressure. That is to say, losing a few pounds may very well save your life. (For more information on the basics of losing weight, see Weight Loss on page 17.)

But healthy eating for diabetes prevention or control is about more than weight loss: You need to eat foods that will, first and foremost, keep your blood sugar stable.

## HIGH-QUALITY CARBOHYDRATES
## (VERSUS LOW-QUALITY CARBOHYDRATES)

During digestion, carbohydrates break down to create glucose, which enters the bloodstream, triggering a rise in insulin, which is necessary for the glucose to enter cells. In people with diabetes, this system is defective, so glucose stays in the blood. This is what you are checking when you test your blood sugar level.

You may know about the concept of the glycemic index (GI). GI is a measure of how fast and how high a particular food will raise blood sugar. Foods with a high GI raise blood sugar faster and higher than foods with a low GI. It's a controversial topic in nutrition because when it comes right down to it, GI values simply aren't very user-friendly. One type of food can have many different GI values, depending on its ripeness (of a fruit or vegetable), method of preparation, and other factors. For example, a ripe banana has a higher GI than a green banana and a baked potato has a different GI than a boiled potato. If you eat a high-GI food with a protein (and/or a food containing fat), the GI value goes down because protein and fat slow down the absorption of carbohydrate. The myriad factors that influence GI values are mind-boggling. There's an easier way to achieve low-glycemic eating without feeling like every meal is an exercise in advanced mathematics.

If you're looking for foods that raise blood sugar levels slowly and gently, like rolling waves, choose high-quality carbohydrates (see the list below) instead of low-quality carbs, and, whenever possible, couple these carbs with protein and/or healthy fat. For example, eat brown rice and vegetables (high-quality carbs) together with grilled chicken or pork tenderloin (lean protein). High-quality carbs are full of vitamins, minerals, and fiber. They are found primarily in plant foods, including whole grain products, brown and wild rice, oats, vegetables, fruits, and legumes. In addition, some of these high-quality carbs also contain soluble fiber, a component of plant cell walls. Soluble fiber slows the absorption of glucose from food in the stomach, which also helps keep blood sugar under control.

HIGH-QUALITY CARBS—NONSTARCHY VEGETABLES: *artichokes, asparagus, beets, bok choy, broccoli, broccoli raab, Brussels sprouts, cabbage, carrots, cauliflower, celery, cucumber, dark leafy greens (such as beet, collard, dandelion, kale, mustard, Swiss chard, turnip), eggplant, fennel, green beans, lettuce (all varieties), mushrooms, okra, onions (all varieties), peppers (all varieties), pumpkin, radishes, rhubarb, snow peas, spaghetti squash, sugar snap peas, summer squash, tomatoes, water chestnuts, zucchini*

HIGH-QUALITY CARBS—LENTILS AND BEANS: *black-eyed peas, lentils, starchy beans (such as black, navy, pinto, garbanzo, kidney), split peas, soybeans (edamame)*

HIGH-QUALITY CARBS—STARCHY VEGETABLES: *corn, green peas, potatoes (sweet and white), winter squash (acorn, butternut)*

HIGH-QUALITY CARBS—FRUIT: *all fresh and frozen whole fruit (avoid dried fruit and fruit juice)*

HIGH-QUALITY CARBS—WHOLE GRAINS: *amaranth, barley, bulgur, millet, oats, quinoa, rice (brown, wild), whole grain breads, cereals, and pastas*

BEST FOODS FOR SOLUBLE FIBER: *psyllium seeds (ground), lima beans, starchy beans (such as black, navy, pinto, garbanzo, kidney), Brussels sprouts, oat bran, winter squash, parsnips, turnips, sweet potatoes, lentils, black-eyed peas, split peas, green peas, okra, eggplant, barley, oats, rice bran, guava, oranges, grapefruit, apples, peaches, plums, nectarines, pears, prunes, mangoes, strawberries, blackberries, raspberries, bananas, apricots, raisins, white potatoes, avocados, broccoli, carrots, green beans, spinach, cabbage, kale, wheat germ, ground flaxseed*

Low-quality carbs, on the other hand, have much less nutritional value. Candy, sweetened drinks (like soda), maple syrup, honey, jam and jelly, cakes, and most other foods we typically think of as sweets or desserts are made up primarily of sugar. Refined starches—the "white" carbs, such as white rice and white bread—are also low-quality carbohydrates because they act very much like sugars once you begin to digest them. You should also avoid drinking fruit juice—even 100 percent pure fruit juice. Although these beverages certainly provide better nutrition than soda, they're concentrated in fruit sugar and raise blood sugar quickly. The same thing goes for dried fruit. Like fruit juice, dried fruit provides ample nutrition and fiber, but when the water content is removed from fresh fruit, the dried, dehydrated version becomes highly concentrated in sugar and can cause a sharp rise in blood sugar. Clearly not worth the spike! Starchy vegetables—such as potatoes, winter squash, peas, and corn—have a higher glycemic index than other, nonstarchy veggies, such as broccoli, cauliflower, cucumbers, peppers, green beans, spinach, and mushrooms. However, you can enjoy moderate amounts of starchy vegetables if you eat them alongside lean protein at meals. For example, a balanced dinner might include broiled salmon, broccoli, and a small baked white or sweet potato topped with reduced-fat sour cream; lunch might include grilled chicken, a tossed salad, and an ear of corn.

Your goal, then, is to choose high-quality carbs whenever possible and limit or avoid low-quality carbs.

## MODERATE ALL CARBOHYDRATES AND COUPLE WITH PROTEIN

If you stick with high-quality carbs, can you eat as much as you want? Unfortunately, no. To best control your blood sugars, you have to moderate *all* carbs. Your total carb intake should be limited to about 40 percent of your daily food intake. That's why on my meal plan you'll notice items like "half a baked white or sweet potato" or "reduced-calorie whole wheat bread." I've picked the best of the best carbs but limited the total amount.

## CARB COUNTING AND THE EXCHANGE SYSTEM

People with diabetes are sometimes told they need to count carbs or follow a food exchange system to standardize their diets.

Counting carbs is particularly important for people who take insulin because their dosage is dependent on the amount of carbohydrate they need to offset. They determine the number of carbs they will eat in a particular meal, calculate the amount of insulin they will need to clear those carbs from their blood, then give themselves an injection (or program the amount into their insulin pump). Every "portion" of food in a carb-counting list is equal to 15 grams of carbohydrate—including grains, fruits, dairy products, and starchy vegetables. All you need to know is that every 15 grams of carbohydrate counts as one carb choice. For example, one medium apple = 15 grams of carbs = one portion. Some doctors and diabetes educators instruct their patients to count either total carb grams or the number of carb portions. If you are a carb counter, I have provided total carbohydrate grams after each of the meals and snacks in the 4-Step Program.

The Food Exchange System organizes foods according to their nutritional content: starch, fruit, vegetable, fat-free/reduced-fat milk (including milk and yogurt), very lean meat, lean meat, medium-fat meat, high-fat meat, and fat. If your doctor has instructed you to follow the exchange system, then follow those recommendations. I have included exchange information alongside carb grams after each of the meals in my 4-Step Program for type 2 diabetes.

To further slow or prevent a blood sugar rise, remember that, in general, carbs should be eaten together with high-quality protein. Some foods—such as lentils, beans, yogurt, milk, split peas, and edamame—naturally contain both high-quality carbohydrate and lean protein. My food plan (page 199) incorporates moderate amounts of high-quality carbohydrate coupled throughout the day with protein. If you like to have a plan laid out for you in detail, it's all there; if you like to add your own flair to meals, use it as a reference guide.

BEST FOODS FOR HIGH-QUALITY PROTEIN: *skinless chicken and turkey, fish and shellfish, pork tenderloin, lean beef, egg whites, yogurt (fat-free, low-fat), milk (fat-free, 1%), cheese (fat-free, reduced-fat), starchy beans (such as black, navy, pinto, garbanzo, kidney), lentils, split peas, tofu, tempeh, soybeans (edamame), soy milk, nuts and nut butters, seeds and seed butters*

## HEALTHY FATS (VERSUS SATURATED AND TRANS FATS)

All fats are not created equal—some can decrease your risk of diabetes and complications, while others are downright dangerous. Let's talk about the bad fats first.

**Avoid saturated fats.** Saturated fats are found in animal products, including fatty meats, butter, whole-milk dairy (including regular yogurt, cheese, and ice cream), and poultry skin. They are also found in some high-fat plant foods, including palm oil. Some studies have shown that eating a diet with a lot of saturated fat can lead to insulin resistance and may increase the risk of diabetes by up to 20 percent. In addition, many studies confirm that saturated fats increase cholesterol levels. People with diabetes already have an increased risk of heart disease, so eating these unhealthy fats can push your risk even higher. Here are a few simple changes that can dramatically reduce the amount of saturated fat in your diet.

◆ Avoid butter, cream cheese, lard, sour cream, doughnuts, cakes, cookies, white and milk chocolate, ice cream, pizza, cream- or cheese-based salad dressings, cheese sauce, cream sauces, animal shortenings, fatty meats (including hamburgers, bologna, pepperoni, sausage, bacon, salami, pastrami, spareribs, and hot dogs), and whole-milk dairy products.

◆ Choose lean meats only (including skinless chicken and turkey, lean beef, and pork tenderloin), fish and shellfish, reduced-fat or fat-free dairy products, and soy foods (tofu, tempeh, soy milk, edamame).

◆ Always remove skin from poultry.

◆ Prepare foods by baking, roasting, broiling, boiling, poaching, steaming, grilling, or stir-frying in heart-healthy oils, such as olive and canola.

**Avoid trans fats.** Trans fats are worse than saturated fats for diabetes and its complications. The main source of trans fat is partially hydrogenated oil, which is found in most stick margarines, as well as some packaged baked goods, snack foods, fried foods, and fast-food items. (Although fortunately, most major fast-food chains have now gone trans-fat-free.) By substituting vegetable oil for trans fats, you may be able to reduce your risk of diabetes by about 40 percent, and you can reduce your risk of heart disease by 53 percent. Whether you already have diabetes or are working to prevent it, there is no amount of trans fats you can safely incorporate into your diet, so try to keep them as far from your plate as possible.

Packaged products always list the amount of trans fat on the Nutrition Facts panel, but there's a loophole to be aware of: The FDA allows companies to "round down" and list zero gram trans fat as long as a product contains less than 0.5 gram of trans fat per serving. Therefore, if a product contains partially hydrogenated oils and you eat *several* servings of that product, you could end up consuming 1 or 2 grams of trans fat—and any amount of trans fat in your diet is detrimental to heart health.

To be a smart consumer, first check a product's nutrition label to ensure that there is zero gram trans fat. Next, browse the ingredients list to confirm that the product does not contain any "partially hydrogenated oils." If it does, put it back on the shelf. Although a trace amount of partially hydrogenated oil here and there certainly isn't life threatening, there are now so many packaged foods that are completely free of these toxic fats that there's no reason to compromise.

**Incorporate healthy fats.** Incorporating healthy fats into your diet is important for blood sugar control. Fat, as well as protein, blunts the rise in blood sugar at meals by slowing down the body's absorption of carbohydrate. For this reason, I've gone out of my way to include healthy fats (and protein) with most meals and snacks in my diabetes meal plan. When it comes to overall health, the best fats are omega-3s and monounsaturated fats. Both improve cholesterol levels and other cardiovascular risk factors, so they're a win-win for people with diabetes. Consider using olive and canola oil for cooking, swapping steak for salmon, adding a thin slice of avocado to your next sandwich, tossing olives into your salad, and snacking on a handful of nuts instead of sweets. (My Best Foods list includes only the fatty fish that have been shown to be low in mercury, PCBs, and dioxins.)

BEST FOODS FOR OMEGA-3 FATTY ACIDS: *wild salmon (fresh, canned), herring, mackerel (not king), sardines, anchovies, rainbow trout, Pacific oysters, chia seeds, ground flaxseed, walnuts, butternuts (white walnuts), seaweed, walnut oil, canola oil, flaxseed oil, soybeans (edamame)*

BEST FOODS FOR MONOUNSATURATED FATS: *olive oil, canola oil, avocados, olives, macadamia nuts, hazelnuts, pecans, almonds, peanuts, cashews, Brazil nuts, pistachios, pine nuts, peanut butter, almond butter, cashew butter, macadamia nut butter, sunflower seed butter*

## OTHER VITAMINS AND MINERALS

**Calcium and vitamin D.** According to the Nurses' Health Study, which followed more than 83,000 women for 20 years, both calcium and vitamin D may help prevent type 2 diabetes. Women who got at least 800 IU of total vitamin D daily from food and/or supplements had a 23 percent lower risk of developing diabetes, compared with those who consumed less than 200 IU daily.

Women who got at least 1,200 milligrams total calcium daily from food and/or supplements had a 21 percent lower risk of developing diabetes, compared with those who consumed less than 600 milligrams per day. Combining vitamin D and calcium was even better—women who got at least 800 IU vitamin D and 1,200 milligrams calcium reduced their risk of diabetes by 33 percent. Strive to add more vitamin D–rich foods to your diet. It can be difficult to get all the vitamin D you need from foods, so consider taking a supplement as well. (See the Supplements section, page 198, for more information.)

Scientists are unclear about exactly what these nutrients do to reduce diabetes risk. It could be that vitamin D regulates the insulin-producing cells of the pancreas, and calcium may improve insulin sensitivity. Of course, the synergy between the two makes sense—the body can't efficiently absorb or use calcium without vitamin D. Improvements in insulin sensitivity are important for everyone with diabetes, but calcium also seems to help control blood pressure, which contributes to heart disease. So whether you have prediabetes or diabetes, calcium and vitamin D are essential to your health.

I recommend that women aim to eat at least three servings of calcium-rich foods daily and consider taking a calcium supplement only if they can't reliably fit calcium into their meals and snacks. (See page 233 in the Osteoporosis chapter for more information on calcium supplements.) Men should never take a calcium supplement without approval from their doctors because some research suggests that high-calcium diets may increase the risk of prostate cancer.

> BEST FOODS FOR CALCIUM: *yogurt (fat-free, low-fat), milk (fat free, 1%), soy milk, cheese (fat-free, reduced-fat), tofu with calcium (check nutrition label), soybeans (edamame), frozen yogurt (fat-free, low-fat), low-fat ice cream, bok choy, kale, white beans, collard greens, broccoli, almonds and almond butter*

> BEST FOODS FOR VITAMIN D: *wild salmon (fresh, canned), mackerel (not king), sardines, herring, milk (fat-free, 1%), soy milk, fortified yogurt (fat-free, low-fat), egg yolks, vitamin D–enhanced mushrooms\**

> *\*These mushrooms are treated with UV light, which dramatically increases their vitamin D content.*

**Magnesium.** A 2010 study found that people who consumed significant amounts of magnesium from food and supplements slashed their risk of diabetes in half, compared with people who took in very little magnesium. Higher magnesium intake was also linked to lower levels of inflammation and better insulin sensitivity, which may explain why magnesium is so beneficial. Whether you currently have diabetes or you're trying to drive down your risk, strive to add more magnesium-rich foods to your diet. Because most people don't get enough magnesium from food alone, consider taking a multivitamin that provides at least 25 percent DV of magnesium. (See the Supplements section, page 198, for more information.)

> BEST FOODS FOR MAGNESIUM: *pumpkin seeds, spinach, Swiss chard, amaranth, sunflower seeds, cashews, almonds, quinoa, tempeh, potatoes (sweet, white), soybeans (edamame), millet, starchy beans (such as black, navy, pinto, garbanzo, kidney), artichoke hearts, peanuts and peanut butter, brown rice, whole grain bread, sesame seeds, wheat germ, flaxseed*

## BONUS POINTS

- ◆ **Get your team together.** Diabetes is a whole-body problem. Although your primary care physician may have been the one to order blood glucose testing, you need a team of professionals to guide you through all the medical details. Ideally, your core team will include your primary care physician, an endocrinologist (a hormone specialist) who understands the intricacies of insulin, and a registered dietitian to help you fine-tune your eating plan. You may also need to consult with the following specialists: an ophthalmologist (eye specialist) who can look for diabetes-related signs of damage to the retina, a podiatrist (foot health specialist) who can help prevent complications from diabetes-related nerve damage and skin sores, and a dentist to keep periodontal disease and other infections under control. Because people with diabetes have a high risk of heart disease, your primary care physician will also be your guide to preventing or managing high blood pressure and/or high cholesterol (or your primary care physician may refer you to a cardiologist).

◆ **Monitor your blood glucose levels every day.** Some people fight against checking their blood sugar levels, but daily monitoring really is the only way to know if blood sugar is under control. Diet, activity level, medications, illness, and even stress can affect blood glucose. Unless you check, you won't know whether your levels are holding steady or spiraling out of control. Your doctor will tell you how often you need to test your sugar. Some people need to check only once a day; others may need to check four or five times per day. In addition, you should ask—in advance—what to do if your blood glucose readings are abnormal.

◆ **If you have diabetes medication, take it as directed.** People who have head-splitting migraines remember to take their medications because pain is a terrific motivator. People who take medication for severe acne have no trouble remembering to take it because they know that if they miss a few doses, the consequences will be written all over their faces. But diabetes symptoms are silent, which makes it easier for people to forget to take prescribed medications. *Don't forget.* Take medications or insulin as directed by your physician. If you have uncomfortable side effects or questions about your medication or treatment plan, talk with your doctor.

◆ **Exercise.** Next to weight control and medical treatment, exercise is the most important step you can take to control diabetes. Exercise decreases body fat and promotes weight loss. But even if you don't lose weight as a result, exercise will improve blood sugar control and your body's response to insulin—it can also improve cholesterol, blood pressure, and triglycerides. So physical activity directly helps control diabetes and also helps prevent heart disease.

For optimal blood sugar control, the American College of Sports Medicine and the American Diabetes Association recommend a combination of aerobic (cardio) and strength-training exercises. Aim for 150 minutes of moderate to vigorous aerobic exercise spread out over at least 3 days each week (that works out to 50 minutes 3 days a week or 30 minutes 5 days a week). Popular forms of aerobic exercise include walking, swimming, biking, using an elliptical machine or stationary bike, and taking step aerobics or fitness dance classes. If you can't commit to 50 or 30 straight minutes of exercise, break it up into 10-minute spurts and space them throughout the day. In addition, incorporate strength-training exercises two or three days a week (about 15 minutes per session). This could involve doing exercises with light hand weights or your own body weight (such as lunges, squats, and planks), using weight machines at the gym, or following a strength-training DVD.

◆ **Keep a food record.** As you get control over your weight and blood sugar, it can be helpful to keep a log that includes some specific information about your eating habits. Every time you eat, jot down (1) where you are, (2) what time it is, (3) how hungry you are before beginning to eat, (4) how hungry you are when you stop eating, (5) the foods and amounts eaten, and (6) your thoughts or feelings at the time. A food log will help you identify undesirable patterns, such as eating in response to anxiety or stress, eating past the point of fullness, or oversnacking at night. It can also help you stay focused on new, beneficial food habits. Some clients enjoy and feel empowered by keeping a food record and continue the process for months. Others do so for only a few weeks, stopping once they understand their personal eating patterns. I strongly recommend keeping a record for at least a week—you may be surprised at what you learn.

◆ **Learn the value of distraction.** Your food record will help you identify the times of day and situations in which you're mostly likely to make poor food choices, and once you know your weak spots, you can plan new activities to take the place of unhealthy habits. One trick that many of my clients use is a combination of delay and distraction. If you get the urge to eat when you're not physically hungry and it isn't a mealtime, set a timer and wait 20 minutes. In that time, do something else to keep your mind off food—clean out a closet or purse, catch up on your e-mail, put on a fresh coat of nail polish, call a friend, schedule your outstanding appointments, pick up that knitting you've been meaning to finish—anything that keeps your hands busy and off food. If you still want to eat when the timer goes off, have a healthy snack. Most people discover, however, that their craving disappears by then.

◆ **If you smoke, quit.** Smoking increases the risk of developing diabetes and, once you have diabetes, makes every problem and complication worse. Smoking raises blood glucose levels, constricts blood vessels, and causes inflammation. As a result, people who smoke have an increased risk of kidney disease, nerve damage, blood vessel damage, and foot and leg infections. One extra piece of advice: Many people gain weight after quitting smoking because they try to satisfy their nicotine cravings by eating more. This is *not* a good strategy for anyone, but it is particularly dangerous for people with diabetes. Talk with your doctor about the best ways to quit smoking without overeating.

◆ **Limit or avoid alcohol intake.** A review of medical literature published in 2004 concluded that moderate alcohol consumption doesn't present a risk for people with diabetes. "Moderate" typically means one serving of alcohol per day for women and no more than two servings for men. (A serving is 12 ounces of beer, 5 ounces of wine, or 1½ ounces of liquor.) If you have diabetes, I also recommend checking with your personal physician to make sure that alcohol is safe for you and to learn how it might affect your blood glucose levels. If you don't already drink alcohol, don't start.

◆ **Brush and floss regularly.** Just as unregulated diabetes leads to high levels of glucose in your blood, it also leads to higher-than-usual levels of glucose in your saliva. This high-glucose environment in your mouth allows bacteria to multiply and thrive, raising the risk of dental decay. Plus, diabetes makes fighting infection harder, so if gum disease develops, you'll have a more difficult time getting rid of it than someone without diabetes. Studies have shown that among people with periodontal disease, those who also have diabetes experience more severe cases than those without diabetes. On the flip side, getting treatment for gum disease may help with diabetes management. Research suggests that diabetics who gain control over their periodontal problems have better glycemic control after gum treatment than before. For healthy teeth and gums, dentists and nutritionists alike recommend that you see your dentist regularly, brush at least twice a day, and remember to floss.

◆ **If you have sleep apnea or daytime sleepiness, seek treatment.** Excessive daytime sleepiness is often a sign of sleep apnea, a disorder that causes interruptions in breathing during sleep. Breathing stops for 10 seconds or more because of faulty signals from the brain or because the soft tissue at the back of the throat relaxes and blocks the

## FAQS

**I used to read a lot about chromium picolinate supplements. Are they valuable for people with diabetes?**

Back in the 1990s, chromium picolinate was popular as a simple treatment that scientists thought might help improve glycemic control and insulin sensitivity. Most of the studies that supported that claim had been done on laboratory animals, which is never the same as investigating the effects of a treatment on people. More recently, the picture for chromium picolinate has turned much less optimistic. In 2006, scientists reported that they were unable to find any benefit of chromium picolinate supplements in people with type 2 diabetes, even when relatively high dosages were tested. A major review of all high-quality studies found that the data were ultimately inconclusive—no one can say with any degree of certainty whether chromium is helpful or not. More research will need to be done, but as of right now, I don't recommend chromium supplements for diabetes control.

airway (called obstructive sleep apnea, or OSA). This can happen several times per night. Each time, the sleeper will partially awaken, begin to breathe again, and then fall back asleep. Most people with sleep apnea don't know what is happening or why they feel so tired after what seemed like a full night's rest. People with diabetes are more likely to have sleep apnea than nondiabetics. Even more intriguing is the possibility that sleep apnea may contribute to diabetes. OSA itself increases the risk of insulin resistance and may be a roadblock to controlling your diabetes. If you have sleep apnea or experience unusual sleepiness during the daytime, talk with your doctor. A full night's sleep is not just a luxury, it's a health necessity.

- ◆ **Be meticulous with your foot care.** The key words are *clean* and *dry*. Wash your feet daily in warm water, and dry them with a clean, soft towel. Do not soak your feet or use hot water. Inspect your feet regularly for sores, blisters, calluses, swelling, bruising, or breaks in the skin, and if you notice anything, talk with your doctor about how to treat it. Don't walk barefoot—always wear shoes or slippers, and wear clean, soft socks with your shoes. Talk with your podiatrist about other ways to keep your feet safe.

- ◆ **Add cinnamon.** Some studies suggest that adding cinnamon to foods may slightly blunt the rise in blood sugar after meals. Try stirring a generous dose of ground cinnamon into oatmeal, cereal, yogurt, or cottage cheese, or sprinkle it on apple, pear, or peach slices.

## SUPPLEMENTS

For years, scientists have been hunting for a "magic bullet" to treat diabetes—one or more nutrients that could be taken in supplement form to improve glycemic control. As of now, the search is still on. Researchers have tested all logical possibilities, including antioxidants, vitamin E, and fish oil. The results are confusing and inconsistent, sometimes showing a benefit and sometimes showing that taking a particular supplement actually makes blood sugar control worse.

At this time, the only supplement I can responsibly recommend for people with diabetes is a **multivitamin.** Look for a brand that contains at least 25 percent DV of magnesium and at least 800 IU of vitamin D. If you are a man or a women who is no longer menstruating, choose a "senior" formula, which doesn't contain iron. I do not recommend taking high doses of any individual vitamins at this point in time.

For more information on how food affects type 2 diabetes, visit www.joybauer.com/diabetes.

# JOY'S 4-STEP PROGRAM
## FOR TYPE 2 DIABETES

Follow this program if you have diabetes or prediabetes.

## Step 1 ... START WITH THE BASICS

These are the first things you should do to regain control over your blood glucose and manage diabetes.

- Begin a program of exercise.
- If you smoke, quit.
- If you have diabetes, be a good patient—monitor your blood glucose levels, take your medications, and gather a great medical team.
- Start keeping a food log.

## Step 2 ... YOUR ULTIMATE GROCERY LIST

A diabetes food plan involves eating high-quality carbs instead of low-quality carbs; healthy proteins and fats; and plenty of foods rich in soluble fiber, vitamin D, calcium, and magnesium. You don't have to purchase every item, but these foods should make up the bulk of what you eat every week. If you find yourself getting bored, try some unfamiliar foods from these groups—they may become new favorites.

For a printable version of this list, visit www.joybauer.com/diabetes.

## FRUIT

All fresh fruit, but especially:

Apples

Apricots (fresh, not dried)

Bananas

Berries (blackberries, blueberries, raspberries, and strawberries)

Cantaloupe

Grapefruit

Honeydew

Oranges

Peaches

Pears

Plums

Watermelon

## VEGETABLES AND LEGUMES

All vegetables, but especially:

Artichokes

Asparagus

Avocados

Beans, starchy (such as black, garbanzo, kidney, navy, and pinto)

Beets

Bok choy

Broccoli

Broccoli raab

Brussels sprouts

Cabbage

Carrots

Cauliflower

Corn

Dark leafy greens (such as beet, collard, dandelion, kale, mustard, Swiss chard, and turnip)

Lentils

Lettuce (all varieties)

Mushrooms

Okra

Olives

Onions

Parsnips

Peas (black-eyed, green, and split)

Peppers (all varieties)

Potatoes (sweet and white)

Pumpkin (fresh and canned 100% pure pumpkin puree)

Soybeans (edamame)

Spinach

Sugar snap peas

Squash, summer

Squash, winter (acorn and butternut)

Tomatoes

Zucchini

## SEAFOOD

All fish and shellfish, but especially:

Anchovies

Herring

Mackerel (not king)

Salmon, wild

Sardines

Trout (rainbow, wild)

## LEAN PROTEINS

Beef, lean

Chicken, ground (at least 90% lean)

Chicken, skinless

Eggs and egg substitutes

Pork tenderloin

Tempeh

Tofu

Turkey, ground (at least 90% lean)

Turkey, skinless

Turkey bacon

Turkey burgers, lean

Veggie burgers

## NUTS AND SEEDS (PREFERABLY UNSALTED)

Almonds and almond butter

Butternuts (white walnuts)

Cashews and cashew butter

Chia seeds

Flaxseed, ground

Hazelnuts

Macadamia nuts

Peanuts and peanut butter

Pecans

Pine nuts

Pistachios

Pumpkin seeds

Sunflower seeds and sunflower butter

Walnuts

## WHOLE GRAINS

Amaranth

Barley

Bread, reduced-calorie whole wheat (50 calories or less per slice)

Bulgur

Cereals, whole grain (at least 3 grams fiber; no more than 8 grams sugar per serving)

English muffins, whole grain

Millet

Oats

Pitas, whole grain, mini (70 calories)

Quinoa

Rice (brown and wild)

Rice cakes

Waffles, whole grain

## DAIRY

Cheese (fat-free or reduced-fat)

Cottage cheese (fat-free or 1%)

Cream cheese (fat-free or reduced-fat)

Milk (fat-free or 1%)

Milk alternatives (almond, rice, and soy)

Sour cream (fat-free or reduced-fat)

Yogurt (fat-free plain or flavored with sugar substitute)

## MISCELLANEOUS

Canola oil

Cinnamon, ground

Garlic

Herbs and spices (fresh, dried, and ground)

Hot sauce

Hummus

Marinara sauce (no more than 6 grams sugar per serving)

Mayonnaise, reduced-fat

Mustard

Olive oil

Salad dressing, reduced-calorie

Salsa

Soft tub spread, trans-fat-free (reduced-fat)

Sugar substitute (such as stevia and sucralose)

Vinegar (all varieties)

# Step 3 . . . GOING ABOVE AND BEYOND

If you want to do everything you can to prevent or control diabetes, here are some additional things you might try.

- ◆ Take a multivitamin.
- ◆ Avoid eating foods high in saturated fats, including butter, ice cream, whole milk, full-fat cheese, and fatty meats. Also, avoid trans fats.
- ◆ Drink alcohol in moderation, if at all.
- ◆ Take extra good care of your teeth and feet.
- ◆ Seek treatment for sleep apnea or excessive daytime sleepiness.
- ◆ Sprinkle cinnamon onto your food and beverages.

## DAYTIME SLEEPINESS

If you find yourself becoming sleepy during the day, don't automatically assume that it is due to insomnia from sleep apnea. I had a client who became unbearably sleepy every day around 3:00 p.m. His blood sugars, which he tested twice each day (once in the morning and once at night), were always well within normal, thanks to his combination of diet, exercise, and glucose-lowering medications. He sought help for sleep apnea and continued with a stellar eating plan, but weeks later, he was still crashing in the afternoon. Finally, he tested his blood sugar at 3:00 p.m. To everyone's surprise, his blood sugar was very low—below 60. His doctor adjusted his medication, and he regained his energy. If you find yourself losing the battle to stay awake in the middle of the day, test your blood sugar. If it is low, work with your physician to find a way to level it out.

# Step 4 . . . MEAL PLANS

These sample menus include foods and specific food combinations that have been shown to help improve glycemic control. Each meal is perfectly balanced with the right mix of high-quality carbs, protein, fat, and calories to help keep your blood sugar level stable. Some people find counting carbs helpful and necessary. Therefore, I provide the total calories and grams of carbohydrate for every meal and snack (each meal contains 45 grams of carbs or less). And for people who are most comfortable using the food exchange system, I also present how each meal breaks down into various exchanges. Make sure you pay close attention to the carbohydrate portions with each meal—my numbers and your blood sugar will count on it. If your blood sugar tests high on any particular day, choose the lower-carb meal options. Please note places where reduced-calorie breads are used.

Every day, choose one option for each of the three meals—breakfast, lunch, and dinner. Then, once or twice each day, choose from my suggested snacks. Approximate calories have been provided to help adjust for your personal weight-management goals. If you find yourself hungry (and if weight is not an issue), feel free to increase the portion sizes for protein and fat only—extra portions of carbohydrate may increase your blood sugar. Beverage calories are not included. If you'd prefer something other than water, stick with sugar-free beverages only.

## BREAKFAST OPTIONS

(300 TO 400 CALORIES, LESS THAN 45 GRAMS CARBOHYDRATE)

### Turkey and Cheese Omelet with Toast

Beat 1 whole egg with 3 egg whites. Cook in a heated pan coated with oil spray. Add 2 ounces diced skinless turkey. When the bottom side is cooked, gently flip. Top with 2 tablespoons shredded reduced-fat cheese. Fold the omelet over and cook until the cheese melts and the egg mixture is firm. Season with ground black pepper and preferred herbs. Enjoy with 1 toasted slice whole wheat bread (or 2 toasted slices reduced-calorie whole wheat bread, 50 calories or less per slice) topped with 2 teaspoons reduced-fat, soft tub, trans-fat-free spread.

335 calories, 16 g carbohydrate

Exchanges: 1 medium-fat meat, 4⅓ very lean meats, 1 starch, ¾ fat

### Toast with Cream Cheese, Tomato, Onion, and Lox

Toast 2 slices reduced-calorie whole wheat bread (50 calories or less per slice) and top each with 1 tablespoon fat-free or light cream cheese, sliced tomato, onion, and 2 ounces smoked salmon.

300 calories, 26 g carbohydrate

Exchanges: 2 lean meats, 1 starch, 1 vegetable, ½ fat

### Cinnamon-Walnut Cottage Cheese with Apple Slices

Mix 1 cup fat-free or 1% cottage cheese with optional cinnamon and top with 1 tablespoon chopped walnuts and 1 tablespoon ground flaxseed. Enjoy with 1 sliced apple.

320 calories, 29 g carbohydrate

Exchanges: 4 very lean meats, 1 fruit, 2 fats

### Scrambled Eggs with Turkey Bacon and Fruit

Beat 1 whole egg with 3 egg whites. Cook in a heated pan coated with oil spray, adding preferred chopped vegetables (onion, red and green bell peppers, or tomato). Enjoy with 2 strips turkey bacon and 1 orange (or ½ grapefruit or ¼ cantaloupe).

320 calories, 30 g carbohydrate

Exchanges: 1 medium-fat meat, 2 lean meats, 1⅓ very lean meats, 1 vegetable, 1 fruit

### Oatmeal with Berries, Flaxseed, and Nuts

Prepare ½ cup dry oats with water and top with 2 tablespoons ground flaxseed (or wheat germ), 2 tablespoons chopped nuts (walnuts, pecans, soy nuts, or slivered almonds), and ½ cup berries (sliced strawberries, raspberries, and/or blackberries). Sweeten with optional sugar substitute and sprinkle with optional cinnamon.

350 calories, 43 g carbohydrate

Exchanges: 1 starch, 1 fruit, 4 fats

### Cereal with Milk and a Hard-Cooked Egg

Mix 1 cup whole grain cereal with 1 cup milk (fat-free, 1%, or soy). Enjoy with 1 hard-cooked egg (or 2 strips turkey bacon).

320 calories, 43 g carbohydrate

Exchanges: 1 medium-fat meat, 1¼ starch, 1 fat-free milk

### Strawberry-Banana Cottage Cheese with Almonds

Mix 1 cup fat-free or 1% cottage cheese with ¼ sliced banana, ½ cup chopped strawberries, and 2 tablespoons slivered almonds. Sprinkle with optional cinnamon.

332 calories, 27 g carbohydrate

Exchanges: 4 very lean meats, 1½ fruits, 2 fats

### Breakfast Burrito

Beat 1 whole egg with 2 egg whites. Cook on a heated griddle coated with oil spray. Mix with ¼ cup black beans and 2 tablespoons reduced-fat shredded cheese. Wrap in 1 whole grain tortilla (150 calories or less), adding optional onions, peppers, salsa, and/or hot sauce.

380 calories, 35 g carbohydrate

Exchanges: 1 medium-fat meat, 1 lean meat, 1 very lean meat, 2¾ starches, optional 1 vegetable

### Whole Grain Waffles with Yogurt and Nuts

Toast 2 frozen whole grain waffles and top with 6 ounces fat-free flavored yogurt (100 calories or less) and 1 tablespoon chopped nuts (walnuts, pecans, soy nuts, peanuts, or slivered almonds). Sprinkle with optional cinnamon.

319 calories, 43 g carbohydrate

Exchanges: 2 starches, 1 fat, 1 fat-free milk

### Vegetable Scramble with Toasted English Muffin

Sauté ½ cup each sliced mushrooms, chopped pepper, chopped onion, and broccoli florets in oil spray until soft. Beat 1 whole egg with 2 or 3 egg whites and pour over the vegetables. Add 2 tablespoons chopped tomato and continue to scramble until the eggs are cooked. Season with black pepper. Enjoy with 1 toasted whole grain English muffin, dry or with optional 2 teaspoons reduced-fat, soft tub, trans-fat-free spread. (For half of English muffin, you may substitute one of the following fruits: 1 orange, 1 plum, ½ cup berries, ½ grapefruit, or ¼ cantaloupe.)

363 calories, 43 g carbohydrate

Exchanges: 1 medium-fat meat, 1 very lean meat, 2 starches (or 1 starch and 1 fruit, optional ¾ fat), 2 vegetables

### Rice Cakes with Cottage Cheese and Tomato

Top 3 rice cakes with sliced tomato, onion, and 1 cup fat-free or 1% cottage cheese mixed with 2 tablespoons ground flaxseed.

330 calories, 33 g carbohydrate

Exchanges: 4 very lean meats, 1½ starches, 1 vegetable, 2 fats

### Peanut Butter Pita and String Cheese

Spread a 70-calorie whole grain pita (or 1 slice whole wheat bread) with 1 level tablespoon peanut butter. Enjoy with 1 or 2 part-skim string cheeses.

320 calories, 18 g carbohydrate

Exchanges: 1 to 2 medium-fat meats, 1 starch, 2 fats

## LUNCH OPTIONS

(400 TO 500 CALORIES, LESS THAN 45 GRAMS CARBOHYDRATE)

### Turkey, Cheese, and Avocado Sandwich

Layer 4 ounces sliced turkey (or chicken), 1 ounce reduced-fat cheese, 2 or 3 thin slices avocado, lettuce, tomato, and onion between 2 slices reduced-calorie whole wheat bread (50 calories or less per slice). Add optional mustard and/or 2 teaspoons reduced-fat mayonnaise or hummus. Enjoy with 1 cup green, red, or yellow pepper strips.

416 calories, 34 g carbohydrate

Exchanges: 1 lean meat, 4 very lean meats, 1 starch, 1 vegetable, 1¾ fats

### Caesar Salad with Grilled Chicken or Shrimp

Top unlimited lettuce leaves with 4 ounces grilled chicken or shrimp, 1 ounce grated Parmesan cheese (4 to 5 level tablespoons), and optional anchovies (4 fillets). Toss with 4 tablespoons reduced-calorie Caesar dressing (40 calories or less per tablespoon) or 2 tablespoons regular Caesar dressing.

413 calories, 22 g carbohydrate

Exchanges: 2 lean meats, 4 very lean meats, 4 fats

### Open-Faced Tuna Melt

Mash 1 can (6 ounces) water-packed light tuna (or chicken or salmon) with 1 tablespoon reduced-fat mayonnaise and minced onion and black pepper and spread on 2 toasted slices reduced-calorie whole grain bread (50 calories or less per slice). Top each half with sliced tomato and 1 slice reduced-fat cheese. Bake in a 350°F oven until the cheese melts. Enjoy with celery stalks and bell pepper strips.

453 calories, 31 g carbohydrate

Exchanges: ¾ lean meat, 6 very lean meats, 1 starch, 1 vegetable, 1 fat

### Turkey Burger with Veggies

Top a 5-ounce lean turkey burger with lettuce, tomato, onion, and 2 tablespoons ketchup and serve on ½ whole grain bun (or in a 70-calorie pita pocket). Enjoy with 1 cup steamed vegetables (broccoli, cauliflower, spinach, etc.) topped with optional 1 tablespoon grated Parmesan cheese.

416 calories, 37 g carbohydrate

Exchanges: ½ lean meat, 5 very lean meats, 2 vegetables

### Edamame with Wild Salmon Dijonnaise

Enjoy 1 cup boiled edamame (green soybeans in the pod) with 5 ounces canned wild salmon, drained, mashed, and mixed with 1 tablespoon reduced-calorie mayonnaise, 1 to 2 teaspoons Dijon mustard, and minced onion and black pepper to taste. Serve on a large bed of leafy greens tossed with unlimited fresh lemon juice or vinegar (or 2 tablespoons low-calorie dressing).

400 calories, 18 g carbohydrate

Exchanges: 1 medium-fat meat, 5 lean meats, 1 starch, 1 vegetable, 1 to 2 fats

### Spinach Salad with Beets, Goat Cheese, and Walnuts

Top a large bed of spinach leaves with ½ cup sliced beets, ½ cup sugar snap peas, 2 ounces soft goat cheese, and 2 tablespoons chopped walnuts. Toss with 2 teaspoons olive oil and unlimited vinegar or fresh lemon juice (or 2 to 4 tablespoons low-calorie dressing).

460 calories, 27 g carbohydrate

Exchanges: 2 medium-fat meats, 5 vegetables, 4 fats

### Mushroom-Cheddar Omelet with Sweet Potato

In a heated pan coated with oil spray, sauté ½ cup sliced mushrooms and ½ cup sliced onion until soft. Beat 1 whole egg with 3 egg whites, pour over the sautéed vegetables, and season with preferred herbs. When the bottom is cooked, gently flip and add 1 ounce reduced-fat cheese. Fold the omelet over and continue cooking until the egg mixture firms and the cheese melts. Enjoy with 2 thin slices avocado plus ½ medium baked sweet or white potato topped with 2 tablespoons fat-free or reduced-fat sour cream.

420 calories and 33 g carbohydrate

Exchanges: 1 medium-fat meat, 1 lean meat, 2⅓ very lean meats, 1 starch, 2 vegetables, 2 fats

### Cottage Cheese with Cantaloupe and Almonds

Fill ½ cantaloupe with 1 cup fat-free or 1% cottage cheese mixed with optional cinnamon, and top with 1 tablespoon slivered almonds (or sunflower seeds).

402 calories, 33 g carbohydrate

Exchanges: 4 very lean meats, 1 fruit, 1 fat

### Grilled Chicken-Pepper Wrap with Avocado

Mix 5 ounces grilled chicken with unlimited chopped onion and red, yellow, and green bell peppers sautéed in oil spray. Wrap in 1 whole grain tortilla (100 calories or less). Enjoy with 3 thin slices avocado and unlimited sliced cucumber.

431 calories, 40 g carbohydrate

Exchanges: 5 very lean meats, 1 starch, 4 vegetables, 2 fats

### Veggie Tuna Salad with Pita

Serve Veggie Tuna Salad (page 271) on a bed of romaine or spinach leaves. Enjoy with mini whole wheat pita (70 calories or less) and 1 cup baby carrots with 2 tablespoons low-calorie salad dressing.

404 calories, 37 g carbohydrate

Exchanges: 6 very lean meats, 6 vegetables, 3 fats

### Baked Fish with Green Beans and Potato

Enjoy 5 ounces grilled or baked fish (Easy! 3-Step Microwave Salmon, page 345, or any other preferred grilled fish) with 1 cup steamed green beans and ½ baked potato topped with 2 tablespoons reduced-fat or fat-free sour cream.

475 calories, 31 g carbohydrate

Exchanges: 5 lean meats, 1 starch, 2 vegetables, 1 fat

### Salad with the Works

Choose one of the following 4-ounce protein options: sardines, canned light tuna in water, wild salmon, chicken, turkey, shrimp, lean roast beef, or tofu. Place on a large bed of leafy greens mixed with ½ chopped pepper (red, yellow, or green), 5 cherry tomatoes, and ¼ cup each sliced mushrooms, chopped cucumbers, sliced beets, chopped red onion, and artichoke hearts. Add 2 tablespoons chickpeas (garbanzo beans), 5 sliced olives, and ¼ chopped avocado. Toss with 2 teaspoons olive oil and unlimited vinegar or fresh lemon juice (or 2 to 4 tablespoons low-calorie dressing).

468 calories, 38 g carbohydrate

Exchanges: 4 very lean meats, 5 vegetables, 4 fats

## DINNER OPTIONS

(500 TO 600 CALORIES, 45 GRAMS OR LESS CARBOHYDRATE)

### Turkey Meatballs in Red Pepper–Tomato Sauce

Enjoy 1 serving Turkey Meatballs in Red Pepper–Tomato Sauce (page 78) with a side salad of 2 cups lettuce, ½ chopped pepper, ¼ sliced onion, ½ cup sliced mushrooms, and ½ chopped cucumber tossed with 2 teaspoons olive oil and unlimited vinegar or fresh lemon juice (or 2 to 4 tablespoons low-calorie dressing).

553 calories, 42 g carbohydrate

Exchanges: 4 lean meats, 1 starch, 6 vegetables, 3 fats

### Pesto Salmon with Roasted Artichoke Hearts and Potato

Enjoy 1 serving Pesto Salmon with Roasted Artichoke Hearts (page 150) or 5 ounces any grilled, baked, poached, or broiled fish with 1 cup steamed vegetables and ½ medium baked sweet potato topped with 1 tablespoon reduced-fat, soft tub, trans-fat-free spread.

550 calories, 39 g carbohydrate

Exchanges: 5 lean meats, 1 starch, 2 vegetables, 2 fats

### Sirloin Steak with Mozzarella and Tomato Salad

Top 5 ounces grilled sirloin steak with optional 2 tablespoons steak sauce or ketchup. Enjoy with mozzarella and tomato salad: Slice ½ red tomato and 1 ounce reduced-fat mozzarella cheese, alternate slices of tomato and mozzarella on a plate, and drizzle with 2 tablespoons low-calorie balsamic vinaigrette. Serve with 12 steamed or grilled asparagus spears.

550 calories, 39 g carbohydrate

Exchanges: 1 medium-fat meat, 5 lean meats, 2 vegetables, 2 fats

### Pork Tenderloin with Cauliflower Mashed "Potatoes"

Enjoy 5 ounces grilled, baked, or broiled lean pork tenderloin with 1 serving Cauliflower Mashed "Potatoes" (page 216) and a side salad of 2 cups lettuce with ¼ cup each chopped bell pepper, onion, cucumber, mushrooms, and grated or chopped carrots tossed with 1 to 2 teaspoons olive oil and unlimited vinegar or fresh lemon juice (or 2 to 4 tablespoons low-calorie salad dressing).

510 calories, 27 g carbohydrate

Exchanges: 5 lean meats, 1 very lean meat, 6 vegetables, 1 to 2 fats

### Orange Pepper Beef Stir-Fry with Cucumber Slices

Enjoy 1 serving Orange Pepper Beef Stir-Fry (page 97) with 1 sliced cucumber.

519 calories, 38 g carbohydrate

Exchanges: 4 lean meats, 1 starch, 4 vegetables, 1½ fats

### Chopped Chicken Salad with Apples and Walnuts

Enjoy 1 serving (page 321).

460 calories, 41 g carbohydrate

Exchanges: 4 very lean meats, ½ starch, 1 vegetable, ½ fruit, 3 fats

### Turkey Tacos with Lettuce, Tomato, and Cheese

Enjoy 3 Turkey Tacos (page 244) with optional salsa and hot sauce.

525 calories, 30 g carbohydrate

Exchanges: 9 very lean meats, 2 starches, 1 vegetable, 1½ fats

### Sweet and Sour Tofu-Veggie Stir-Fry with Edamame

Enjoy 1 serving Sweet and Sour Tofu-Veggie Stir-Fry (page 245) with 1 cup boiled edamame (green soybeans in the pod).

526 calories, 42 g carbohydrate

Exchanges: 1 medium-fat meat, 3 lean meats, 2 starches, 2 vegetables, 1 fat

### Cheddar Burger with Baked Potato

Top a 5-ounce lean hamburger (or turkey or veggie burger) with 1 ounce melted reduced-fat Cheddar cheese, sliced tomato, onion, and optional 2 tablespoons ketchup. Serve on a bed of unlimited leafy greens tossed with 2 tablespoons low-calorie salad dressing. Enjoy with ½ medium plain baked potato topped with 1 tablespoon reduced-fat, soft tub, trans-fat-free spread. (For the potato, you may substitute ½ hamburger bun, preferably whole wheat.)

520 calories, 42 g carbohydrate

Exchanges: 6 lean meats, 1 starch, 2 vegetables, 3 fats

### Satay Chicken with Broccoli and Brown Rice

Enjoy 5 ounces chicken breast, grilled or pan-fried in oil spray, with satay dipping sauce (1 level tablespoon creamy peanut butter mixed with 1 tablespoon reduced-sodium soy sauce and 1 teaspoon minced garlic), 1 cup steamed broccoli, and ½ cup cooked brown rice.

442 calories, 38 g carbohydrate

Exchanges: 5 very lean meats, 1 starch, 2 vegetables, 2 fats

### Shrimp Cocktail with Grilled Fish, Brussels Sprouts, and Brown Rice

Enjoy 5 large shrimp with 1 tablespoon cocktail sauce and 5 ounces fish fillet (wild salmon, flounder, sole, tilapia, or trout), grilled with 1 teaspoon olive oil and preferred seasonings, 1 cup steamed Brussels sprouts, and ½ cup cooked brown rice tossed with 1 tablespoon toasted, slivered almonds.

531 calories, 40 g carbohydrate

Exchanges: 8 very lean meats (if you choose salmon, 3 very lean meats and 5 lean meats), 1 starch, 2 vegetables, 2 fats

### Hearty Turkey Meat Loaf with Cauliflower Mashed "Potatoes"

Enjoy 1 serving Hearty Turkey Meat Loaf (page 149) with 1 serving Cauliflower Mashed "Potatoes" (page 216) or 1 cup steamed cauliflower topped with 1 to 2 tablespoons Parmesan or Romano cheese. Serve with 1 cup steamed green beans (or asparagus or broccoli) tossed with 1 tablespoon reduced-fat, soft tub, trans-fat-free spread and 2 tablespoons toasted slivered almonds.

500 calories, 42 g carbohydrate

Exchanges: 1 lean meat, 4 very lean meats, 1 starch, 5 vegetables, 3 fats

## LOW-CARB SNACK OPTIONS

100 CALORIES OR LESS

- ◆ 1 part-skim string cheese

    80 calories, 0 g carbohydrate

    Exchanges: 1 medium-fat meat

- ◆ 4 hard-cooked egg whites

    80 calories, 0 g carbohydrate

    Exchanges: 2 very lean meats

- ◆ 2 ounces turkey wrapped in lettuce leaves

    70 calories, 2 g carbohydrate

    Exchanges: 2 very lean meats

- ◆ 10 almonds

    80 calories, 3 g carbohydrate

    Exchanges: 2 fats

◆ Celery sticks with 2 tablespoons fat-free cream cheese

  40 calories, 4 g carbohydrate

  Exchanges: 1 very lean meat

◆ Celery sticks with 1 level tablespoon peanut butter

  100 calories, 4 g carbohydrate

  Exchanges: 2 fats

◆ 1 slice reduced-fat cheese on 1 plain rice cake

  100 calories, 7 g carbohydrate

  Exchanges: 1 medium-fat meat, ½ starch

◆ 8 baby carrots with 2 level tablespoons guacamole

  90 calories, 10 g carbohydrate (substitute pepper strips for the carrots
  and carbs drop to 6 grams)

  Exchanges: 2 vegetables, 1 fat

◆ ½ apple, sliced, with 1 level teaspoon peanut butter

  70 calories, 11 g carbohydrate

  Exchanges: ½ fruit, 1 fat

◆ 8 baby carrots and 2 level tablespoons hummus

  85 calories, 13 g carbohydrate (substitute pepper strips for the carrots
  and carbs drop to 9 grams)

  Exchanges: 1½ vegetables, 1 fat

◆ 6 ounces fat-free yogurt (plain or flavored with sugar substitute)

  90 calories, 17 g carbohydrate

  Exchanges: 1 fat-free milk

100 TO 200 CALORIES

◆ ½ cup fat-free or 1% cottage cheese mixed with 1 tablespoon chopped nuts

  130 calories, 4 g carbohydrate

  Exchanges: 2 lean meats, 1 fat

◆ Whole nuts: 1 ounce (¼ cup) almonds, cashews, pecans, walnuts, or peanuts

  180 to 200 calories, 5 g carbohydrate

  Exchanges: 4 fats

◆ ¼ cup roasted edamame

  130 calories, 10 g carbohydrate

  Exchanges: 2 lean meats, 1 starch

◆ ½ cup fat-free or 1% cottage cheese mixed with 2 tablespoons ground flaxseed

  140 calories, 7 g carbohydrate

  Exchanges: 2 lean meats, 2 fats

◆ ½ cup pistachios nuts in the shell

  165 calories, 8 g carbohydrate

  Exchanges: 3 fats

◆ 8 baby carrots dipped in ½ cup fat-free or 1% cottage cheese

  110 calories, 10 g carbohydrate

  Exchanges: 2 lean meats, 1½ vegetables

◆ 1 bell pepper, cut up, with ¼ cup guacamole

  144 calories, 11 g carbohydrate

  Exchanges: 2 vegetables, 2 fats

◆ 1 cup boiled edamame (green soybeans in the pod)

  105 calories, 8 g carbohydrate

  Exchanges: 1 lean meat, ½ starch

◆ 1 bell pepper, cut up, with ¼ cup hummus

  118 calories, 13 g carbohydrate

  Exchanges: 2 vegetables, 2 fats

◆ 10 almonds with 1 apple

  150 calories, 21 g carbohydrate

  Exchanges: 1 fruit, 2 fats

◆ 1 slice reduced-calorie whole wheat toast (50 calories or less) with 1 level tablespoon peanut butter

  140 calories, 14 g carbohydrate

  Exchanges: ½ starch, 2 fats

◆ 6 ounces fat-free yogurt (plain or flavored with sugar substitute) mixed with 2 tablespoons ground flaxseed (or 1 tablespoon chopped nuts)

150 calories, 20 g carbohydrate

Exchanges: 2 fats, 1 fat-free milk

◆ 1 apple, sliced, with 1 level tablespoon peanut butter

180 calories, 23 g carbohydrate

Exchanges: 1 fruit, 2 fats

◆ 1 ounce plain soy crisps

Check labels; nutrition information will vary

Exchanges: 1 lean meat, 1 starch

## SPECIAL SUGAR-FREE RECIPES

◆ Chocolate-Hazelnut Biscotti (page 217)

40 calories, 6 g carbohydrate

Exchanges: ½ starch

◆ Chocolate Angel Food Cake (page 219)

70 calories, 15 g carbohydrate

Exchanges: 1 starch

◆ Sour Cream Coffee Cake with Cinnamon and Walnuts (page 218)

240 calories, 29 g carbohydrate

Exchanges: 2 starches, 2 fats

# CAULIFLOWER MASHED "POTATOES"

*Whether you're watching your carbs or trying to lose weight, or if you simply love hot, creamy comfort food, this recipe is calling your name. It's very popular in my house, and 1 serving provides only 78 calories and 9 grams of carbs.*

**MAKES 4 SERVINGS (¾ CUP EACH)**

1 head cauliflower, cut into florets

¾ cup low-sodium chicken or vegetable broth

1 tablespoon cornstarch

4 ounces fat-free cream cheese

2 tablespoons grated Romano or Parmesan cheese

½ teaspoon garlic powder

¼ teaspoon onion powder

¼ teaspoon paprika

Kosher salt

Ground black pepper

Steam the cauliflower for 15 to 20 minutes, or until tender. Drain. Place in a food processor or blender along with ½ cup of the broth. Puree on high until smooth. Transfer to a medium saucepan.

In a cup, dissolve the cornstarch in the remaining ¼ cup broth and add to the cauliflower puree. Add the cream cheese, Romano or Parmesan, garlic powder, onion powder, and paprika. Cook over medium heat, stirring, for 2 to 3 minutes, or until the puree begins to thicken. Season with salt and pepper to taste. Serve immediately.

**Per serving:** 78 calories, 8 g protein, 9 g carbohydrate, 3 g total sugar, 1 g fat (1 g saturated), 0 mg cholesterol, 262 mg sodium, 3 g fiber

**Exchanges:** 1 very lean meat, 2 vegetables

# CHOCOLATE-HAZELNUT BISCOTTI

*When it came time to test recipes, I knew biscotti had to be included—they are among my personal favorite desserts. I made two batches, one with white flour and one with whole wheat pastry flour, completely expecting the white flour version to taste better. But lo and behold, they were equally fantastic! Take the time to make a batch of these crunchy sugar-free cookies; they're well worth it.*

**MAKES 20**

1½ cups whole wheat pastry flour

1 cup sugar substitute

½ cup unsweetened cocoa powder

1½ tablespoons instant espresso powder

1 teaspoon baking soda

¼ teaspoon kosher salt

2 eggs

2 egg whites

2 teaspoons vanilla extract

1 teaspoon almond extract

¼ cup hazelnuts, toasted and coarsely chopped

Preheat the oven to 300°F. Line a large baking sheet with parchment or waxed paper.

Sift the flour, sugar substitute, cocoa, espresso powder, baking soda, and salt onto a piece of waxed paper or foil. In a large bowl, combine the eggs, egg whites, vanilla, and almond extract. Beat with an electric mixer set on medium speed. Reduce the speed to low and gradually add the flour mixture until a stiff dough forms, adding the hazelnuts after the flour has all been added to the bowl and about half of it is incorporated into the dough.

On a floured surface, divide the dough in half. Form each half into a 12"-long log, pressing the tops down to make the logs about 3" wide. Transfer the logs to the prepared baking sheet, placing them an inch or two apart. Bake for about 40 minutes, or until almost firm to the touch. Remove from the oven and let cool for 10 minutes.

Using a spatula, carefully transfer the logs to a work surface. Using a serrated knife, cut the logs on the diagonal into ½"- to ¾"-thick slices. Arrange the slices, cut sides down, on the baking sheet. Return to the oven and bake for 30 minutes longer, turning once halfway through. Cool completely on a wire rack. Store in an airtight container in the refrigerator for up to 2 weeks.

**Per biscotti:** 40 calories, 2 g protein, 6 g carbohydrate, 0 g total sugar, 1 g fat (0 g saturated), 14 mg cholesterol, 73 mg sodium, 1 g fiber

**Exchanges:** ½ starch

# SOUR CREAM COFFEE CAKE WITH CINNAMON AND WALNUTS

*This is a perfect dessert to bake when you're looking to enjoy something special. It's a bit more caloric and carb-heavy than my other sugar-free sweet treats, but it is definitely lighter and safer for your diet than traditional coffee cake. The walnuts, eggs, and fat-free sour cream lend great taste and help slow the absorption of carbs in the blood.*

**MAKES 8 SERVINGS**

**Topping**

⅔ cup all-purpose flour

⅓ cup sugar substitute

1 teaspoon ground cinnamon

½ teaspoon freshly grated nutmeg

¼ cup reduced-fat, soft tub, trans-fat-free spread, frozen for 15 minutes

**Cake**

¾ cup whole wheat pastry flour

¾ cup all-purpose flour

1¼ cups sugar substitute

1½ teaspoons baking powder

1 teaspoon baking soda

¼ teaspoon kosher salt

1 cup fat-free sour cream

2 eggs

¼ cup canola oil

2 teaspoons vanilla extract

1 teaspoon maple extract

½ cup walnuts, coarsely chopped

Preheat the oven to 350°F. Coat a 9" round springform pan with oil spray.

**To make the topping:** In a small bowl, stir together the flour, sugar substitute, cinnamon, and nutmeg. Add the spread and use a pastry cutter or your fingers to quickly cut or rub in the spread until coarse crumbs form. Cover and refrigerate.

**To make the cake:** On a piece of waxed paper, sift the whole wheat flour, all-purpose flour, sugar substitute, baking powder, baking soda, and salt. In a large bowl, whisk together the sour cream, eggs, oil, vanilla, and maple extract until well blended. Add the flour mixture. Using an electric mixer on medium speed or a wire whisk, beat for 1 to 2 minutes, or until smooth and creamy.

Spoon half of the batter into the prepared pan and spread evenly. Sprinkle evenly with half of the topping. Cover evenly with the remaining batter. Sprinkle evenly with the nuts, gently pressing them into the batter. Cover with the remaining topping.

Bake for 40 to 45 minutes, or until the topping is golden brown and a wooden pick inserted into the center of the cake comes out clean. Transfer the pan to a wire rack and let cool for 20 minutes. Remove the sides of the springform pan. Serve the cake warm or at room temperature, cut into wedges.

**Per serving:** 240 calories, 6 g protein, 29 g carbohydrate, 0 g total sugar, 12 g fat (2 g saturated), 45 mg cholesterol, 323 mg sodium, 2 g fiber

**Exchange:** 2 fats, 2 starches

# Chocolate Angel Food Cake

*You won't believe that there are just 70 calories in one slice of this light, airy cake—and no sugar at all! Serve it at your next dinner party and no one will know the difference.*

**MAKES 8 SERVINGS**

¾ cup whole wheat pastry flour

1½ cups sugar substitute

¼ cup unsweetened cocoa powder

2 teaspoons instant espresso powder

1½ cups egg whites (from about 10 eggs)

¼ teaspoon kosher salt

2 teaspoons vanilla extract

Preheat the oven to 350°F. Coat a 10" angel food cake pan with oil spray.

In a large bowl, sift the flour, sugar substitute, cocoa powder, and espresso powder three times. Set aside.

In a large metal bowl, beat the egg whites with the salt on high speed for 4 to 6 minutes, or until they become stiff but not lumpy. They should cling firmly to the side of the bowl when tilted. Add the vanilla but do not mix.

With a spatula, gently fold one-third of the egg whites into the flour mixture. Repeat twice, until all of the egg whites are just combined but not deflated.

Gently spread the batter into the prepared pan. Bake for 35 to 40 minutes, or until the cake springs back when touched. Remove from the oven and invert the pan onto its feet or the neck of a wine bottle. Let cool completely.

Gently run a long knife between the cake and the outer rim of the pan, pressing it firmly against the pan to prevent tearing the cake. Run the knife or a skewer around the inside of the tube. Invert the pan and remove the cake.

**Per serving:** 70 calories, 7 g protein, 15 g carbohydrate, 0 g total sugar, 0 g fat, 0 mg cholesterol, 144 mg sodium, 2 g fiber

**Exchange:** 1 starch

# CHAPTER 10

# OSTEOPOROSIS

All too often, the first sign of osteoporosis is a broken bone. For my client Janice, it was her wrist. At age 64, her overall good health was the envy of more than one of her close friends—she felt good, looked younger than her age, and regularly saw her internist and gynecologist for routine checkups. Then she slipped and fell in the snow, and osteoporosis, which had been silently developing for years, made itself known.

Osteoporosis is defined by low bone mineral density (BMD), as measured by an x-ray bone density scan. If a scan shows your bone density is a bit low, your diagnosis is osteopenia, or preosteoporosis. If your BMD is quite low, the diagnosis is osteoporosis. The results of bone density scans are expressed in terms of T-scores. Scores ranging from –1.0 to –2.5 indicate osteopenia; less than –2.5 means osteoporosis.

Regardless of the cause, if you have low bone density, you're facing a higher-than-average risk of breaking a bone. If you are lucky, your doctor will recognize some of the risk factors and send you for a bone density scan before you have to endure the pain and recovery of a break. Unfortunately for Janice, the first clue was that sickening crunch of her wrist.

When I first saw Janice, she had just started taking osteoporosis medication, but her doctor wanted her to have an intensive nutrition intervention as well. During our first meeting, I found out why she needed my help. She ate terribly, making meals from whatever food was on hand—generally, lots of processed foods—without giving a thought to what nutrients she might be missing.

I rose to the challenge. I gave Janice a thorough lesson in osteoporosis and a comprehensive meal plan filled with food choices rich in nutrients that would help her condition (more about these in the pages to follow). I also recommended that she start taking a calcium supplement with vitamin $D_3$ (cholecalciferol, the most potent form of vitamin D). I explained the benefits of exercise and how to alternate strength training and weight-bearing aerobic exercises. I suggested that she walk on the treadmill five times per week, 40 minutes per session, at a speed of 3.5 miles per hour. By the time Janice left, I felt confident that she had all the tools she needed to turn a corner.

## FAQS

**I know I need to get more calcium in my diet because my diet is pretty bad. I don't exercise much, and I've always been on the thin side, so I guess I could be at risk of developing osteoporosis. If I'm taking a multivitamin with calcium in it, do I really need to take a separate calcium supplement, too?**

Calcium is bulky, so there is no way to fit a day's supply in a multivitamin. Most multivitamins have, at most, 100 to 200 milligrams of calcium—much less than the 1,000 to 1,200 milligrams you'll need. So yes, you really should be taking a separate calcium supplement. But if you radically change your diet, you can definitely get enough calcium from diet alone.

Start counting your servings of high-calcium foods. If you consistently eat at least three servings of a high-calcium food every day, you're probably safe. But if your diet is erratic, then take 500 to 600 milligrams of calcium with vitamin $D_3$ once a day, either in the morning or afternoon. By the evening, think back to how you ate during the day: If you ate two or more servings of a high-calcium food, then you can skip the evening dose. If not, take an additional 500 to 600 milligrams with a snack before bed. (However, if you have been diagnosed with osteoporosis or osteopenia, always follow your doctor's instructions, which may be to take the second dose of calcium regardless of how much calcium you've consumed from food.) Your body can only absorb about 500 milligrams of calcium at one time, so if you require a large amount from supplements, it's important to split your calcium into two daily doses rather than taking 1,000 to 1,200 milligrams in a single tablet.

If you find that taking calcium supplements causes constipation, try taking a supplement that includes magnesium, as well as vitamin D. The magnesium acts as a gentle laxative and helps keep you regular.

Two weeks later, Janice returned to the office with her food journal filled out and ready for my evaluation. She had done nothing! Well, next to nothing. She took the calcium supplements, but she didn't exercise, and, most distressing of all, she had made no changes to her diet.

Janice understood my instructions, but when it came time to implement them, she felt overwhelmed. Embracing a new way of eating meant breaking the eating habits she'd established decades ago. She'd never been that interested in planning and cooking meals anyway. To my eyes—brutal honesty alert!—her eating life was just so boring. Every day for breakfast Janice ate a toasted English muffin with peanut butter and washed it down with a cup of black coffee. Every morning. For years! The thing was, it didn't matter to her. She ate the same foods day in and day out because it was just easier that way. I have nothing against peanut butter or whole wheat English muffins—that's a fine quick breakfast—but it didn't supply her with essential nutrients, and it did nothing to help her fight low BMD.

I learned an important lesson from Janice. I know I advised her well nutritionally, but there's a second, sometimes greater challenge to tackle beyond that: changing a lifetime of apparently harmless eating habits. Janice felt healthy. Janice looked terrific. But all the while, Janice's bones had quietly been losing mass, becoming thinner and thinner. Breaking her wrist was frightening and painful, but it didn't mean she could instantly embrace a whole new way of eating.

I decided to try another tactic. This time, I gave Janice three specific goals to focus on. First, I told her that if she wanted to eat the same foods for breakfast day after day, that was fine, but she had to switch to foods that would specifically address her needs—namely, cereal with fat-free milk, sliced banana, and a glass of calcium-fortified orange juice. Second, she could eat whatever she wanted for dinner, but she had to eat a high-calcium appetizer. She decided on a predinner salad of leafy greens topped with 1 ounce of feta or shredded Cheddar cheese and, in signature Janice fashion, ate that every day. And third, I instructed her to eat a snack of yogurt before bed. Those changes alone gave her four hits of high-calcium, bone-strengthening foods (plus potassium from the orange juice, dairy, and banana; vitamin C from orange juice; vitamin K from leafy greens; and vitamin D from the morning milk). Thanks to Janice being such a creature of habit, she was consistently getting so much calcium from her diet that her physician and I decided to put a halt on her calcium supplement. (She continued to take a solid multi with ample vitamin D.) In addition, Janice joined a local gym and started doing strength-training exercises there with a friend three days a week.

At the end of a year, these few changes (with medication) helped Janice do more than arrest bone loss—she actually increased bone density in her spine.

Initially, Janice was one of the least-compliant people I've ever seen in my practice. So why am I telling you her story? Because you don't have to be perfect right off the bat or at every meal to see real results. By the end of this chapter, you'll have all the tools you need to make your bones healthier. It's a lot of information. If you can't do it all right away, that's perfectly fine. Take one step. Then another. Eventually, all those little steps add up. But you have to take action—your bones are too important to ignore.

## WHAT AFFECTS OSTEOPOROSIS?

Children are taught that bones are like steel girders, the framework of the glorious structure that is the human body. The problem with that analogy is that girders are designed to last hundreds of years without losing strength. In reality, bones are more like the interstate highway system: They fall apart, crack, get potholes, and then get patched up again so we can continue using them.

Nor are our bones uniformly dense. The outer layer is called compact bone, and it is relatively solid. But just under the compact bone is another layer called spongy bone, which is porous, with holes like a sponge or Swiss cheese. And because bone is live tissue, there are also nerves and blood vessels to feed the cells, as well as other structures. Bones also contain specialized cells that help form it (osteoblasts) and break down or resorb it (osteoclasts). Osteoclasts and osteoblasts work like little construction crews, constantly remodeling, working to keep the bones healthy and strong. If your overall health is good and you eat nutritionally sound meals, there is a balance—for every bit of bone lost, an equal amount is created.

With osteoporosis, though, more bone is lost than formed. As you might imagine, the spongy bone, with all its holes and slender walls, becomes weak and compromised more quickly than compact bone does. Breaks can occur anywhere, but the most common sites are the hip and wrist, which are more likely to bear the impact of a fall. The bones of the back (vertebrae) are also affected, but they don't break—they are crushed. The weight of the body is enough to compress the back bones, causing a multitude of tiny fractures in the spongy bone. Over time, people with osteoporosis can become shorter—they lose a little height each time a vertebra compresses.

No one knows definitively what causes some people to develop osteoporosis, but several factors are clear.

## HORMONAL CHANGES

Estrogen and testosterone are important for bone health because they regulate bone loss, or resorption. Both these hormones seem to inhibit the formation of osteoclasts (the cells that break down bone), so when hormone levels are high, there are more bone-building cells than bone-destroying cells. If hormone levels fall, the balance shifts and bone density is lost.

The question, then, is what causes levels of estrogen or testosterone to fall? The most common cause is aging. Men can develop osteoporosis when they get older as testosterone levels slowly decline. For women, menopause causes an extreme drop in estrogen, and their greatest bone loss occurs within the first ten years after menopause.

## FAQS

### I've heard that coffee makes your body lose calcium. Is that true?

Yes, it is true that the caffeine in coffee can slightly decrease calcium absorption, but research has shown that the effect is minimal. In fact, the amount of calcium lost is so small that it can be completely offset simply by adding 1 to 2 tablespoons of milk to each cup of joe. (For overall health, choose fat-free or 1% milk or soy milk.) Even if you drink your coffee black, experts have concluded that moderate amounts of caffeine from coffee or tea do not negatively impact bone health or increase the risk of osteoporosis, *as long as you consume adequate calcium in your diet.* (That's 1,000 mg a day for adults under 50 and 1,200 mg a day for adults over 50.) So, provided that you eat a calcium-rich diet—and take in at least 800 IU of vitamin D, which is just as critical to bone health as calcium—you can continue to enjoy moderate amounts of coffee without concern.

That's why many physicians recommend that women get a bone density scan when they turn 50 or when they enter menopause, whichever comes first. That first test acts as a baseline. The scan should be repeated one or two years later to get a sense of the rate of bone loss.

Menopause isn't the only female condition that triggers osteoporosis. Unfortunately, eating disorders can take a toll on the bones, too. When a woman's weight drops too low, her hormones get out of whack, her estrogen levels fall, and she stops menstruating. In terms of bone health, a too-thin woman in her twenties looks a lot like a postmenopausal woman in her sixties. The only real cure is for the young woman to gain enough weight to start menstruating again and then to maximize her bone density while she can—that is, until about age 30, when bone density reaches its peak.

## CORTICOSTEROIDS

Corticosteroid medications are used to treat a number of common illnesses, including asthma and some autoimmune disorders. But steroids seem to inhibit bone-building activity and may also increase bone resorption. It has been estimated that up to half of all people who take steroids long-term will end up with osteoporosis. Significant bone loss can occur after even a relatively short course of corticosteroids—taking common steroid medications for two to three months may require treatment to prevent bone loss.

## BODY WEIGHT

Bones get stronger if they get more use. In the earlier stages of life, exercise helps build bone. And as much as it pains me to say it, weight builds bone. When it comes to osteoporosis, thin women have a greater risk than heavy women. Think about it: Bones that support a 170-pound woman work harder than bones that carry a 110-pound woman. Studies have shown that lean muscle mass helps strengthen bone density more than fat does, but overall weight still contributes to strong bones.

Of course, my advice is not for you to put on a few pounds for the sake of strengthening your bones! Being overweight puts you at greater risk for so many life-threatening diseases that it is never a wise choice. But women who diet excessively to keep their weight fashionably low are hurting their bones, now and in the future.

## OTHER DISEASES

Any disorder that reduces the body's ability to absorb calcium and other nutrients can cause osteoporosis. The most common is celiac disease, an autoimmune disorder that causes the small intestines to lose their absorption capability. Previously thought to be a rare childhood disease, celiac disease is now known to affect about 1 percent of Americans and can strike at any age. (For more information, see Celiac Disease, page 414.)

## HOW FOOD AFFECTS OSTEOPOROSIS

Next to genetic predisposition, poor nutrition is the most common cause of osteoporosis. Making healthy food choices can help prevent dangerous bone loss, and food is one of the most important treatments recommended by physicians and nutritionists alike once osteopenia or osteoporosis is diagnosed.

## GOOD FOODS TO CHOOSE

It is important to ensure that you're getting the right amount of calcium, vitamin D, and other bone-building vitamins and minerals. Protein also plays an important role in the prevention and management of osteoporosis.

### Calcium and Vitamin D

When it comes to osteoporosis prevention or treatment, the two most important nutrients are calcium and vitamin D.

Bone is made mostly of calcium. In addition, calcium fuels many other bodily functions, such as muscle movement, nerve operation, and immune activation. Typically, we get our daily dose of calcium from food. But if your diet isn't the greatest, your body will use your bones as a lending institution, borrowing the calcium it needs from the abundant supply in your bones. This creates a kind of calcium debt, and if you eat enough high-calcium foods to keep functioning, any excess will be used to pay back the debt. But if you eat poorly, the debt

## FAQS

### I've heard that calcium can be leached from bones by the phosphorus in soda. Is that true?

Soda is definitely bad for your bones, but scientists haven't yet figured out if the phosphoric acid found in it is partly to blame. Some researchers believe phosphoric acid leaches calcium from our bones or interferes with calcium metabolism in other ways, but our understanding is still limited. Others hypothesize that the overall ratio of calcium to phosphorus intake in the diet has a bigger impact on bone health than phosphorus intake on its own.

Another plausible explanation for the link between high soda intake and low bone mass is that soda often elbows out calcium-rich milk as our drink of choice. Back in the "good old days," kids drank milk with lunch and dinner (and they often started the day with a bowl of cereal and milk rather than a sugary-sweet toaster pastry!). Some studies have shown that kids who drink soda instead of milk have lower bone density than kids who get plenty of calcium in their diets. The same is true for adults. So while soda appears to be partially to blame for low bone density, we'll have to wait and see *why* this is the case. Causality aside, I highly encourage you to cut soda out of your diet and replace it with healthy beverages like water, fat-free or 1% milk, naturally flavored seltzer, and unsweetened coffee and tea.

never gets repaid. While you can skate by for a few years, eventually the debt will catch up with you in the form of weakened, thinning bones.

As we physically develop, our bones get denser and denser if we supply them with calcium by eating calcium-rich foods. After about age 30, our bones are as dense as they will ever be. That's why it is so important for children and young adults to get enough calcium in their diets; if they later need to "borrow" calcium from their bones, strong, dense bones are the equivalent of a high spending limit on a credit card. After menopause, all women lose bone density because of hormonal changes. A woman with dense bones will be able to lose some density without developing osteoporosis. After menopause, it is still important to get enough calcium so that you don't run up a larger calcium debt than is necessary.

On the other hand, it is possible to get too much of good thing. Most people struggle to get the recommended 1,000 to 1,300 milligrams of calcium daily. But some folks can't help but go overboard when they finally see the light about bone health—they change their diets and take excessive amounts of supplements. Unfortunately, you can't make up for lost calcium overnight. The upper recommended limit for calcium consumption is 2,500 milligrams per day for women under 50 and 2,000 milligrams per day for women over 50. Taking more than this amount can reduce your body's ability to absorb other minerals and may lead to kidney stones.

One interesting note: Some foods—most notably, spinach and rhubarb—contain lots of calcium, but they also contain oxalates, substances that bind to the calcium, making it unavailable to your body. My list of calcium-rich foods includes only the absolute best sources, so every serving serves your bones.

**BEST FOODS FOR CALCIUM:** *yogurt (fat-free, low-fat), milk (fat-free, 1%), soy milk, cheese (fat-free, reduced-fat), tofu with calcium (check nutrition label), soybeans (edamame), frozen yogurt (fat-free, low-fat), low-fat ice cream, bok choy, kale, white beans, collard greens, broccoli, almonds and almond butter*

Calcium is useless without vitamin D. Vitamin D allows calcium to move from the gastrointestinal tract to the parts of the body that need it—including the bones. Without enough vitamin D, a child's bones can become so weak that they bow under the body's own weight, a condition called rickets. In adults, lack of vitamin D means that the body borrows calcium from bones to feed the rest of its needs. Eventually, osteoporosis will set in.

Vitamin D can be made in the body when the skin is exposed to sunlight. Just 10 to 15 minutes of sun on the bare skin of the arms three or four times a week is enough to keep most of us healthy. Of course, too much sunlight causes skin damage and premature aging and may lead to skin cancer. That's why I recommend getting vitamin D primarily from food sources and supplements. Since few foods are rich in vitamin D, you may need to take a supplement (or a multivitamin that contains vitamin D) in order to take in at least 800 IU of vitamin D daily (my personal recommendation for healthy adults).

BEST FOODS FOR VITAMIN D: *wild salmon (fresh, canned), mackerel (not king), sardines, herring, milk (fat-free, 1%), soy milk, fortified yogurt (fat-free, low-fat), egg yolks, vitamin D-enhanced mushrooms**

**These mushrooms are treated with UV light, which dramatically increases their vitamin D content.*

## Other Nutrients

Although calcium and vitamin D are the superstars of osteoporosis prevention and treatment, there are many other nutrients that play supporting roles.

**Magnesium:** You don't need a chemistry class to know that acids can be corrosive. The same is true for acids formed in your body during the process of metabolism. These metabolic acids need to be balanced and neutralized by alkaline compounds; otherwise, they can cause bone loss. Magnesium can help neutralize these acids. Furthermore, magnesium plays an integral role in bone crystal growth, thereby helping to strengthen bone structure.

In addition, magnesium helps your body absorb calcium. For calcium to be absorbed in the body, it needs vitamin D (as we already discussed) and parathyroid hormone (PTH). Because magnesium affects PTH, it indirectly—but very critically—affects how much calcium is available for building and maintaining bone.

While the scientific research is mixed, some studies show that a high magnesium intake can increase bone density or decrease the risk of fractures. You don't necessarily need to reach for a supplement, though. Magnesium is found in a wide variety of healthy foods, so you can definitely reach your daily quota if you make an effort to load up on magnesium-rich ingredients.

BEST FOODS FOR MAGNESIUM: *pumpkin seeds, spinach, Swiss chard, amaranth, sunflower seeds, cashews, almonds, quinoa, tempeh, potatoes (sweet, white), soybeans (edamame), millet, starchy beans (such as black, navy, pinto, garbanzo, kidney), artichoke hearts, peanuts and peanut butter, brown rice, whole grain bread, sesame seeds, wheat germ, flaxseed*

**Potassium** aids in bone formation, improves calcium balance, increases bone mineral density, and reduces bone resorption by neutralizing metabolic acids. Researchers from the United Kingdom looked at the effects of dietary potassium on the bone mineral density of more than 3,000 pre- and postmenopausal women. For women who were still menstruating, eating lots of potassium-rich foods increased bone mineral density by 8 percent—a relatively modest gain but one that the researchers estimated could translate into a 30 percent reduced risk of fracture in later years.

## FAQS

### My kids won't drink milk, and I can't stand drinking it myself. Should I worry about the amount of calcium we're getting?

Milk is an easy source of calcium, but it is certainly not the only one. All dairy foods contain calcium, and many kids enjoy eating yogurt and cheese. Whenever possible, substitute foods your kids already eat with calcium-fortified versions. For example, there are calcium-fortified waffles and orange juice.

For children ages 1 to 3, aim for 500 milligrams of calcium per day, which equates to about two servings of calcium-rich foods. Kids 4 to 8 years old require 800 milligrams per day, or three servings of calcium-rich foods. Older children and teens (ages 9 to 18) need 1,300 milligrams per day, which equates to about four servings of calcium-rich foods. If your children consistently fall short on calcium, you can try one of the candy-flavored calcium chews. In my experience, most kids don't like the chocolate flavors that adults are drawn to; they may eat them for a couple of days, but then the appeal wears off. Instead, choose one of the other flavors, such as caramel or fruity flavors. (Always be careful to store supplements where your children can't get them. If they think of them as candy, you can bet they'll be looking for opportunities to grab extras, and too much calcium can be dangerous.)

Another way to slip some calcium and vitamin D into your kids' diets is to buy a pill crusher at your local pharmacy and mix one crushed calcium pill into yogurt, pudding, or another soft food your kids eat regularly.

Of course, it is difficult to separate the effects of potassium specifically from the effects of fruits and vegetables in general. Fruits and veggies, many of which contain significant quantities of potassium, have a whole rainbow of nutrients that contribute to bone health. They also contain compounds that can neutralize the acid load in the body. A diet void of produce generates a high acidity level in the body, which can weaken bones over time. The important takeaway is that produce, rich in potassium and other beneficial nutrients, can help keep your bones as healthy and strong as possible.

BEST FOODS FOR POTASSIUM: *white potatoes, yogurt (fat-free, low-fat), soybeans (edamame), Swiss chard, all fish, sweet potatoes, avocados, cantaloupe, artichokes, bananas, spinach, lettuce, honeydew, pumpkin, milk (fat-free, 1%), carrots, starchy beans (such as black, navy, pinto, garbanzo, kidney), lentils, lima beans, apricots, papayas, split peas, pistachios, winter squash (acorn, butternut), soy milk, watermelon, beets, tomatoes, kale, mushrooms, raisins, peanuts, plums, almonds, sunflower seeds, prunes, oranges, broccoli*

**Vitamin K** is essential for the formation of osteocalcin, a type of protein found only in bone. High intake of vitamin K has been linked to lower risk of fractures in some populations. Therefore, I highly recommend loading up on foods rich in vitamin K. One caveat: Vitamin K is a natural blood thinner, so people taking blood-thinning medication (such as warfarin) should talk with their doctors before eating vitamin K–rich foods.

BEST FOODS FOR VITAMIN K: *kale, spinach, collard greens, Swiss chard, turnip greens, endive, escarole, mustard greens, lettuce (all varieties), parsley, broccoli, broccoli raab, Brussels sprouts, watercress, asparagus, okra*

**Vitamin C** is essential for the health of collagen, a key protein that contributes strength and resilience to bone tissue. Some studies have shown that eating lots of foods high in vitamin C increases bone mineral density and results in fewer fractures. A Tufts University study found that older men who consumed the most vitamin C experienced less bone loss over a four-year period, but the same relationship was not seen in women. More research is needed to understand the relationship between vitamin C and bone health during aging, but regardless of future findings, it's a good idea to consume plenty of vitamin C–rich produce.

BEST FOODS FOR VITAMIN C: *guava, bell peppers (all colors), oranges and orange juice, grapefruit and grapefruit juice, strawberries, pineapple, kohlrabi, papayas, lemons and lemon juice, broccoli, kale, Brussels sprouts, kidney beans, kiwifruit, cantaloupe, cauliflower, cabbage (all varieties), mangoes, white potatoes, mustard greens, tomatoes, sugar snap peas, snow peas, clementines, rutabagas, turnip greens, raspberries, blackberries, watermelon, tangerines, okra, lychees, summer squash, persimmons*

**Protein:** For many years, conventional wisdom was that protein increased the risk of osteoporosis because people who ate large amounts of it had a large amount of calcium in their urine. Scientists thought that protein was somehow leaching calcium from the bones, which then found its way out of the body through urine. Excessive amounts of protein may indeed pose a problem. However, more recent research suggests that eating too little protein is just as harmful to bone health, if not more so, than overdoing it.

Protein is an important component of bone and absolutely necessary for bone strength. Studies show that people who don't get adequate protein may have reduced calcium absorption, lower bone density, and higher rates of bone loss. People who eat relatively large amounts of protein have a reduced risk of fractures and higher bone mineral density. Older women, the primary group affected by osteoporosis, are especially at risk and need to take extra care to make sure they're incorporating quality proteins into meals and snacks.

Although more research needs to be done to unravel the complicated relationship between protein intake and bone health, a few studies suggest that vegetarian proteins (like beans, lentils, and whole soy foods) may be more beneficial to bone health than animal proteins. But, as mentioned earlier, too much protein from any source may still be harmful, so don't go protein crazy: no high-protein/carb-free diets or excessive amounts of protein bars or shakes.

The bottom line is that you need to ensure that you're getting an appropriate amount of protein through lean meats, skinless poultry, fish, eggs, beans, lentils, dairy, soy foods, and nuts. What defines "appropriate" depends on your weight.

Here's a simple rule of thumb: Take your weight and divide it in half—that's approximately how many grams of protein you need to eat every day for good bone health. For example, if you weigh 140 pounds, you need about 70 grams of protein each day. And remember that lean animal proteins—such as skinless poultry, seafood, and lean steak—are incredibly rich sources of protein, meaning that just a small 3-ounce cooked portion (about the size of your palm) can provide between 20 and 25 grams. Depending on your size, that can be one-third of your daily protein needs.

Also keep in mind that fattier cuts of beef will provide *less* protein per ounce than leaner cuts will. That's because the fat content takes up space and displaces protein. Reduced-fat and fat-free milk, cheese, and yogurt can sometimes even provide *more* calcium per ounce than their full-fat counterparts do, for the same reason. When fat is removed, the lost volume is replaced with more calcium-rich, reduced-fat dairy. Double bonus—less saturated fat, more calcium!

BEST FOODS FOR PROTEIN: *yogurt (fat-free, low-fat), milk (fat-free, 1%), cheese (fat-free, reduced-fat), starchy beans (such as black, navy, pinto, garbanzo, kidney), lentils, split peas, tofu, tempeh, soybeans (edamame), soy milk, nuts and nut butters, seeds and seed butters, egg whites, skinless turkey, skinless chicken, fish and shellfish, pork tenderloin, lean beef*

| FOOD | APPROXIMATE GRAMS OF PROTEIN |
|---|---|
| 1 egg | 6 |
| 1 cup milk (fat-free, 1%) | 8 |
| 1 ounce cheese (fat-free, reduced-fat) | 7–14 |
| ½ cup cottage cheese (fat-free, 1%) | 14 |
| 1 cup fat-free yogurt | 8–14 |
| ½ cup beans | 7–9 |
| 1 ounce almonds | 6 |
| 1 ounce peanuts | 8 |
| 1 ounce soy nuts | 12 |
| 6 ounces tofu | 15 |
| 1 ounce lean beef, poultry, or fish | 7 |
| 5 ounces skinless chicken breast or fish fillet | 35 |
| 3 ounces sirloin steak (size of a deck of cards) | 21 |

## FOODS TO LIMIT

While plenty of nutrients help your bones, there are some that may cause harm when consumed in excessive amounts. Here's what you need to know about limiting your intake of vitamin A and salt.

### Vitamin A

Too much vitamin A can harm bones, increasing the risk of fractures. Although more research needs to be done, it looks as though too much vitamin A may stop vitamin D from doing its job of making calcium available to bones. In food, vitamin A comes from beta-carotene and retinol, and recent studies suggest that only retinol causes problems. To avoid overdosing on retinol, the troublesome form of vitamin A, do not regularly eat liver or foods that are fortified with vitamin A. In addition, your multivitamin should provide no more than 100 percent DV for vitamin A, and at least half of that should come from beta-carotene or mixed carotenoids. Look for this information on your bottle's nutrient listing, right next to vitamin A.

### Salt

Salt causes the body to lose a little bit of calcium through what scientists call renal excretion and what everyone else calls peeing. The actual amount is very small, but if you are already fighting a calcium deficiency or if you have bone density problems, every little bit counts. In addition, salt seems to increase bone resorption. Limit your salt intake, and on those days when salt can't be avoided, just try to eat an extra serving of reduced-fat dairy to make up for it.

## BONUS POINTS

◆ **Talk with your doctor about osteoporosis prevention.** Because every individual is different, it is important to learn about your particular risk of osteoporosis as soon as possible. Topics to discuss include whether you need to get a bone density scan, whether your personal medical history and genetic makeup increase your likelihood of developing osteoporosis in the future, and whether some of the new bone-building medications might be right for you.

◆ **Exercise.** When you're younger, exercise helps build and maintain strong bones by turning on bone-building activities. When you move your muscles (and, by extension, your bones), the action stimulates osteoblasts to create more bone. That's why it's critical for children and young adults to get plenty of exercise during their bone-building years. However, exercise remains vital to maintaining your bone health even in later years. Regular strength-training has been shown to preserve or even slightly increase bone density in older adults. Physical activity also maintains muscle tone and strength surrounding the bone and will help prevent falls and injuries that could lead to breaks and fractures. Weight-bearing exercises—those that require you to move against gravity while standing upright, such as walking, jogging, and low-impact aerobics—are very helpful. Even better, however, are strength-training or resistance exercises like lunges, planks, pushups, and exercises that require resistance bands, dumbbells, free weights, or weight machines. (Even water jugs and soup cans make great weights.) These types of exercises build healthy lean muscle mass, which in turn protects your precious bone tissue underneath.

◆ **Maintain a healthy weight.** Although many women believe that there is no such thing as "too thin," there is. Eating disorders, gastrointestinal issues, and other medical problems can cause weight to drop to levels that are unhealthy for bones. Check your BMI on page 19 to see if you fall into the category called underweight. If so, you might want to consider talking with your doctor about how to bring your weight up to a healthy level.

◆ **Stop smoking.** For more than 20 years, smoking has been linked with a higher risk of osteoporosis, but the reasons why aren't clear. It could be that people who smoke have other risk factors that make them more likely to have low bone density, such as lower body weight, infrequent exercise, or poor food choices. It could also be that cigarette smoke spurs changes in some body hormones that might trigger bone loss. Some research with laboratory animals suggests that nicotine may have a direct effect on bone—namely, inhibiting the production of bone-building osteoblasts.

◆ **Encourage those you love to stop smoking.** You want the people you love to protect their health, but on a more selfish level, their smoking may be hurting your bones. Harvard researchers studied bone health in more than 14,000 people in China and discovered that nonsmoking women who were exposed to secondhand smoke were three times more likely to develop osteoporosis than women who had no exposure to smoke. The theory is that cigarette smoke may affect levels of estrogen, a hormone that regulates bone turnover. If you can't persuade the smoker in your life to quit the habit, try to establish house rules (such as only smoking outdoors) that will minimize your exposure.

◆ **Drink alcohol only in moderation.** Drinking alcohol to excess is undeniably harmful to your bones. Heavy drinkers are more prone to bone loss and accidental falls, which can result in fractures. That said, preliminary research suggests that light drinking may actually help preserve bone strength. In a study of hundreds of women ages 65 to 77, researchers discovered that women who did not drink alcohol at all had the lowest bone density of all. Bone density was highest in women who drank two to four alcoholic drinks per week (not per day!). Women who drank more than four alcoholic drinks per week had lower total body bone mineral density (although it was still higher than for nondrinkers). Scientists believe that small amounts of alcohol may reduce bone breakdown, perhaps by increasing levels of estrogen. I *don't* recommend that nondrinkers start imbibing as a way to maintain bone density. However, if you do drink, you can continue to do so in moderation without fear of weakening your bones. For overall good health, women should limit their intake to no more than one drink per day; men should have no more than two drinks per day.

♦ **Yo-yo no more.** Even though thin women are generally more susceptible to osteoporosis than overweight women are, women who are chronic dieters may also be at increased risk of weak bones regardless of how much they weigh. Researchers believe that years of dieting cause women to eat so poorly that they don't get the nutrients needed to build bones up to a healthy, strong level. Dieting by severely restricting food intake is never a good idea. If you want a better way to lose weight, see Weight Loss on page 17.

## SUPPLEMENTS

If you are concerned about osteoporosis or have been diagnosed with osteopenia and want to consider supplements in addition to food fixes, I have some recommendations.

1. **A multivitamin.** Because so many micronutrients are important for bone health, I always recommend taking a multivitamin. Look for a brand that contains at least 800 IU vitamin D in the form of $D_3$ (cholecalciferol, the most potent form) and at least 100 milligrams (25 percent DV) of magnesium. Your multi should also provide no more than 100 percent DV of vitamin A (with at least half of that coming from beta-carotene or mixed carotenoids). Avoid iron in your supplement, unless you are a premenopausal woman.

2. **Calcium with vitamin D (and optional magnesium).** I always prefer that women get their calcium from food, but if you're not consistently consuming at least three daily servings of calcium-rich foods or beverages, you may want to consider taking a separate supplement. When buying supplements, remember that calcium is worthless without vitamin D, so make sure you're getting a total of at least 800 IU vitamin $D_3$ through your multi and/or calcium supplement. Also consider buying a brand with additional magnesium, especially if you're not eating magnesium-rich foods.

   If you and your doctor decide that you're a good candidate for calcium supplements, here's a good strategy to follow: Take 500 to 600 milligrams of calcium every morning with breakfast. (Check your specific brand label to see how many individual pills you need to get that dose.) Then, right after dinner, tally up how many servings of calcium-rich foods you've consumed that day. If you've consumed at least two servings, you can skip the evening supplemental dose of calcium. The following foods count as one serving: 1 cup milk, 1 cup yogurt, 1 ounce cheese, 1 cup cooked collard greens, and 1 cup calcium-fortified beverages (such as soy milk, almond milk, or orange juice). If you haven't had at least two servings, go ahead and take the second dose right after dinner. If your doctor is adamant that you take a full supplemental dose of 1,000-plus milligrams every day (regardless of how much calcium you've taken in through food), be sure to split the total amount into two doses taken several hours apart, because your body can absorb up to only 600 milligrams of calcium at one time.

The two most common forms of calcium supplements are calcium carbonate and calcium citrate. Calcium carbonate supplements must be taken with food to be well absorbed, so you should always take them with or just after a meal. Calcium citrate supplements can be absorbed on an empty stomach, so you don't need to take them with food—you can take them whenever is most convenient. Also, calcium citrate supplements are generally better tolerated by individuals with gastrointestinal issues. The drawback to calcium citrate supplements is that you typically need to take twice as many pills as you would of calcium carbonate to get the same amount of calcium.

**Special note for men:** I never recommend calcium supplements to men. Some studies have shown a link between high calcium intake and increased risk of prostate cancer. Men should have no trouble meeting their recommended calcium intake if they stick with dietary sources of calcium only (foods and beverages).

For more info on foods that promote strong, healthy bones, visit www.joybauer.com/osteoporosis.

# JOY'S 4-STEP PROGRAM
## FOR OSTEOPOROSIS

Follow this program if you have osteopenia, osteoporosis, or a family history of bone density problems.

## Step 1 . . . START WITH THE BASICS

These are the first things you should do to help preserve bone density.

◆ See your doctor for advice about osteoporosis prevention and treatment if you are a menopausal woman who has never had a bone density scan, if you have ever had an eating disorder, or if you have taken corticosteroid medications for three or more months at any time in your life.

◆ Take a multivitamin. See guidelines on page 233.

◆ Consider taking calcium supplements with vitamin $D_3$ and optional magnesium. If you're a man, speak with your physician before taking calcium supplements.

◆ Start an exercise program.

◆ If you smoke, quit. Encourage people in your life to quit smoking, too.

## Step 2 . . . YOUR ULTIMATE GROCERY LIST

A nutrition plan is only as good as the foods you choose. This list contains foods with high levels of nutrients that help strengthen bones, as well as other overall healthy foods to round out your grocery list. You don't have to purchase every item, but these foods should make up the bulk of what you eat for the week. If you find yourself getting bored, try some unfamiliar foods from the list—they may become new favorites.

For a printable version of this list, visit www.joybauer.com/osteoporosis.

## FRUIT

*All* fruit, but especially:

Apricots

Bananas

Berries (blackberries, blueberries, boysenberries, raspberries, and strawberries)

Cantaloupe

Clementines

Fruit juice, calcium-fortified

Grapefruit

Guava

Honeydew

Kiwifruit

Lemons

Limes

Lychees

Mangoes

Oranges

Papayas

Persimmons

Pineapple

Plums

Prunes

Raisins

Tangerines

Watermelon

## VEGETABLES AND LEGUMES

*All* vegetables, but especially:

Artichokes

Asparagus

Avocados

Beans, starchy (such as black, navy, garbanzo, kidney, pinto, and white)

Beets

Bok choy

Broccoli

Broccoli raab

Brussels sprouts

Cabbage

Carrots

Cauliflower

Dark leafy greens (such as beet, collard, dandelion, kale, mustard, Swiss chard, and turnip)

Kohlrabi

Lentils

Lettuce (all varieties)

Mushrooms (especially vitamin D-enhanced*)

Okra

Parsnips

Peas (black-eyed, green, and split)

Peppers (all varieties)

Potatoes (sweet and white)

Pumpkin

Rutabagas

Snow peas

Soybeans (edamame)

Spinach

Squash, summer

Squash, winter (acorn and butternut)

Tomatoes

Zucchini

*These mushrooms are treated with UV light, which dramatically increases their vitamin D content.

## SEAFOOD

*All* fish and shellfish, but especially:

Herring

Mackerel (not king)

Salmon, wild

Sardines

## LEAN PROTEINS

Beef, lean

Chicken, ground (at least 90% lean)

Chicken, skinless

Eggs and egg substitutes

Pork tenderloin

Tempeh

Tofu

Turkey, ground (at least 90% lean)

Turkey, skinless

Turkey bacon

Turkey burgers, lean

Veggie burgers

## NUTS AND SEEDS (PREFERABLY UNSALTED)

Almonds and almond butter

Butternuts (white walnuts)

Cashews and cashew butter

Chia seeds

Flaxseed, ground

Hazelnuts

Macadamia nuts

Peanuts and peanut butter

Pecans

Pine nuts

Pistachios

Pumpkin seeds

Sunflower seeds and sunflower butter

Walnuts

## WHOLE GRAINS

Amaranth

Barley

Bread, whole grain (buns, crackers, English muffins, pitas, tortillas, and wraps)

Bulgur

Cereals, whole grain

Millet

Oats

Pasta, whole grain

Quinoa

Rice (brown and wild)

Waffles, whole grain (preferably calcium-fortified)

Wheat germ

## DAIRY

Cheese (fat-free or reduced-fat)

Cottage cheese (fat-free or 1%)

Cream cheese (fat-free or reduced-fat)

Frozen yogurt

Ice cream (low-fat)

Milk (fat-free or 1%)

Milk alternatives (almond, rice, and soy)

Ricotta cheese (part-skim)

Sour cream (fat-free or reduced-fat)

Yogurt (fat-free or low-fat)

## MISCELLANEOUS

Canola oil

Garlic

Herbs and spices (fresh, dried, and ground)

Hot sauce

Hummus

Marinara sauce

Mayonnaise, reduced-fat

Mustard (all varieties)

Olive oil

Salad dressing, reduced-calorie

Salsa

Soft tub spread, trans-fat-free (reduced-fat, or regular)

Vinegar (all varieties)

# Step 3 ... GOING ABOVE AND BEYOND

If you want to do everything you can to prevent or control osteoporosis, here are some additional things you might try.

◆ Limit the amount of salt you eat.

◆ If you drink alcohol, be sure to drink in moderation (no more than one drink per day for women and two drinks per day for men).

◆ If you need to diet for weight loss, do it in a way that is smart for your bones. See Weight Loss, page 17, for more information.

◆ If you are underweight, talk with your doctor to learn the healthiest ways to bring your weight up. Also, see "How to Pile on the Pounds," below.

## HOW TO PILE ON THE POUNDS

If you need to gain weight as part of your bone-building strategy, it is important to add healthy pounds, as opposed to "ice cream and doughnut" pounds. Start by substituting products that are higher in healthy fats. For example, sauté vegetables in olive oil instead of steaming them, and use full-fat vinaigrette salad dressing. Also, add avocado to salads and sandwiches. Incorporate two or three healthy snacks each day, in addition to breakfast, lunch, and dinner. Hummus, guacamole, seeds, nuts (and nut and seed butters), trail mix, nutrition bars, dried fruit, fruit-yogurt smoothies, granola, and wholesome homemade muffins add good calories to your daily count. If your appetite is poor or if you cannot gain weight, talk with your doctor.

# Step 4 ... MEAL PLANS

These sample menus include foods that have been shown to strengthen bones—specifically, foods high in calcium, vitamin D, magnesium, vitamin K, potassium, protein, and vitamin C.

Every day, choose one option for each of the three meals—breakfast, lunch, and dinner. Then, once or twice per day, choose from my suggested snacks. Approximate calories have been provided to help adjust for your personal weight-management goals. If you find yourself hungry (and weight is not an issue), feel free to increase the portion sizes for meals and snacks. Beverage calories are not included.

## BREAKFAST OPTIONS

(300 TO 400 CALORIES)

### Strawberry-Nut Yogurt Parfait

Spoon ⅓ cup vanilla fat-free yogurt into a parfait glass. Top with ¼ cup sliced strawberries (or raspberries or blackberries) and 1 tablespoon nuts or seeds. Repeat the layers two more times for a total of three layers (yogurt, berries, and then nuts/seeds).

### Cereal with Milk and Fruit

1 cup whole grain cereal with 1 cup milk (fat-free, 1%, or soy, almond, or rice). Enjoy with 1 cup sliced pineapple (or 1 cup berries, ½ grapefruit, ½ banana, or 1 orange).

### Melon with Cottage Cheese and Sunflower Seeds

Mix ½ cantaloupe or ¼ honeydew (about 1½ cups cubed) with 1 cup fat-free or 1% cottage cheese and top with 1 tablespoon sunflower seeds (or 2 tablespoons wheat germ).

### Oatmeal with Milk and Fresh Berries

Prepare ½ cup dry oats with 1 cup milk (fat-free, 1%, or soy, almond, or rice) and sprinkle with 1 to 2 tablespoons wheat germ or chopped nuts and ½ cup berries (sliced strawberries, blueberries, raspberries, and/or blackberries). Sweeten with optional 1 teaspoon sugar, honey, or sugar substitute.

### Breakfast Potato and Yogurt

Enjoy 1 medium baked sweet potato with a 6-ounce container fat-free vanilla yogurt (or ½ cup fat-free or 1% cottage cheese) mixed with cinnamon.

### Scrambled Eggs with Broccoli and Cheese

Beat 1 whole egg and 2 egg whites. Cook in a small skillet coated with oil spray. When the eggs are almost cooked, add 1 cup cooked broccoli florets and 1 ounce shredded reduced-fat cheese. Enjoy with ½ grapefruit (or ½ banana or 1 orange).

### Strawberry-Kiwi Smoothie with Peanut Butter Toast

Enjoy 1 serving (2 cups) Strawberry-Kiwi Smoothie (page 114) with 1 slice whole grain toast topped with 1 level tablespoon peanut butter (or 2 heaping tablespoons fat-free or 1% cottage cheese sprinkled with 1 tablespoon slivered almonds and optional cinnamon).

## LUNCH OPTIONS

(400 TO 500 CALORIES)

### Turkey and Cheese Sandwich

Layer 4 to 5 ounces sliced turkey or chicken, 1 slice reduced-fat cheese, lettuce, tomato, and onion between 2 slices whole grain bread or in a pita. Spread with 2 teaspoons reduced-fat mayonnaise or hummus and optional mustard. Serve with unlimited baby carrots or bell pepper strips.

### Artichoke Salad with Grilled Chicken and Feta Cheese

Mix 1 cup canned, drained artichoke hearts with 2 to 3 cups leafy greens (spinach, romaine, arugula, etc.), ½ cup cherry tomatoes, 1 ounce (¼ cup) crumbled feta cheese (preferably reduced-fat), and 2 ounces grilled chicken or turkey. Toss with 2 teaspoons olive oil and unlimited vinegar or fresh lemon juice and seasonings.

### Baked Potato with Broccoli and Cheese

Top 1 baked white potato with steamed, chopped broccoli and 1 ounce (¼ cup) shredded reduced-fat cheese (or ½ cup fat-free or 1% cottage cheese). Serve with 1 cup vegetable soup or Vegetable Oatmeal Bisque (page 322).

### Edamame with Wild Salmon Dijonnaise

Enjoy 1 cup boiled edamame (green soybeans in the pod) with 5 ounces canned wild salmon, drained, mashed, and mixed with 1 tablespoon reduced-fat mayonnaise, 1 to 2 teaspoons Dijon mustard, and minced onion and black pepper to taste. Serve on a large bed of leafy greens (spinach, romaine, etc.) tossed with fresh lemon juice or 2 tablespoons reduced-calorie dressing.

### Broccoli-Cheese Soufflé with Cottage Cheese and Almonds

Enjoy 1 serving Broccoli-Cheese Soufflé (page 113) with ½ cup fat-free or 1% cottage cheese topped with 1 tablespoon slivered almonds (or any preferred nut or seed).

### Tomato-Cheese Omelet with Tropical Mango-Citrus Smoothie

Beat 1 whole egg with 2 or 3 egg whites and cook in a heated small skillet coated with oil spray. When the bottom is cooked, gently flip and add a few tablespoons chopped tomato, optional dried basil, and 1 ounce (¼ cup) shredded reduced-fat cheese. Fold the omelet in half and continue cooking until the egg mixture firms and the cheese melts. Enjoy with 1 serving (2 cups) Tropical Mango-Citrus Smoothie (page 114).

### Mixed Vegetable Salad with Sardines

Toss 4 ounces (about 8) sardines with unlimited leafy greens, chopped tomato, carrots, mushrooms, bell pepper and onion and ½ cup starchy beans. Drizzle with 2 to 4 tablespoons reduced-calorie salad dressing (or 1 teaspoon olive oil and unlimited vinegar or fresh lemon juice). Season with ground black pepper.

## DINNER OPTIONS

(500 TO 600 CALORIES)

### Whole Wheat Pita Pizza with the Works

Toast 1 split whole wheat pita (or use 200 calories' worth of prebaked whole wheat pizza crust). Top each half with 2 to 3 heaping tablespoons marinara sauce and ¼ cup part-skim ricotta cheese, plus ½ cup cooked peppers and unlimited chopped broccoli florets sautéed in oil spray until soft. Top each half with 2 tablespoons shredded reduced-fat mozzarella cheese and optional crushed red pepper and oregano. Heat in a 350°F oven until the cheese melts and bubbles.

### Turkey Chili with Cheese

Enjoy 1 serving (2 cups) Turkey Chili (page 363), topped with 1 ounce shredded reduced-fat Cheddar cheese, with ½ cup cooked brown rice or quinoa and a salad of leafy greens (optional peppers, carrots, and artichokes) tossed with 1 teaspoon olive oil and unlimited vinegar or fresh lemon juice.

### Tofu Salad with Snow Peas, Almonds, and Mandarin Oranges

Toss 6 to 8 ounces extra-firm tofu, cubed and chilled, with 2 to 3 cups baby spinach leaves, 1 cup steamed and chilled snow peas, ½ chopped tomato, and ½ cup mandarin orange sections (canned in juice or light syrup). Drizzle with 1 to 2 teaspoons sesame oil and 1 tablespoon reduced-sodium soy sauce and top with 2 tablespoons slivered almonds.

### Healthy Chicken Parmesan and Broccoli

Enjoy 1 serving (page 246).

### Sweet and Sour Tofu-Veggie Stir-Fry with Brown Rice

Enjoy 1 serving Sweet and Sour Tofu-Veggie Stir-Fry (page 245) with 1 cup cooked brown rice (or plain medium baked sweet or white potato).

### Red Snapper with Fresh Herbs and Brussels Sprouts

Poach 6 ounces red snapper fillet in ⅔ cup water and ⅓ cup chicken stock or white wine. Add 2 tablespoons each fresh parsley, dill, thyme, and rosemary and drizzle with fresh lemon or lime juice just before serving. (Or season fish with a pinch of kosher salt and ground black pepper and lightly brush with olive oil, then grill or pan roast on medium-high for about 3 minutes on each side, or until golden brown. You may substitute any favorite fish, but cooking times will vary.) Serve with unlimited steamed Brussels sprouts (or Swiss chard or asparagus) and 1 medium baked sweet or white potato.

### Turkey Tacos

Enjoy 3 Turkey Tacos (page 244) with optional salsa and hot sauce.

## SNACK OPTIONS

100 CALORIES OR LESS

◆ *Best Vegetable Snacks:* up to 2 cups raw or cooked bell peppers (red, green, yellow), broccoli, sugar snap peas, cherry tomatoes, mushrooms, carrots, asparagus, cauliflower

- *Best Fruit Snacks:* 1 orange, tangerine, persimmon, kiwifruit, or guava; 2 clementines or plums; ½ papaya, mango, grapefruit, or cantaloupe; 1 cup cherries or berries (boysenberries, blackberries, blueberries, raspberries, or sliced strawberries); 1 cup cubed watermelon, honeydew, or pineapple; ½ cup lychees; 4 apricots or prunes; 20 whole strawberries; 2 tablespoons raisins

- 1 cup milk (fat-free)

- 1 part-skim string cheese or 1 ounce fat-free or reduced-fat cheese

- 1 hard-cooked egg

- 8- to 12-ounce skim latte or skim cappuccino

- 6 ounces fat-free plain or flavored yogurt

- ½ cup fat-free or 1% cottage cheese, mixed with optional cinnamon

- 1 cup low-fat hot cocoa

### 100 TO 200 CALORIES

- 1 small bag soy crisps

- 8 ounces fat-free or low-fat yogurt

- ½ cup frozen yogurt or light ice cream

- Low-fat ice cream pop, bar, or sandwich

- 2 cups Tropical Mango-Citrus Smoothie (page 114)

- 2 cups Strawberry-Kiwi Smoothie (page 114)

- 1 cup fat-free milk or soy/almond/rice milk with 1 tablespoon chocolate syrup

- 1 ounce (about ¼ cup) nuts (almonds, pecans, walnuts, cashews, peanuts)

- ½ cup sunflower seeds or pistachios in the shell

- 1 cup boiled edamame (green soybeans in the pod)

- ¼ cup roasted edamame

- 4 cups light or air-popped popcorn topped with 2 tablespoons grated Parmesan cheese

# TURKEY TACOS

*In my house, Turkey Tacos are a sure thing—they're nothing fancy, but we never have leftovers. They're even a hit with my kids' picky-eater friends. And nobody has ever suspected the slimming swaps: lean ground turkey meat and reduced-fat shredded cheese. If you have extra time, set up bowls with chopped peppers, carrots, and sweet corn that your kids and their friends can add on their own. Or pick your favorites—any vegetable can go into a taco.*

**MAKES 8 TACOS**

1¼ pounds ground turkey (at least 90% lean)

1 packet taco seasoning, preferably lower-sodium

Chopped or shredded lettuce

1 large tomato, finely chopped

1 cup shredded reduced-fat Cheddar cheese

8 hard or soft taco shells

Salsa and/or hot sauce (optional)

In a large skillet, cook the turkey over medium-high heat until browned. Drain the fat. Stir in the taco seasoning (plus water, as indicated in package directions). Bring to a boil. Reduce the heat and simmer, stirring occasionally, for 5 to 6 minutes.

Evenly divide the turkey mixture, lettuce, tomato, and cheese among the taco shells. Top with salsa and/or hot sauce if you like.

**Per serving (1 taco):** 175 calories, 21 g protein, 10 g carbohydrate, 5 g fat (2 g saturated), 40 mg cholesterol, 350 mg sodium, 2 g fiber; plus 150 mg calcium (15% DV)

# SWEET AND SOUR TOFU-VEGGIE STIR-FRY

*If you haven't tried tofu or just assume you won't like it, this dish may surprise your tastebuds. It's loaded with nearly every bone-strengthening ingredient known to nutritionists and tastes just as good cold if you have leftovers! Serve over brown rice or whole wheat pasta.*

**MAKES 4 SERVINGS (1½ CUPS PER SERVING)**

½ cup low-sodium chicken or vegetable broth

¼ cup apple cider vinegar or rice wine vinegar

¼ cup reduced-sodium soy sauce

2 tablespoons apple or orange juice

1 tablespoon cornstarch

1 package (14 ounces) extra-firm tofu with calcium (check nutrition label), pressed and drained

2 tablespoons canola oil

1 large red bell pepper, seeded and thinly sliced

1 cup shredded cabbage

¼ pound green beans, quartered

2 cloves garlic, minced

1 teaspoon minced fresh ginger

1 small jalapeño chile pepper, seeded and minced

1 cup baby corn or frozen corn kernels, rinsed under hot water

1 cup frozen, shelled edamame, rinsed under hot water

In a small bowl, combine the broth, vinegar, soy sauce, juice, and cornstarch. Mix well and set aside. Pat the tofu dry with a paper towel and cut it into 1" chunks.

Spray a large wok or nonstick skillet with oil spray. Place over high heat and add 1 tablespoon of the oil. When the oil shimmers, add the tofu and brown for 3 to 4 minutes on one side, then turn and brown the opposite side for 3 to 4 minutes. Transfer to a plate.

Reduce the heat to medium and add the remaining 1 tablespoon oil to the wok. Add the bell pepper, cabbage, and green beans. Cook, stirring occasionally, for 4 to 5 minutes, or until the vegetables begin to soften but are still crisp. Stir in the garlic, ginger, and chile pepper, and cook for an additional minute, until the mixture becomes fragrant. Add the corn and edamame and cook for 2 to 3 minutes longer. Reduce the heat to low and add the reserved broth mixture, stirring for 1 to 2 minutes, or until it thickens. Turn off the heat, return the tofu to the wok or skillet, and stir gently to coat with the sauce.

**Per serving:** 320 calories, 22 g protein, 23 g carbohydrate, 17 g fat (1 g saturated), 0 mg cholesterol, 669 mg sodium, 6 g fiber; plus 341 mg calcium (34% DV), 827 mg potassium (24% DV), 21 mcg vitamin K (27% DV), 120 mg magnesium (30% DV)

# HEALTHY CHICKEN PARMESAN AND BROCCOLI

*This is my husband's absolute favorite recipe from this book. My youngest daughter, Ayden Jane, agrees. If you need more reasons to dig in, one serving provides your bones with more than one-third of your daily calcium requirements, more than 20 percent each of daily requirements of magnesium and potassium, and an entire day's worth of vitamin K. Great taste and stellar nutrition—home run!*

**MAKES 4 SERVINGS**

2 tablespoons olive oil

1 medium onion, chopped

1 bay leaf

3 cloves garlic, minced

1 can (28 ounces) no-salted-added diced tomatoes

¼ cup fresh basil leaves, torn, plus 1 whole sprig

Kosher salt

Ground black pepper

1 large bunch broccoli, cut into florets

¼ cup whole wheat or all-purpose flour

2 egg whites

1 cup whole wheat bread crumbs

¼ teaspoon dried oregano

¼ teaspoon dried rosemary

3 tablespoons grated Parmesan cheese

4 skinless chicken breasts (6 ounces each), pounded very thin

1 cup shredded reduced-fat mozzarella cheese

Coat a large skillet with oil spray. Place over medium heat and add the oil. When the oil is hot, add the onion, the bay leaf, and two-thirds of the garlic. Cook, stirring, for 6 to 7 minutes, or until the onion begins to soften and become translucent. Reduce the heat to medium and add the tomatoes and basil sprig. Cook, stirring occasionally, for about 10 minutes, or until the sauce starts to thicken. Season with a pinch of kosher salt and pepper. Cover and simmer over low heat while you prepare the broccoli and chicken.

Preheat the oven to 450°F. Cover a large baking sheet with aluminum foil or parchment paper. Sprinkle the remaining garlic over the broccoli and season with a pinch of kosher salt and pepper. Wrap tightly in the foil. Set aside.

Place the flour on a piece of waxed paper or aluminum foil. In a shallow bowl, beat the egg whites. On another piece of waxed paper or aluminum foil, mix the bread crumbs with the oregano, rosemary, and 2 tablespoons of the Parmesan and season with pepper.

Lightly dredge the pounded chicken breasts in the flour, then dip in the egg whites, shaking off any excess egg, and then dredge in the bread crumb mixture. Coat both sides of each chicken breast with oil spray and place on the prepared baking sheet.

Bake the chicken and foil packet of broccoli for 8 to 10 minutes, or until the chicken breasts are golden and the broccoli is tender. Remove from the oven.

Preheat the broiler. Sprinkle the chicken with the mozzarella and remaining 1 tablespoon Parmesan. Place under the broiler for 1 to 2 minutes, or until the cheese is golden. (Watch carefully—they can burn easily!) Transfer the chicken and broccoli to a platter. Remove the bay leaf from the tomato sauce and ladle the sauce around the chicken. Sprinkle with the torn basil and serve immediately.

**Per serving:** 569 calories, 59 g protein, 41 g carbohydrate, 16 g fat (4 g saturated), 111 mg cholesterol, 600 mg sodium, 7 g fiber; plus 365 mg calcium (36% DV), 86 mg magnesium (22% DV), 97 mcg vitamin K (122% DV), 1,017 mg potassium (29% DV)

# CHAPTER 11

# VISION

For more than 75 years, Nat was a glutton for the printed word. He read everything—newspapers, magazines, even instruction manuals—but he loved books best. He was active, with plenty of friends and a terrific family, but he was happiest when he could relax with a good novel. So it was particularly devastating when Nat lost most of his sight to macular degeneration. Now, when he finally has all the leisure time in the world, he can't read much more than the large type of the newspaper headlines. Instead of reading novels, he settles for listening to television and radio. It breaks his family's heart. It breaks my heart, because I'm a part of Nat's family: He is my husband's grandfather.

Vision loss and its tragic implications are all too common—cataracts affect more than half of all Americans over age 80, and as many as 11 million Americans have some form of macular degeneration. In the past decade, research has pointed to nutrition as one of the factors that might reduce the risk and slow the progression of these disorders. I wish that this information had been available back when Nat was still in his prime, when it might have helped to preserve at least some of his sight. I'm sure he would have embraced the changes discussed in this chapter if it meant he could have spent even one more quiet hour with the mystery novels he loves so much.

## WHAT AFFECTS CATARACT DEVELOPMENT?

The process allowing us to see begins with light entering our pupils, the round, black openings at the center of our eyeballs. Our lenses, located behind each pupil, catch the incoming light and focus it onto the retinas at the back of our eyes.

A cataract is formed when protein fibers in the lens change shape and clump together, clouding the normally transparent lens. This is similar to the process that turns the protein in egg whites from clear to white when the egg is cooked. In fact, most well-developed cataracts look milky white, although in some cases, the lens can turn yellow or brown.

Cataracts usually take years to develop, and before they can be seen from the outside, the sufferer's vision can become blurry or cloudy, like looking through a fogged windshield. Other possible symptoms include worsened night vision, faded color vision, and starburst or halo effects around bright lights. Because cataracts can be surgically removed, these symptoms are only temporary. If you undergo cataract surgery, you may need glasses to see detail afterward, but your sight will be clear.

No one knows exactly what causes eye proteins to clump and create a cataract. Many scientists blame unstable molecules known as free radicals, which can wreak havoc throughout the body, causing destruction and disease wherever they go through a complex chemical process called oxidative stress. Natural metabolic processes from normal body functions like breathing and digesting food generate a lot of free radicals that, unless they are neutralized, build up over time. Accumulated damage from years of free radical attacks causes our bodies to slowly deteriorate with age.

Two large contributors to free radical damage are smoking and ultraviolet radiation from sunlight. Thus, all cataract prevention strategies must include a commitment to stop smoking and reduce exposure to sunlight. Cataracts can also be caused by surgery for other eye problems, traumatic eye injury, or long-term use of corticosteroids. In very rare circumstances, genetic anomalies can create cataracts in newborn babies or infants.

## HOW FOOD AFFECTS CATARACTS

The ultimate prevention for cataracts is simple: Never grow old.

For those of you who can't stop time, nutrition and lifestyle changes are your best bets for preventing or slowing the development of cataracts. Although research has not absolutely, positively proved nutrition's role in cataract prevention, science provides ample evidence that eating the right foods could help—and I know for certain it can't hurt!

For cataract prevention, increasing your intake of foods rich in antioxidants and B vitamins is your best line of defense. You'll also want to dramatically limit your intake of low-quality carbs—sugary foods and beverages and refined, white starches.

### ANTIOXIDANTS: VITAMIN C AND VITAMIN E

As the name suggests, antioxidants fight the oxidative stress caused by free radicals. There is no single antioxidant—rather, it is a broad category that includes vitamin C, vitamin E, lutein, beta-carotene, and a number of other substances that can neutralize free radicals. All vegetables and fruits contain antioxidants, so eating a diet rich in those foods may help prevent cataracts.

The Nurses' Health Study revealed that women who ate a very healthy diet full of all kinds of antioxidants from vegetables, fruits, and whole grains were half as likely to develop cataracts as women who did not eat such a healthy diet. In addition, numerous studies have observed that people with high dietary intakes or blood levels of antioxidants—particularly vitamins C and E—are at a significantly lower risk of cataracts. But when researchers took the studies to the next level by giving people supplements of individual antioxidants or combination pills with a mix of antioxidants, the results were disappointing. In most trials, antioxidant supplements did not prevent or slow cataract development.

These results aren't as contradictory as they seem at first glance—there are many plausible reasons why supplements seem to have struck out. Antioxidants found in foods may act synergistically with other nutrients, and you miss out on those potential benefits when you take isolated antioxidants in pill form. In addition, people with higher intakes of antioxidants likely consume a nutritious, produce-rich diet and have healthier lifestyle habits, both of which may put them at lower risk of cataracts. Regardless, the big-picture message is clear: Antioxidant supplements do not ward off cataracts, but eating plenty of vegetables, fruit, and whole grains, including those rich in vitamins C and E, may be protective (and will benefit the rest of your body, as well!).

BEST FOODS FOR VITAMIN C: *guava, bell peppers (all colors), oranges and orange juice, grapefruit and grapefruit juice, strawberries, pineapple, kohlrabi, papaya, lemons and lemon juice, broccoli, kale, Brussels sprouts, kidney beans, kiwifruit, cantaloupe, cauliflower, cabbage (all varieties), mangoes, white potatoes, mustard greens, tomatoes, sugar snap peas, snow peas, clementines, rutabagas, turnip greens, raspberries, blackberries, watermelon, tangerines, okra, lychees, summer squash, persimmons*

BEST FOODS FOR VITAMIN E: *almonds and almond butter, sunflower seeds and sunflower butter, wheat germ, hazelnuts, spinach, dandelion greens, Swiss chard, pine nuts, peanuts and peanut butter, turnip greens, beet greens, broccoli, canola oil, flaxseed oil, red bell pepper, collard greens, avocados, olive oil, mangoes*

## ANTIOXIDANTS: LUTEIN AND ZEAXANTHIN

The antioxidants lutein and zeaxanthin are of tremendous interest to eye health researchers. The pair belongs to a family of nutrients called carotenoids (along with their more popular sister carotenoid, beta-carotene). Lutein and zeaxanthin stand out because they're the only carotenoids found in the lens of the eye, and they may play a key role in keeping the lens clear of protein buildup. Like all antioxidants, lutein and zeaxanthin can defuse potentially damaging free radicals. In addition, they may also prevent the development of some free radicals by absorbing blue light—part of the cataract-causing, short-wave spectrum of sunlight.

Using data from the Woman's Health Study, researchers at Harvard University determined that women who consumed the highest combined amount of lutein

BEST SOURCES OF FOOD ANTIOXIDANTS: TOP 20 FRUITS, VEGETABLES, AND NUTS (AS MEASURED BY TOTAL ANTIOXIDANT CAPACITY PER SERVING SIZE)

| RANK | FOOD ITEM | SERVING SIZE | TOTAL ANTIOXIDANT CAPACITY PER SERVING SIZE |
|------|-----------|--------------|---------------------------------------------|
| 1 | Small red bean (dried) | ½ cup | 13,727 |
| 2 | Wild blueberry | 1 cup | 13,427 |
| 3 | Red kidney bean (dried) | ½ cup | 13,259 |
| 4 | Pinto bean | ½ cup | 11,864 |
| 5 | Blueberry (cultivated) | 1 cup | 9,019 |
| 6 | Cranberry | 1 cup (whole) | 8,983 |
| 7 | Artichoke (cooked) | 1 cup (hearts) | 7,904 |
| 8 | Blackberry | 1 cup | 7,701 |
| 9 | Prune | ½ cup | 7,291 |
| 10 | Raspberry | 1 cup | 6,058 |
| 11 | Strawberry | 1 cup | 5,938 |
| 12 | Red Delicious apple | 1 | 5,900 |
| 13 | Granny Smith apple | 1 | 5,381 |
| 14 | Pecan | 1 ounce | 5,095 |
| 15 | Sweet cherry | 1 cup | 4,873 |
| 16 | Black plum | 1 | 4,844 |
| 17 | Russet potato (cooked) | 1 | 4,649 |
| 18 | Black bean (dried) | ½ cup | 4,181 |
| 19 | Plum | 1 | 4,118 |
| 20 | Gala apple | 1 | 3,903 |

Source: USDA; *Journal of Agricultural and Food Chemistry*, 2004

plus zeaxanthin had an 18 percent reduced risk of cataracts when compared with women with the lowest intake. Similar results were reported from the Nurses' Health Study, the US Male Health Professionals Study, and the Beaver Dam Eye Study. These results are encouraging, but I can't recommend lutein and zeaxanthin supplements at this time because no one knows everything there is to know about the effects of individual nutrients, and it could be that lutein and zeaxanthin work best only when paired with other antioxidants or with certain vitamins and minerals. Right now, the only solid information we have supports eating a diet full of lutein- and zeaxanthin-rich leafy green vegetables, plus an abundance of other antioxidant-rich vegetables and fruits.

> BEST FOODS FOR LUTEIN AND ZEAXANTHIN: *kale, spinach, Swiss chard, collard greens, turnip greens, dandelion greens, mustard greens, beet greens, radicchio, summer squash (all varieties), watercress, green peas, persimmons, winter squash (acorn, butternut), pumpkin, broccoli, Brussels sprouts, lettuces (especially dark lettuces), asparagus, corn, green beans, okra, artichokes, green bell peppers*

## B VITAMINS

There is strong evidence that two of the B vitamins—riboflavin (vitamin $B_2$) and niacin (vitamin $B_3$)—may help prevent cataracts, and early research suggests that other Bs may also contribute to eye health.

Although these vitamins are not antioxidants, they provide some of the building blocks the body needs to make antioxidant compounds. So without enough riboflavin and niacin, the risk of cataracts increases. Indeed, several scientific studies have shown that people who eat a diet containing plenty of foods rich in riboflavin and niacin can slash their risk of cataracts by about half, compared with people who eat a diet with very little of those vitamins.

As with antioxidants, the information about the benefits of B vitamin supplements is less clear. The Blue Mountain Eye Study, a large Australian study with about 2,900 participants, found that those who took riboflavin supplements had a 20 percent lower risk of cataracts, compared with people who didn't take supplements. Niacin supplements lowered risk by 30 percent, and supplements of other B vitamins—thiamin, folate, and vitamin $B_{12}$—also seemed to show some benefit. Combining these vitamins may have an even greater effect. A large study conducted by the National Eye Institute in Bethesda, Maryland, showed that people who took a dual supplement containing both riboflavin and niacin reduced their risk of cataracts by 44 percent. Even general multivitamins providing 100 percent DV of these B vitamins seem to decrease risk by more than 30 percent. As promising as these results sound, the jury is still out on exactly how much of which types of B vitamins is necessary or optimal for cataract prevention. I can recommend only food sources, not pills (with the exception of a multivitamin providing 100 percent DV of riboflavin and niacin).

> BEST FOODS FOR RIBOFLAVIN: *lean beef and lamb, venison, yogurt (fat-free, low-fat), milk (fat-free, 1%), mushrooms, almonds, eggs, spinach, coffee*

> BEST FOODS FOR NIACIN: *tuna (canned light), skinless chicken and turkey, lean beef and lamb, pork tenderloin, mackerel (not king), wild salmon (fresh, canned), anchovies, kidney beans, peanuts and peanut butter, mushrooms, sunflower seeds and sunflower butter*

## LOW-QUALITY CARBS

Most studies have focused on nutrients that can help *protect* the eyes from cataracts, but emerging research suggests that certain foods—most notably, low-quality carbohydrates—may increase the risk of developing them. Low-quality carbohydrates include sugar, honey, and other sweeteners; soda and other sugary drinks; candy; baked goods; sugary cereals; anything made with white flour (including white bread and regular pasta); and white rice. Most of these foods are classified as high-glycemic carbs, which means they are quickly digested and absorbed by the body, causing a rapid, unhealthy surge in blood sugar levels. Glucose eventually moves from the blood into the eye, and scientists believe that exposure to high sugar concentrations in the eye's lens may accelerate protein damage and clumping, thus contributing to cataract formation. A few studies have shown that people who eat a lot of high-glycemic foods have an increased risk of developing cataracts. These findings may also explain why the incidence of cataracts is substantially higher in people with diabetes, who have chronically elevated blood sugar levels.

We're only beginning to understand the impact of low-quality carbs on eye health, but we already know for sure that they're not doing our hearts, blood vessels, or waistlines any good. In the meal plans on page 265, I've bypassed junky, nutrient-poor carbs and filled your daily menus with high-quality carbohydrates like vegetables, fruits, beans, and whole grains.

## TEA

Tea contains powerful antioxidants, and some research suggests that drinking relatively large amounts of tea—the equivalent of about five cups daily—may help prevent or delay cataract development. But antioxidants may tell only part of the story. While investigating the effects of tea on blood sugar in diabetic laboratory rats, researchers from the University of Scranton discovered that the animals that were given tea had lower blood sugar than those that did not get tea. But there was also a side benefit: Drinking tea reduced the level of glucose in the eye lens, and there was a lower incidence of cataracts. In fact, the tea-drinking rats had about half the risk of cataracts as the others. We're still waiting to see if these results hold up in humans, but tea is an incredibly healthy drink all around, so I encourage you to sip both green and regular black tea to your heart's content. What's more, unsweetened tea is a terrific substitute for sugary beverages like soda, sweetened waters, fruit drinks, and sugary coffee concoctions.

## WHAT AFFECTS MACULAR DEGENERATION?

The retina is the part of the eye that receives light and images from the world and sends them to the optic nerve to be processed in the brain. The macula is the center, most sensitive part of the retina. It fine-tunes focus at the center of our visual field, allowing us to recognize faces, read words on a page, and discern detail in anything we look at. Macular degeneration, then, is a deterioration of the macula, gradually leading to central blindness. Peripheral vision remains clear, so it isn't a total lack of sight, but, as Nat's story demonstrates, the loss of detailed vision is a life-altering change all the same.

There are two types of macular degeneration: dry (also called atrophic), caused by a gradual breakdown of light receptors, and wet (also called exudative), caused by leaks in the blood vessels of the retina, which in turn cause scarring and tissue death. With both types, people usually begin to notice vision distortions, such as straight lines appearing wavy, and have difficulty reading and recognizing faces. Then, as more and more receptors die, their central vision disappears. Fortunately, major advances have been made in treating the wet form of macular degeneration. For example, doctors can now prescribe injectable drugs that stop the leaky blood vessels from growing. There is currently no medical treatment for dry macular degeneration.

Macular degeneration happens most often in people—primarily women—over age 70. Although it can run in families, no one knows exactly why some people experience macular degeneration or how to stop it once it begins.

## HOW FOOD AFFECTS MACULAR DEGENERATION

The Age-Related Eye Disease Study (AREDS), a research project conducted by the National Eye Institute, has given us some clues about how nutrition might help prevent macular degeneration or at least delay the progression to blindness. AREDS results showed that certain antioxidant vitamins and zinc helped to slow the progression of advanced macular degeneration by about 25 percent over a six-year period. The antioxidants—vitamins C and E and beta-carotene—are thought to prevent damage caused by free radicals. The mineral zinc is important for the health of all body tissues, but it is found in unusually high concentrations in tissues of the retina.

The results of AREDS were so impressive that in the wake of the study's publication, several supplement manufacturers created special macular degeneration-fighting formulas. These supplements are a great treatment option for some, but they don't appear to be as effective at slowing the progression of macular degeneration from the early to intermediate stage, so most doctors don't recommend them for people that fall into this group. On top of that, high supplemental doses of antioxidants, especially vitamin E, may pose health risks. Only your eye doctor can determine whether your condition has progressed to a point where supplements may be beneficial. If your condition is still in the early phases, or if you have a family history of macular degeneration but no signs of disease, your best bet is to follow my plan and load up on food sources packed with vision-friendly nutrients.

## VITAMIN C, VITAMIN E, BETA-CAROTENE

A study led by researchers from Erasmus Medical Centre in Rotterdam, the Netherlands, followed a group of more than 4,000 people to see how diet affected the risk of developing macular degeneration. After eight years, the scientists compared the diets of people who developed the condition with the diets of those who did not. The results were encouraging: People who ate a diet rich in vitamins C and E, beta-carotene, and zinc had a 35 percent reduced risk of developing macular degeneration, compared with people who ate an average diet. And those who ate worse-than-normal diets, with low levels of those nutrients, actually had a 20 percent increased risk of disease. A 2009 study by Tufts University researchers confirmed the links between diets rich in C, E, and zinc (plus lutein and

**FAQS**

**I understand that there may be a risk to taking high doses of certain antioxidants for macular degeneration. Should I still take a multivitamin?**

Yes. High levels of vitamin E supplements can be problematic, but a daily multivitamin with only 100 percent DV of vitamin E is fine (and it will provide at the very least 100 percent DV of zinc and vitamin C, along with some beta-carotene). Unless your doctor has recommended specially formulated high-dose antioxidant supplements for macular degeneration, it's safer to get these nutrients from food. Try making one of my Smooth-SEE recipes (pages 270 and 272), which are chock-full of the best nutrients for your eyes.

zeaxanthin) and decreased risk of macular degeneration. The Tufts study, however, failed to show any benefit from beta-carotene. (That said, I figure it's best to include extra beta-carotene–rich foods in your diet until we know more.) I highly recommend that anyone with a family history of macular degeneration follow the food plan for high-antioxidant, high-zinc foods to reduce their risk. For an easy way to get a large dose of all the nutrients, try one of my Smooth-SEE recipes (pages 270 and 272).

BEST FOODS FOR VITAMIN C: *guava, bell peppers (all colors), oranges and orange juice, grapefruit and grapefruit juice, strawberries, pineapple, kohlrabi, papaya, lemons and lemon juice, broccoli, kale, Brussels sprouts, kidney beans, kiwifruit, cantaloupe, cauliflower, cabbage (all varieties), mangoes, white potatoes, mustard greens, tomatoes, sugar snap peas, snow peas, clementines, rutabagas, turnip greens, raspberries, blackberries, watermelon, tangerines, okra, lychees, summer squash, persimmons*

BEST FOODS FOR VITAMIN E: *almonds and almond butter, sunflower seeds and sunflower butter, wheat germ, hazelnuts, spinach, dandelion greens, Swiss chard, pine nuts, peanuts and peanut butter, turnip greens, beet greens, broccoli, canola oil, flaxseed oil, red bell pepper, collard greens, avocados, olive oil, mangoes*

BEST FOODS FOR BETA-CAROTENE: *sweet potatoes, carrots, kale, butternut squash, turnip greens, pumpkin, mustard greens, cantaloupe, red bell pepper, apricots, Chinese cabbage, spinach, lettuces (especially darker lettuces), collard greens, Swiss chard, watercress, grapefruit (pink, red), watermelon, cherries, mangoes, tomatoes, guava, asparagus, red cabbage*

## ZINC

AREDS and the Rotterdam study confirmed zinc's role in eye health. Zinc is concentrated in the retina and is required for the functioning of enzymes that keep vision sharp. In people with macular degeneration, levels of zinc in the retina can be very low, so eating zinc-rich foods is a logical first step toward preventing and treating macular degeneration.

BEST FOODS FOR ZINC: *oysters, lobster, lean beef, crab, ostrich, wheat germ, skinless chicken and turkey (especially dark meat), lean lamb, clams, mussels, pumpkin seeds, yogurt (fat-free, low-fat), pork tenderloin, starchy beans (such as black, navy, pinto, garbanzo, kidney), lentils, black-eyed peas, soybeans (edamame), lima beans, pine nuts, cashews, peanuts and peanut butter, sunflower seeds and butter, pecans*

## LUTEIN AND ZEAXANTHIN

Lutein and zeaxanthin are a matched pair of antioxidants—almost without exception, foods that contain one also contain the other. These antioxidants are found in high concentrations in the tissue of the macula, and because they absorb 40 to 90 percent of blue light intensity, they act like sunscreen for your eyes. Our bodies can't make lutein and zeaxanthin on their own, so we have to get them from food. Studies have shown that eating foods rich in lutein and zeaxanthin can increase the pigment density in the macula, and greater pigment density means better retina protection and possibly a lower risk of macular degeneration. A few studies have found that eating foods with high amounts of these antioxidants reduces the risk of developing macular degeneration. A second AREDS trial, now under way, is currently testing whether supplemental lutein and zeaxanthin is more effective than beta-carotene at slowing the progression of macular degeneration and should soon provide more clarity on the benefits of this nutrient duo.

BEST FOODS FOR LUTEIN AND ZEAXANTHIN: *kale, spinach, Swiss chard, collard greens, turnip greens, dandelion greens, mustard greens, beet greens, radicchio, zucchini, watercress, green peas, persimmons, winter squash (acorn, butternut, etc.), pumpkin, broccoli, Brussels sprouts, lettuces (especially dark lettuces), asparagus, corn, green beans, okra, artichokes, green bell peppers*

## OMEGA-3 FATTY ACIDS

Retinal pigment cells contain a type of omega-3 called docosahexaenoic acid (DHA), which helps protect light receptor cells in the eye from damage by sunlight and free radicals. Researchers are excited by recent findings that omega-3 fats may help stave off macular degeneration. One study found that people who ate just one weekly serving of fish, generally a good source of omega-3 fats, cut their risk of macular degeneration by over 30 percent. The good news doesn't stop there: It turns out that omega-3 fats may be just as effective for those already at high risk. In a 2009 study of people who already showed early signs of disease in their retinas, eating a diet rich in omega-3s reduced the risk of developing advanced macular degeneration by about 30 percent. If you want to take advantage of this promising research, I recommend eating fatty fish at least two times each week and striving to incorporate other omega-rich foods into your daily diet, too. (My Best Foods list includes only the fatty fish that have been shown to be low in mercury, PCBs, and dioxins.)

> BEST FOODS FOR OMEGA-3 FATTY ACIDS: *wild salmon (fresh, canned), herring, mackerel (not king), sardines, anchovies, rainbow trout, Pacific oysters, chia seeds, ground flaxseed, walnuts, butternuts (white walnuts), seaweed, walnut oil, canola oil, flaxseed oil, soybeans (edamame)*

## B VITAMINS

It seems the whole alphabet of vitamins promotes healthy vision! B vitamins are the latest to show potential for protection from macular degeneration. In a recent study, Harvard researchers tested whether a combination B vitamin supplement containing $B_6$, $B_{12}$, and folic acid reduced the risk of cardiovascular disease in a group of over 5,000 women. The B vitamins didn't provide any heart protection, but (surprise!) they *did* dramatically reduce the risk of macular degeneration. Scientists speculate that B vitamins may help by lowering blood levels of homocysteine, an amino acid that may damage the eye in some way. This is the first trial to look at the benefits of B vitamins for macular degeneration, and though the results are encouraging, it's definitely too soon to recommend supplements. While we wait for the science to catch up, I recommend loading up on healthy foods naturally rich in $B_6$, $B_{12}$, and folate (and consider taking a standard multi with 100 percent DV of each).

> BEST FOODS FOR VITAMIN $B_6$: *wild salmon (fresh, canned), trout (rainbow, wild), skinless chicken and turkey, pork tenderloin, starchy beans (especially chickpeas and pinto beans), bananas, pistachios, tuna (canned light), fish (especially haddock, halibut, cod), sweet and white potatoes, spinach, winter squash (especially acorn), lentils, avocados, bell peppers (all colors)*

**BEST FOODS FOR VITAMIN B$_{12}$:** *shellfish (clams, oysters, crab), wild salmon (fresh, canned), soy milk, trout (rainbow, wild), tuna (canned light), lean beef, veggie burgers, cottage cheese (fat-free, 1%), yogurt (fat-free, low-fat), milk (fat-free, 1%), eggs, cheese (fat-free, reduced-fat)*

**BEST FOODS FOR FOLATE:** *lentils, black-eyed peas, soybeans (edamame), oats, turnip greens, spinach, mustard greens, green peas, artichokes, okra, beets, parsnips, broccoli, broccoli raab, sunflower seeds, wheat germ, oranges and orange juice, Brussels sprouts, papayas, seaweed, berries (boysenberries, black-berries, strawberries), starchy beans (such as black, navy, pinto, garbanzo, kid-ney), cauliflower, Chinese cabbage, corn, whole grain bread, whole grain pasta*

## LOW-QUALITY CARBS

Sugary foods and refined starches such as white bread, white rice, and baked goods may be double trouble for your eyes. High amounts of low-quality (high-glycemic) carbs may increase your chances of developing cataracts, and new findings also implicate them in the progression of macular degeneration. Researchers at Tufts University discovered that people who ate a diet with a high glycemic index score faced a greater risk of developing macular degeneration. High-glycemic foods cause a dramatic rise in blood sugar, which also increases the sugar concentration in the eye. Long-term exposure to high sugar loads may damage the retina and tiny capillaries in the eye by promoting oxidative stress and inflammation. Avoiding sugary foods and refined carbs is a smart strategy for overall health, so protecting your vision is just one more good reason to sweep these foods out of your kitchen. Low-quality carbs to limit include sugar, honey, and other sweeteners; soda and other sugary drinks; candy; baked goods; sugary cereals; anything made with white flour (including white bread and regular pasta); and white rice.

## BONUS POINTS

♦ **Get regular eye exams.** It is important to get a regular comprehensive checkup by an optometrist or ophthalmologist—every one to two years if you're over age 60. Be sure that the exam includes eye dilation so that any changes in your lenses and retinas can be spotted easily and early.

♦ **Protect your eyes from the sun.** One of the leading causes of cataracts is radiation from the sun. Take steps to protect your eyes by wearing sunglasses and, when possible, a hat with a brim whenever you are out in bright daylight.

♦ **Stop smoking.** Smoking increases your risk of both cataracts and macular degeneration because it creates free radicals and decreases the amount of oxygen to the eye.

◆ **If you smoke, don't drink alcohol or take beta-carotene supplements.** I strongly encourage you to stop smoking, but if you haven't yet quit entirely, you should follow these guidelines. Although drinking alcohol in moderation doesn't appear to increase the risk of cataracts on its own, smokers who drink alcohol have a greater risk than smokers who don't drink. And beta-carotene supplements may increase the risk of lung cancer in smokers, so that's a dangerous combination.

◆ **Maintain a healthy weight.** People with early-stage macular degeneration who are also overweight have double the risk of moving on to the advanced stage, so losing weight may help keep the disease from progressing. Plus, if you are overweight, you have a greater risk of developing type 2 diabetes, which increases the risk of cataracts. (See Weight Loss on page 17 for more information.)

◆ **Avoid eating foods high in saturated and trans fats.** Butter, stick margarine, marbled red meat, cream, whole milk, ice cream, lard, cheese, products made with hydrogenated oil, and other damaging fats can cause a buildup of plaque in blood vessels, which can then choke off blood flow—including blood flow to the eye. Any decrease in oxygen can harm the eye and promote tissue damage.

## SUPPLEMENTS

### FOR CATARACTS

If you are concerned about cataracts and want to consider supplements in addition to food fixes, I have only one recommendation.

◆ **A multivitamin.** It is important to get the necessary amounts of the cataract-fighting B vitamins, along with a basic amount of vitamin C and E. Look for a standard multivitamin that contains 100 percent of vitamins C and E, as well as riboflavin ($B_2$) and niacin ($B_3$). Supplements with "mega" doses of any vitamin or mineral are not recommended.

### FOR MACULAR DEGENERATION

For people who are at risk for macular degeneration, the following supplements may help prevent or delay the onset of the disease.

### I RECOMMEND THAT EVERYONE TAKE

◆ **A multivitamin** that provides 100 percent DV of vitamin C, zinc, vitamin $B_6$, vitamin $B_{12}$, and folic acid, as well as some beta-carotene. In addition, make sure your multivitamin provides *only* 100 percent DV of vitamin E. (This amount is safe, but higher dosages have been linked to certain health risks.)

## AND SPEAK WITH YOUR DOCTOR
## ABOUT THESE ADDITIONAL SUPPLEMENTS

◆ **Omega-3 fish oil.** If you can't get enough omega-3 fats through diet alone, you may want to consider fish oil supplements. I recommend 1,000 milligrams daily coming from a combination of EPA (eicosapentaenoic acid) and DHA (docosa-hexaenoic acid), the two most beneficial types of omega-3 fats. Because the amount of EPA plus DHA per capsule varies widely among brands, you'll need to read labels and add up the individual milligrams yourself to determine how many pills it will take to reach that dosage. Store pills in the fridge to prevent the fish oils from going rancid. To avoid fishy burps and aftertaste, take these with food, and choose enteric-coated varieties, which are designed to dissolve in the intestines instead of the stomach. Because fish oil acts as a blood thinner, do not take it if you have hemophilia or are already taking blood-thinning medications or aspirin.

◆ **Specially formulated "antioxidant plus zinc" supplements for macular degeneration.** If you're at high risk of advanced macular degeneration or already have the disease, your doctor may recommend taking a specific high-dose formula of antioxidants plus zinc—the same formulation found to be effective in the AREDS trial. These formulations provide 500 milligrams of vitamin C; 400 IU of vitamin E; 15 milligrams of beta-carotene (often labeled as equivalent to 25,000 IU of vitamin A); 80 milligrams of zinc as zinc oxide; and two milligrams of copper as cupric oxide. (Copper is added to balance out the high level of zinc, which can block the body's ability to absorb copper.)

> For more information on food cures for eye health, visit www.joybauer.com/vision.

# JOY'S 4-STEP PROGRAM
## FOR VISION

Follow this program if you have macular degeneration, cataracts, or a family history of these diseases.

## Step 1 ... START WITH THE BASICS

These are the first things you should do to address eye problems.

◆ See an optometrist or ophthalmologist for a comprehensive eye exam. If you are over age 60, have an exam every one to two years. If you notice any vision changes, see a doctor immediately—don't wait for your next appointment.

◆ If you have macular degeneration, talk with your physician about whether you are a good candidate for the AREDS supplements.

◆ If you smoke, quit.

◆ Protect your eyes from the sun whenever you're outdoors by wearing sunglasses, and, when possible, a brimmed hat.

## Step 2 ... YOUR ULTIMATE GROCERY LIST

A nutrition plan is only as good as the foods you choose. This list contains foods with high levels of nutrients that contribute to eye health, including antioxidants, B vitamins, and omega-3 fats. You don't have to purchase every item, but these foods should make up the bulk of what you eat each week.

## FRUIT

*All* fruits, but especially:

Apples

Apricots

Bananas

Berries (blackberries, blueberries, raspberries, and strawberries)

Cantaloupe

Cherries

Clementines

Cranberries, fresh and dried

Grapefruit

Guava

Kiwifruit

Lemons

Lychees

Mangoes

Oranges

Papayas

Persimmons

Pineapple

Plums

Prunes

Tangerines

Watermelon

## VEGETABLES AND LEGUMES

*All* vegetables, but especially:

Artichokes

Asparagus

Avocados

Beans (especially chickpeas, kidney, and pinto)

Beets

Bell peppers

Broccoli

Broccoli raab

Brussels sprouts

Cabbage

Carrots

Cauliflower

Corn

Green beans

Dark leafy greens (such as collard, dandelion, kale, mustard, Swiss chard, and turnip)

Kohlrabi

Lentils

Lettuce (especially dark lettuces)

Lima beans

Mushrooms

Okra

Parsnips

Peas (black-eyed and green)

Potatoes (sweet and white)

Pumpkin

Rutabagas

Snow peas

Soybeans (edamame)

Spinach

Squash, summer (all varieties)

Squash, winter (acorn and butternut)

Sugar snap peas

Tomatoes

Zucchini

## SEAFOOD

*All* fish and shellfish, but especially:

Anchovies

Clams

Cod

Crab

Haddock

Halibut

Herring

Lobster

Mackerel (not king)

Mussels

Oysters (especially Pacific)

Salmon, wild (fresh and canned)

Sardines

Trout (rainbow, wild)

Tuna (canned light)

## LEAN PROTEINS

Beef, lean

Chicken, ground (at least 90% lean)

Chicken, skinless

Eggs

Lamb, lean

Pork tenderloin

Tempeh

Tofu

Turkey, ground (at least 90% lean)

Turkey, skinless

Turkey bacon

Turkey burgers, lean

Veggie burgers

Venison

## NUTS AND SEEDS (PREFERABLY UNSALTED)

Almonds and almond butter

Butternuts (white walnuts)

Cashews and cashew butter

Chia seeds

Flaxseed, ground

Hazelnuts

Macadamia nuts

Peanuts and peanut butter

Pecans

Pine nuts

Pistachios

Pumpkin seeds

Sunflower seeds and sunflower butter

Walnuts

## WHOLE GRAINS

Amaranth

Barley

Bread, whole grain (buns, crackers, English muffins, pitas, tortillas, and wraps)

Bulgur

Cereals, whole grain (at least 3 grams fiber; no more than 8 grams sugar per serving)

Millet

Oats

Pasta, whole grain

Quinoa

Rice (brown and wild)

Waffles, whole grain

Wheat germ

## DAIRY

Cheese (fat-free or reduced-fat)

Cottage cheese (nonfat or 1%)

Milk (fat-free or 1%)

Milk alternatives (almond, rice, and soy)

Yogurt (fat-free or low-fat)

## MISCELLANEOUS

Canola oil

Garlic

Guacamole

Herbs and spices (fresh, dried, and ground)

Hummus

Marinara sauce

Mayonnaise, reduced-fat

Mustard (all varieties)

Olive oil

Salad dressing, reduced-calorie

Salsa

Soft tub spread, trans-fat-free (reduced-fat or regular)

Tea (black and green)

Vinegar (all varieties)

# Step 3 . . . GOING ABOVE AND BEYOND

If you want to do everything you can for eye health, here are some additional things you might try.

- ◆ If you like, feel free to take a multivitamin with 100 percent DV of B vitamins, folic acid, vitamin C, and zinc. Look for a supplement that contains *only* (no more than) 100 percent DV of vitamin E.

- ◆ If you're at risk of macular degeneration, consider taking an omega-3 fish oil supplement if you don't regularly eat fatty fish.

- ◆ If you have macular degeneration (not cataracts), consult with your physician about taking a specially formulated, high-dose "antioxidant plus zinc" supplement for macular degeneration. These are treatment-level dosages; if you do not have macular degeneration, do not take these supplements. If you are a smoker, high doses of beta-carotene pose health risks and are generally not advised.

- ◆ Avoid eating foods high in saturated and trans fats, including butter, stick margarine, marbled red meat, ice cream, whole milk, cheese, and products made with hydrogenated oils.

## SUNGLASSES

Your choice of sunglasses makes a fashion statement, but please don't let that statement include the words *eye damage*. Not all designer models protect the eyes. Don't be fooled into thinking that large or dark lenses necessarily protect against radiation. The American Academy of Ophthalmology recommends choosing sunglasses that are certified to block 99 to 100 percent of UVA and UVB radiation. Glasses should fit well so they don't slide down your nose. If possible, look for models that wrap all the way around to your temples. Wear your sunglasses every time you go outside, even on cloudy days. (Radiation is still there, even if the sun is hidden.) If you wear contact lenses with UV protection, it is still important to wear sunglasses because contacts cover only a small portion of your eyes.

# Step4 . . . MEAL PLANS

These sample menus include foods high in nutrients that have been shown to protect against cataracts and macular degeneration—specifically, vitamins C and E, lutein, zeaxanthin, beta-carotene, zinc, B vitamins, and omega-3 fats.

Every day, choose one option for each of the three meals—breakfast, lunch, and dinner. Then, once or twice per day, choose from my suggested snacks. Approximate calories have been provided to help adjust for your personal weight-management goals. If you find yourself hungry (and if weight is not an issue), feel free to increase the portion sizes for meals and snacks. Beverage calories are not included.

## BREAKFAST OPTIONS

(300 TO 400 CALORIES)

### Cottage Cheese and Cantaloupe

Fill ½ cantaloupe with 1 cup fat-free or 1% cottage cheese and top with 1 tablespoon sunflower seeds and 1 tablespoon chopped walnuts (or slivered almonds).

### Cereal with Milk and Fruit

Mix 1 cup whole grain cereal with 1 cup milk (fat-free, 1%, or soy) and top with 1 tablespoon wheat germ. Enjoy with ½ pink grapefruit (or 1 orange or 1 cup berries).

### Peanut Butter Pita

Top a whole wheat pita, split and toasted, with 1 level tablespoon peanut butter (or almond butter).

### Scrambled Eggs with Peppers, Mushrooms, and Onion

Sauté ½ cup each sliced onion, mushrooms, and bell peppers in a skillet coated with oil spray (or 1 to 2 teaspoons canola oil) until soft. Beat 1 whole egg with 2 egg whites. Add to the vegetables and cook, stirring, until the eggs are cooked. Serve with 1 slice whole wheat bread, toasted, with optional 1 teaspoon soft tub, trans-fat-free spread.

### Yogurt with Chopped Mango and Berries

Mix 1 cup fat-free or low-fat vanilla yogurt with ½ chopped mango (fresh or thawed from frozen), ½ cup berries, and 1 to 2 tablespoons wheat germ (or chopped walnuts, almonds, pecans, or sunflower seeds).

## LUNCH OPTIONS

(400 TO 500 CALORIES)

### Turkey Sandwich with Baby Carrots

Layer 4 ounces sliced turkey (or chicken), unlimited baby spinach leaves, and sliced tomato between 2 slices whole grain bread. Add optional 2 thin slices avocado and/or 2 teaspoons reduced-fat mayonnaise or hummus. Enjoy with a large handful of baby carrots.

### Butternut Squash Soup with Mixed Vegetables and Salad

Enjoy 2 to 3 cups butternut squash, lentil, or split-pea soup (canned, no cream or whole milk used in preparation) with a large mixed vegetable salad (unlimited dark leafy greens, tomato, pepper, onion, carrots, cucumber, mushrooms, etc.) tossed with 1 teaspoon olive oil and unlimited vinegar or fresh lemon juice (or 2 tablespoons reduced-calorie salad dressing).

### Edamame with Wild Salmon Dijonnaise

Enjoy 1 cup boiled edamame (green soybeans in the pod) with 5 ounces canned wild salmon, drained, mashed, and mixed with 1 tablespoon reduced-fat mayonnaise, 1 to 2 teaspoons Dijon mustard, and minced onion and black pepper to taste. Serve on a large bed of baby spinach leaves drizzled with lemon juice and your choice of seasonings (or 1 to 2 tablespoons reduced-calorie dressing).

### Veggie Tuna Salad with Fresh Fruit

Enjoy 1 serving Veggie Tuna Salad (page 271) with 150 calories' worth of whole wheat pita or whole grain crackers and 1 orange or kiwi (or ½ mango).

### Spinach Omelet and Sweet Potato

Beat 1 whole egg with 2 or 3 egg whites. Cook in a heated skillet coated with oil spray. When the bottom is cooked, gently flip over. Top with unlimited spinach (raw or sautéed) and 1 ounce reduced-fat cheese. Fold the omelet over and cook until the egg mixture is firm and the cheese melts. Enjoy with a plain baked sweet potato (or 2 cups hearty vegetable soup).

## DINNER OPTIONS

(500 TO 600 CALORIES)

### Pork Tenderloin with Cranberry Couscous and Sautéed Greens

Enjoy 5 ounces baked, grilled, or broiled pork tenderloin (or turkey, chicken, wild salmon, cod, haddock, shrimp, or tofu) with 1 cup cooked whole wheat couscous mixed with 2 tablespoons dried cranberries and unlimited steamed or sautéed greens (kale, Swiss chard, collard greens, spinach, etc.).

### Pasta with Chicken and Broccoli

Enjoy 1 serving (2 cups) Whole Wheat Penne with Chicken and Broccoli (page 364) with a salad of dark leafy greens, tomatoes, peppers, carrots, and 1 tablespoon chopped walnuts tossed with 2 teaspoons olive oil and unlimited vinegar or fresh lemon juice.

### Grilled Salmon with Veggies and Sweet Potato

Enjoy 5 ounces grilled, baked, broiled, or poached salmon (or cod, halibut, haddock, or shrimp) with fresh lemon juice and preferred seasonings. Serve with unlimited steamed or sautéed Brussels sprouts, asparagus, or dark leafy greens and 1 plain baked sweet potato.

### Vegetarian Chili and Salad

Enjoy 2 cups vegetarian chili with a large salad of dark leafy greens, peppers, tomato, artichokes, and carrots tossed with 2 teaspoons olive oil and unlimited vinegar or fresh lemon juice (or 2 to 4 tablespoons reduced-calorie salad dressing).

## Grilled Sirloin with Sautéed Spinach and Butternut Squash

Enjoy 5 ounces grilled sirloin or beef tenderloin (or any other lean beef) with unlimited spinach sautéed in 1 teaspoon olive oil and garlic, plus ½ cup baked butternut squash.

## SNACK OPTIONS

100 CALORIES OR LESS

- ◆ *Best Vegetable Snacks:* up to 2 cups raw or cooked bell peppers (any color), broccoli, cauliflower, asparagus, carrots, green beans, sugar snap peas, snow peas, or cherry tomatoes
- ◆ *Best Fruit Snacks:* 1 guava, apple, peach, orange, banana, or persimmon; 2 plums, kiwifruit, clementines, or tangerines; 4 prunes or apricots; 1 cup blueberries, blackberries, raspberries, sliced strawberries, or cherries; 1 cup cubed watermelon or pineapple; 20 strawberries; ½ mango, papaya, cantaloupe, or grapefruit
- ◆ 1 level tablespoon peanut butter (or other nut butter) with celery sticks
- ◆ 10 almonds
- ◆ 25 pistachios in the shell
- ◆ 1 part-skim string cheese or 1 ounce any reduced-fat cheese
- ◆ ½ cup fat-free cottage cheese with bell pepper strips (red, green, or yellow)

100 TO 200 CALORIES

- ◆ 10 almonds (or 25 pistachios) plus 1 serving fruit (see Best Fruit Snacks)
- ◆ Whole nuts: 1 ounce (about ¼ cup) of your choice of almonds, cashews, pecans, walnuts, or peanuts
- ◆ ½ cup pistachios or sunflower seeds in the shell
- ◆ ½ cup fat-free or 1% cottage cheese mixed with 1 tablespoon chopped nuts (or pumpkin seeds or sunflower seeds)
- ◆ 1 slice whole grain toast with 1 level tablespoon peanut butter (or other nut butter)
- ◆ Bell pepper strips (red, green, or yellow) with ¼ cup hummus or guacamole
- ◆ 1 cup whole grain cereal with ½ cup skim or soy milk
- ◆ 6 to 8 ounces any fat-free plain or flavored yogurt
- ◆ ½ cup chickpeas (garbanzo beans)

◆ 1 cup boiled edamame (green soybeans in the pod)

◆ 1 sliced apple with 1 level tablespoon nut butter (or 1 ounce reduced-fat cheese)

◆ Berry smoothie: In a blender, mix ½ cup fat-free milk (or soy milk), ½ cup fat-free yogurt, ¾ cup fresh or frozen raspberries or 8 whole strawberries, and 3 to 5 ice cubes.

◆ Vanilla Pumpkin Pudding: Mix 1 cup fat-free vanilla yogurt with ½ cup canned 100% pure pumpkin puree and a dash of ground cinnamon.

◆ 1 Ginger-Spiced Pumpkin Muffin (page 180)

200 CALORIES OR MORE

◆ Vision Mix (below)

# VISION MIX

*This packable snack provides more than 90 percent of your daily requirement for vitamin E. For more antioxidants, try adding ½ cup dried cranberries, blueberries, or cherries. But be sure to watch portions—calories can add up quickly with this crunchy concoction.*

**MAKES 6 SERVINGS**

4 cups whole grain cereal

½ cup whole almonds

½ cup unsalted oil-roasted peanuts

¼ cup unsalted sunflower seeds

In a large bowl, combine the cereal, almonds, peanuts, and sunflower seeds and mix thoroughly. Divide evenly among 6 zip-top bags.

**Per serving:** 237 calories, 8 g protein, 21 g carbohydrate, 15 g fat (2 g saturated), 0 mg cholesterol, 198 mg sodium, 5 g fiber

# Green Smooth-See

*My smoothies each provide a great big blast of eye-fighting nutrients—vitamins C and E, zinc, lutein, and beta-carotene. They're the perfect treat for people who want to go that extra mile, as well as people who aren't interested in popping extra supplemental pills.*

*Calories always count, so remember to factor these smoothies into your plan's total calories. If weight is an issue, split this smoothie into two servings and enjoy each as a snack, or count one full serving as your breakfast—either way, the math is a snap. If weight is not an issue, enjoy a daily serving whenever you wish.*

**MAKES 1 SERVING (ABOUT 1¾ CUPS)**

1 carrot, peeled and grated

2 kiwifruit, skin removed

1 cup baby spinach leaves

½ cup watercress

½ cup fat-free plain yogurt

¼ cup avocado, mashed (3 tablespoons)

2 tablespoons wheat germ

2 tablespoons water

1 tablespoon fresh lemon juice

1 teaspoon Worcestershire sauce

¼ teaspoon prepared horseradish

Pinch of salt

In a blender or food processor, combine the carrot, kiwi, spinach, watercress, yogurt, avocado, wheat germ, water, lemon juice, Worcestershire, horseradish, and salt. Blend until smooth.

**Per serving:** 323 calories, 16 g protein, 50 g carbohydrate, 9 g fat (1 g saturated), 0 mg cholesterol, 254 mg sodium, 14 g fiber; plus 172 mg vitamin C (287% DV), 8 IU vitamin E (26% DV), 220 mcg folate (55% DV), 0.6 mg vitamin $B_6$ (30% DV), 4,118 mcg beta-carotene, 1,520 mcg lutein + zeaxanthin, 4 mg zinc (29% DV)

# VEGGIE TUNA SALAD

*Use light instead of albacore white canned tuna in this recipe to get all the nutrition without too much mercury. Chopped peppers and carrots add vitamin C and beta-carotene. Serve the tuna mixture on a bed of fresh baby spinach leaves for an added blast of lutein.*

**MAKES 1 SERVING**

1 can (6 ounces) chunk light tuna in water, drained

½ carrot, peeled and diced

½ celery stalk, diced

½ bell pepper (red, green, or yellow), diced

½ scallion, minced

1 tablespoon reduced-fat mayonnaise

½ teaspoon lemon juice

3 cups baby spinach leaves

4 medium-thick slices red tomato

In a medium bowl, flake the tuna into small pieces with a fork. Add the carrot, celery, bell pepper, scallion, mayonnaise, and lemon juice and mix well with a fork.

Line a plate with the spinach and place the tuna mixture on top. Arrange the tomato slices around the tuna.

> **Per serving:** 227 calories, 40 g protein, 9 g carbohydrate, 4 g fat (1 g saturated), 43 mg cholesterol, 755 mg sodium, 9 g fiber; plus 100 mg vitamin C (167% DV), 20 mg niacin (100% DV), 249 mcg folate (62% DV), 0.9 mg vitamin $B_6$ (45% DV), 2.4 mcg vitamin $B_{12}$ (40% DV)

# CITRUS SMOOTH-SEE

*As with my Green Smooth-See (page 270), you'll need to factor the caloric value for this beverage into your plan's total calories. If weight is an issue, split this smoothie into two servings and enjoy each as a snack, or count one full serving as your breakfast. If weight is not an issue, enjoy a daily serving whenever you wish.*

**MAKES 1 SERVING (ABOUT 1¾ CUPS)**

1 orange, zested, then peeled and cut into sections

½ medium pink grapefruit, peeled and cut into sections

1 carrot, peeled and grated

½ cup fat-free plain yogurt

¼ cup raspberries (fresh or frozen)

¼ cup cubed papaya or mango chunks (fresh or frozen)

2 tablespoons wheat germ

1 tablespoon fresh lemon juice

1 tablespoon granulated sugar

In a blender or food processor, combine ¼ teaspoon of the orange zest and the sections, grapefruit, carrot, yogurt, raspberries, papaya, wheat germ, lemon juice, and sugar. Blend until smooth.

**Per serving:** 340 calories, 15 g protein, 71 g carbohydrate, 2 g fat (0 g saturated), 0 mg cholesterol, 138 mg sodium, 12 g fiber; plus 150 mg vitamin C (251% DV), 6 IU vitamin E (18% DV), 145 mcg folate (36% DV), 4,568 mcg beta-carotene, 482 mcg lutein + zeaxanthin, 4 mg zinc (27% DV)

# CHAPTER 12

# MEMORY

No one has ever come to me specifically looking for nutritional help for a memory problem, but the topic comes up more often than you might think. For example, a client who has trouble recalling what she ate for breakfast the day she comes to see me might mention that she's been noticing more and more memory lapses. I once had a client who kept forgetting to put gas in his car and had to call AAA roadside assistance three times in a single month, and a client who was forever losing her cell phone, only relocating it when the ringing led her to the pantry . . . or the refrigerator . . . or the laundry hamper . . . or a basket of bathroom cleaning supplies.

Of course, memory changes aren't always so obvious. They can be subtle and hardly worth mentioning—until they interrupt the rhythm and flow of our daily lives. We waste valuable time looking for keys, shoes, or important documents filed away somewhere at home or at work. Memory problems can infuriate and frustrate you when that elusive thought is on the tip of your tongue—or the tip of your brain, in this case—but you just can't access it. And if you've seen a friend or family member descend into dementia, your own memory problems might trigger fear for your own future.

My absentminded clients and friends are thrilled when they learn that there are nutritional and lifestyle strategies that may keep them from sliding down the slippery slope of memory loss. Every single suggestion listed here will also help improve overall health, so it's win-win, with no downside. Better memory and better health.

## WHAT AFFECTS MEMORY?

Memory is tricky. So many factors can affect how it functions, and, on top of that, how well it works on any given day is purely subjective. You know when "brain freeze" happens, but with very few exceptions, there are no physical signs that doctors can look for to pinpoint the cause. Even the memory disorder people fear most—Alzheimer's disease—can't be definitively diagnosed except at autopsy after death. (For more on Alzheimer's disease, see page 277.) For the most part, physicians make educated guesses about the cause of memory loss based on your medical history, physical examination results, and lifestyle.

Memory is carried in a network of brain cells called neurons. Each neuron contains a cell body, which houses the cell's information-processing machinery, and a long fiber called an axon, which connects and sends messages to other neurons in the brain. Clusters of cell bodies make up the gray matter in the brain. The gray matter is the brain's computer—the section that allows people to make decisions, form thoughts, plan movements, recognize sensations, and store and recall memories. Clusters of axons make up the white matter in the brain. White matter is like a network of cables that connect neurons and allow them to communicate with one another. The human brain is the epitome of organized chaos—it contains roughly 100 billion neurons, and each one has around 1,000 connections. Memory depends on your total number of brain cells and their connections, the smooth flow of communication between them, and their overall health. That means that it is relatively easy for something somewhere in the brain to go on the fritz. There are several major factors that can affect memory.

## VASCULAR HEALTH

Every cell in your body needs a steady supply of oxygen and nutrients in order to stay alive and work properly, but brain cells are especially needy, like hungry infants that require feeding regularly and often. Because oxygen and nutrients are carried in the bloodstream, anything that impedes blood flow will starve those all-important memory cells. The plain truth is that a healthy heart makes for a healthy brain.

Developing major cardiovascular risk factors like high blood pressure and high cholesterol during your thirties, forties, and fifties raises the risk of memory problems later in life. Here's what you need to watch for.

**High blood pressure (hypertension).** Physicians recommend that you maintain blood pressure at or below 120/80 mmHg. If your numbers are significantly higher than that, your health is generally at risk and your memory can suffer. High blood pressure damages the tiny blood vessels that nourish brain cells. Over time, interruptions in bloodflow cause tiny lesions in the white matter (the brain's communication network), and these pockets of damage may interfere with the brain's ability to send signals and process memories. When researchers at the University of Pittsburgh compared brain scans of people with and without hypertension, they found that those with high blood pressure had significantly more white matter lesions, which could very well indicate a higher risk of memory loss and cognitive decline.

In another study, a different group of researchers at the University of Pittsburgh compared people who had normal blood pressure with people who had high blood pressure on two different measures of memory. Verbal memory was tested by having the participants remember words, and spatial memory was tested by having the participants remember the position of items on a computer screen. While they were performing the tasks, the participants had their brains scanned to see where the blood was flowing. The results were surprising: The participants with hypertension had less blood flowing to the parts of the brain that controlled these types of memory—even though they performed just as well on the tests as the participants with normal blood pressure. The researchers predicted that, over time, the hypertension sufferers' neurons would become damaged and their memories would be severely compromised. The lesson is that high blood pressure starts wreaking havoc before you notice it, so it is hugely important to take action early.

**High LDL, low HDL cholesterol.** Cholesterol comes in two main varieties: the "bad" variety known as low-density lipoprotein (LDL) cholesterol and the "good" variety known as high-density lipoprotein (HDL) cholesterol. LDL cholesterol is one of the components of blood vessel plaque, so the higher your LDL cholesterol, the greater the chance your blood vessels are narrowing. The optimal level of LDL cholesterol is below 100 mg/dL.

HDL cholesterol, on the other hand, acts almost like a plaque magnet, picking up the vessel-clogging cholesterol and carrying it away to the liver. So the higher your HDL levels, the better and healthier your blood vessels—and by extension, your memory—will be. In one study, researchers gave over 3,500 people a simple word recall test and took a blood sample to measure their HDL levels (the "good" cholesterol). They then asked them to return five years later to repeat both measurements. Those people whose HDL levels decreased between visits were 61 percent more likely to see a decline in their memory score than people whose HDL remained high throughout the study. Health experts consider HDL levels below 40 mg/dL for men and 50 mg/dL for women too low to be healthy.

(For more on heart health, see Cardiovascular Disease, page 117.)

## BLOOD SUGAR

Insulin and blood sugar appear to play such integral roles in memory and cognitive health that some researchers are now referring to dementia as "type 3" diabetes. New research suggests that elevated blood sugar may speed up the pace of memory decline with aging.

The most common form of diabetes, type 2, is caused when the body produces too much insulin, a hormone that regulates blood sugar, and the body's cells become resistant to insulin's effects. High blood sugar results as insulin becomes less efficient at shepherding glucose molecules out of the blood and into cells. Chronic exposure to high blood sugar or insulin levels may impair brain function and memory in any number of ways. Carrying an unhealthy sugar load may damage the

**FAQS**

## I'm dieting to lose weight, and now my memory is shot. Did I diet away my brain cells?

No, no, a thousand times no. Your brain cells are all still there. However, it's not surprising that you're noticing changes. When you diet, you have to change the way you shop for food, prepare food, and think about food. British psychologists from the University of Bristol found that diet-related thoughts took over dieters' brains, effectively pushing out all other thoughts. Second, if you go overboard, skip meals, and think that you should eat as little as humanly possible, you will probably feel foggy-brained and forgetful due to lack of energy getting to your brain cells. My advice is to eat controlled portions of healthy foods every four to five hours so that you keep your blood sugar levels as steady as possible.

network of blood vessels that feed the brain and promote inflammation and oxidation, processes that prematurely age brain tissue. In addition, recent findings suggest that insulin resistance may speed the development of sticky plaques in the brain, which play a role in Alzheimer's disease.

For detailed information on managing blood sugar and reducing diabetes risk, see the Type 2 Diabetes chapter, page 183.

## BELLY FAT

Studies show that adults who carry a lot of weight around the midsection during middle age face an increased risk of developing dementia later in life. Abdominal fat is more dangerous than excess fat around your hips and thighs because it specifically triggers a chain of harmful metabolic reactions that increase inflammation, raise insulin and blood sugar levels, promote plaque formation in the arteries, and increase the risk of developing cardiovascular disease and type 2 diabetes. As you've read, all of these undesirable changes can accelerate memory and cognitive loss.

Waist circumference is a quick and simple indicator of abdominal fat, so you should measure yourself to gauge whether you have an unhealthy amount. To do so, wrap a flexible tape measure around your waist just above your hip bone. Make sure the tape is parallel to the floor all the way around. To take your measurement, relax, exhale, and pull the tape measure so it is snug but not squeezing into your skin. (No sucking in or holding your breath allowed!)

For men, a waist circumference greater than 40 inches is considered high risk. For women, a waist circumference over 35 inches is high risk. If your waist falls above these cutoffs, you should make weight loss a priority.

High blood pressure, high cholesterol, high blood sugar, and a large waist are all indicators that you should begin taking steps to protect your memory *now*, whether you're 20 or 60. Making healthy food choices and staying trim and physically active as a young and middle-aged adult can help prevent diabetes and cardiovascular disease in the near future and promote sharper memory and clearer thinking as you grow older.

## AGING

Almost everyone over age 40 has experienced memory problems due in large part to changes in general health. As we get older, there is more that can go wrong with our bodies. Heart and blood flow problems, type 2 diabetes or prediabetes, and some autoimmune disorders can cause memory to decline. But there are other, less

## COULD IT BE ALZHEIMER'S DISEASE?

The horror of Alzheimer's disease (AD) is that it slowly strips away everything that makes us who we are. A lifetime of memories can disappear, leaving a mother unable to recognize her own children or a brother convinced he's never met his own twin. Day-to-day moments, those little kindnesses and conversations that make relationships possible, are gossamer fragile. Walk out of a room and the room no longer exists.

When their memory problems start becoming obvious, many people first wonder if they have the beginnings of AD. It is impossible to know for certain.

Most cases of AD begin after age 60, and the risk increases as the years continue. Estimates suggest that about 5 percent of people under age 75 have AD, but up to 50 percent of those older than age 85 may have it. These numbers are only educated guesses because age-related dementia can look very similar to the symptoms of AD. The only way to get a definitive, 100 percent accurate diagnosis of AD is to examine the brain after death for the abnormal telltale signs of the disease: waxy-looking chunks called amyloid plaques and knotted clumps of fibers called neurofibrillary tangles.

Doctors may tentatively diagnose an elderly person with AD after ruling out other problems, including blood vessel disease, depression, drug interactions, and brain tumors. Although AD begins with mild memory lapses, they typically become far more serious as the disease progresses. People in the middle stages of AD can forget how to perform simple, routine tasks, such as opening a window or tying their shoes. So the time to worry isn't necessarily when you keep losing your cell phone but when you forget what the cell phone is used for.

People suspected of having AD can take medications to slow the progression of the disease, but I think some of the most exciting research focuses on risk reduction. All of the dietary and lifestyle changes recommended in this chapter to help improve general memory function also seem to help prevent or delay the worst symptoms of AD. For example, scientists have discovered links between AD and heart disease. High blood pressure, high cholesterol, and uncontrolled type 2 diabetes all damage blood vessels, and all increase the risks of cardiovascular disease and AD. Cholesterol medications called statins also slow the progression of AD. And from a nutrition perspective, regular exercise, antioxidant-rich produce, and omega-3 fatty acids in fish have all have been associated with decreased risk of heart disease, memory loss, and AD.

If you are worried about AD, see your doctor. But you can also help yourself by following the nutrition advice in this chapter and in the Cardiovascular Disease chapter (page 117).

apparent reasons for age-related memory loss. Beginning in our twenties, we typically start to lose brain cells, which means that we lose the very structures that hold our memories. In addition, older brains make less of certain brain chemicals necessary for memory encoding, so no matter how hard we try to commit something to memory, it may not stick. It would be like putting your keys in a briefcase that had a big hole in the bottom: You may think your keys are safe, but your storage system is leaky.

Some memory experts believe that older brains store information in a qualitatively different way than younger brains. Older brains have built up a complex network of information and memories over time. Every new piece of information has to get wired into the existing network, and sometimes random bits of trivia get lost. While this may mean that we get better at distinguishing between relevant and irrelevant information as we get older, it also does tend to make it more difficult to recall specific pieces of information, such as names or appointments. (See there, it's not just you!)

Just as good nutrition and an active lifestyle can protect your body from looking dumpy before its time, eating healthy and exercising are huge factors in preventing memory loss in middle and old age. During a recent study at the University of California, Los Angeles, participants ate a memory-healthy diet, exercised for cardiovascular training, learned relaxation strategies, and challenged their brains with memory games. After just two weeks, brain scans showed that their minds were working with greater efficiency than they had before starting the regimen, allowing them to remember with less effort. It's not a stretch to imagine that these same lifestyle changes could, over the long term, keep 60- or 70-year-old brains functioning at the level of 20- or 30-year-old brains.

## STRESS

These days, stress seems to have become an unpleasant but inescapable part of life. Until it causes insomnia, overeating, or illness, most of us don't give it much thought—and we give even less thought to its possible effects on memory. However, when you're stressed, your brain releases a steroid hormone called cortisol, which can damage your brain. It doesn't take long—just a week or so of ongoing stress can be toxic.

Chronic stress can also make you feel depressed or anxious, and these feelings can interfere with the way your brain processes memories. Every emotion, positive or negative, causes a shift in brain chemicals. Happiness, for example, is usually associated with increased levels of serotonin, while depression is associated with decreased levels of serotonin. Anytime you change the chemical soup in your brain, you risk changing the way memories are encoded and retrieved. In some cases, the damage can be serious, leading to permanent memory disorders. For example, people who are clinically depressed throughout their lives have a greater risk of developing Alzheimer's disease. (For more information on mood and stress, see Mood on page 301.)

Stress, anxiety, and depression can also affect memory by simply distracting you. These emotions take over your life, push all other thoughts out of your mind, and make everything seem less important. And whatever you don't consider important, you won't remember.

## FATIGUE

Sleep is necessary for the body to recuperate after the physical and mental activities of the day, and recent studies have discovered that it is critically important for learning and memory. European researchers found that during sleep, we organize and consolidate our memories—it's the brain's equivalent of burning a memory DVD. Without enough sleep, our memories don't settle in as well, so we are more likely to forget. Make getting a good night's rest a priority, and aim for 7 to 9 hours of sleep per night.

# HOW FOOD AFFECTS MEMORY

A woman I know told me that when she was young and balked at eating her vegetables, her mother would command, "Eat it—it's brain food." I told my friend to call her mom and thank her because she's absolutely right. Vegetables, fruits, whole grains, and fish can all be considered brain food. And not just because mom says so—memory experts say so, too!

## GOOD FOODS TO CHOOSE

All of the nutrients in this section are important to memory.

### Antioxidants

The colors of fruits and vegetables—red apples, purple blackberries, green broccoli—are caused by natural compounds called phytochemicals. There are thousands of phytochemicals in the world, and each fruit or vegetable can contain more than 100 of them. You know about the importance of vitamins and minerals, right? Well, phytochemicals are a whole new class of nutrients that deserve your respect.

Many phytochemicals are antioxidants, which nourish and defend body cells—including neurons—against the damage of oxidative stress that occurs during normal metabolism. Antioxidants may also help prevent the buildup of plaque in the arteries and ensure good, strong bloodflow to the brain. Overall, general studies of the effects of phytochemicals on memory suggest that the more of them you eat, the better. For example, a 25-year Harvard Medical School study of more than

## FAQS

### I know dark leafy greens like kale and Swiss chard are great memory boosters, but I still walk right by them in the grocery store because I have no idea how to prepare them. Any tips?

Cooking greens is a lot easier than you might think. My preferred method of attack is braising because it's a simple technique, requires only one pan, and helps cut down on the bitterness of the greens. Start by rinsing one or two bunches of greens (spinach, chard, kale, collards, turnip greens, mustard greens, or dandelion greens). If the stems are large or tough (as with chard, kale, and collards), you'll want to strip and discard them to cut down on cooking time. Slice the leaves into 1-inch-wide ribbons and set them aside. Place 1 to 2 teaspoons of olive oil in a skillet over medium heat. Add a few cloves of minced or thinly sliced garlic and, if you like heat, a pinch of red-pepper flakes. Sauté the garlic for about 1 minute, or until the garlic just starts to turn golden. Then add the prepped greens, along with about ⅓ cup water or reduced-sodium broth. Cover and cook until the greens are tender, adding more liquid if the pan begins to dry out. (Cook time varies significantly depending on the type of green. More delicate greens, like spinach and chard, cook up quickly, taking no more than 5 minutes. Sturdier greens like kale take a bit longer, and collards, the toughest of them all, taste best when they've simmered for at least 30 minutes.) Remove the lid, turn the heat up to high, and cook off any liquid remaining in the skillet. To cut down on any residual bitterness, serve the greens dressed with the juice of ½ lemon or a splash of rich, sweet balsamic vinegar.

13,000 women showed that the participants who ate relatively high amounts of vegetables over the years had less age-related decline in memory. Cruciferous vegetables and leafy greens (including spinach and kale) had the biggest effect on helping women retain their memories during the course of the study.

BEST CRUCIFEROUS AND LEAFY GREEN VEGETABLES: *spinach, kale, Swiss chard, mustard greens, turnip greens, collard greens, dandelion greens, broccoli, broccoli raab, Brussels sprouts, cauliflower, cabbage (all varieties), bok choy, arugula, watercress*

Certain phytochemicals have been specifically shown to help improve memory or prevent memory loss. The phytochemicals anthocyanin and quercetin actually reversed some of the age-related memory deficits in laboratory animals. Preliminary research in people also supports a link between antioxidants and improved mental function. In a very small but encouraging study, older adults with early memory problems who drank about 2 cups of blueberry juice daily showed improvements on standard memory tests after just three months on the juice regimen. Exciting results for sure, but I recommend getting your antioxidants in the form of whole berries and other fruits and vegetables, rather than fruit juice. Whole fruit is more filling, lower in sugar, and rich in fiber, making it a better choice for overall health.

> BEST FOODS FOR ANTHOCYANIN: *blackberries, black currants, blueberries, eggplant, elderberries, raspberries, cherries, boysenberries, grapes (red, black, purple), strawberries, plums, cranberries, rhubarb, red onions, red apples, peaches, cabbage (red, purple), red beets, blood oranges*

> BEST FOODS FOR QUERCETIN: *onions, kale, leeks, cherry tomatoes, broccoli, blueberries, black currants, elderberries, lingonberries, cocoa powder (unsweetened), apricots, apples with skin, grapes (red, black, purple), tomatoes, tea, green beans, lettuces, hot chile peppers, celery, chives, red cabbage, lemons, grapefruit*

## Omega-3 Fatty Acids

There are good fats and bad fats, and omega-3 fatty acids fall solidly on the side of good. The most potent forms of omega-3s are DHA (docosahexaenoic acid) and EPA (eicosapentaenoic acid). The human brain is about two-thirds fat by weight, and the most abundant type present is DHA. Neurons' outer membranes are teeming with DHA, and it's this fatty lining that allows for the smooth conductivity of brain signals. Fatty fish are by far the best sources of omega-3s, which explains why they often win the title of ultimate brain food. A study conducted by researchers at the Rush University Medical Center in Chicago followed more than 3,000 men and women for six years to see how diet affected memory. People who ate fish at least once a week had a 10 percent slower decline, compared with those who did not eat fish, which effectively means that the brains of fish eaters were three years younger than the brains of non-fish eaters at the end of the study. Additional studies have linked frequent fish consumption, as well as high blood levels of DHA and EPA, to a slower rate of cognitive decline, but some reports failed to see a benefit. To date, studies on fish oil supplements and

**FAQS**

**What about ginkgo? I've seen it in teas and in supplements, and it seems to be everywhere. Is it helpful for memory?**

Unfortunately, no. Ginkgo biloba is one of the most popular herbal supplements sold in the United States, thanks in large part to claims that it can sharpen memory, but most of the scientific studies testing its effectiveness have shown no benefit. Published in 2009, the longest and largest trial of ginkgo found no difference in memory or cognitive ability when comparing individuals taking capsules of ginkgo extract twice a day with those not taking the supplement. In light of these negative findings, I don't recommend ginkgo for memory.

memory haven't panned out, so I recommend getting your omega-3 fats from food sources. (They taste better than pills, anyway!) To ensure a hearty dose, go out of your way to eat fatty fish at least twice a week, and sprinkle in other sources, like walnuts and ground flaxseed, where you can.

BEST FOODS FOR OMEGA-3S: *wild salmon (fresh, canned), herring, mackerel (not king), sardines, anchovies, trout (wild, rainbow), Pacific oysters, chia seeds, ground flaxseed, walnuts, butternuts (white walnuts), seaweed, walnut oil, canola oil, flaxseed oil, soybeans (edamame)*

## Coffee and Tea

Any coffee lover will tell you they think more clearly after a good strong cup of caffeinated coffee. Now they have proof. Researchers from the University of Innsbruck in Austria used functional magnetic resonance imaging (fMRI) to examine the brain activity of people working on a memory task. The volunteers were tested twice, once after receiving the caffeine equivalent of about 2 cups of coffee and once without any caffeine. Caffeine improved the memory skills and reaction times of the volunteers and increased neuron signaling in the areas of their brains that facilitate memory and attention. Without caffeine, there was no increase in brain activity.

Happily, the benefits of coffee—and tea—seem to extend well beyond a temporary boost in mental clarity. European researchers followed a group of 676 older men with no cognitive problems at the start of the study. After tracking participants for ten years, the researchers found that men who averaged 3 cups of coffee per day experienced significantly less mental decline than nondrinkers did. Similar studies have focused on tea and found that it, too, helps preserve memory and mental function as people age. Regular coffee and tea drinkers may also be at lower risk of Alzheimer's disease and other forms of dementia. Scientists still aren't sure if it's the caffeine that's driving these memory benefits or the

**FAQS**

**I don't think dieting is a good idea for me. I feel like I'm walking around in a fog all the time.**

Don't give up yet. You may just be trying to lose weight too quickly and not eating enough to get you through the day. Read about weight loss (page 17) to make sure you follow a sensible plan. If eating every four to five hours doesn't keep you clear-headed, you could be experiencing hypoglycemia, so try eating every two to three hours. If low blood sugar is the problem, your between-meal snacks should be very small, ideally containing a mix of protein and high-quality carbohydrate. For example, try a handful of walnuts and an orange, ½ cup of low-fat cottage cheese with a quarter wedge of cantaloupe, a 6-ounce container of low-fat yogurt with 1 tablespoon of slivered almonds, or an apple with a slice of low-fat cheese.

potent mix of antioxidants and other bioactive plant compounds found in coffee beans and tea leaves. In any case, this is good news for people who love their morning cup of java or afternoon tea. (Of course, if you have a medical condition that precludes caffeine, opt for the decaf version of your favorite brew.) Unsweetened coffee or tea is the best way to go, but if you need a little sugar, use at most two packets (or 2 teaspoons) per day. Skim or soy cappuccinos, lattes, or cafés au lait are also smart beverage choices. They're low in calories and fat, and the milk provides a nice hit of calcium and protein.

**BEST MEMORY-BOOSTING BEVERAGES:** *coffee, espresso, skim or soy latte, skim or soy cappuccino, skim or soy café au lait, tea*

## FOODS TO AVOID

To protect your brain, you'll want to limit your intake of saturated fat and avoid trans fats at all costs.

### Saturated and Trans Fats

Researchers at the University of Toronto fed laboratory rats either standard chow or an unhealthy, high-fat diet for three months and then tested them to see if there were any effects on memory. It probably won't surprise you to learn that the rats that ate the unhealthy, high-fat food did worse on all aspects of the memory test. Bad fats don't do human brains any good, either. A diet high in major sources of saturated fat, including red meat, full-fat dairy, butter, and organ meats, has been associated with an increased risk of Alzheimer's disease. Trans fats, notoriously dangerous for your heart, have also been linked to a faster rate of cognitive decline in aging adults.

Bolster your memory by sidestepping the worst sources of saturated and trans fats: butter, lard, marbled cuts of beef and pork, fatty meats (including bologna, pepperoni, sausage, bacon, salami, pastrami, spareribs, hot dogs, and hamburgers), full-fat dairy products (whole milk, cheese, sour cream, cream cheese, yogurt, and ice cream), baked goods, creamy and/or cheesy sauces and dressings, stick margarine, and packaged foods containing partially hydrogenated oils. These foods clog the blood vessels that deliver key nutrients to your brain, plus they can crowd out healthier foods in your diet.

## PUTTING IT ALL TOGETHER: THE MEDITERRANEAN DIET

Plenty of specific food groups have been linked to better brain function, but researchers are now more interested in—and enthusiastic about—whole dietary patterns that may slow mental decline as we age. A Mediterranean-style diet appears to be particularly effective at preserving memory and cognitive function.

The "Mediterranean diet" isn't a commercial weight-loss plan or diet book; it's a general way of eating modeled after the way residents of Spain, southern Italy, coastal Greece, and other countries traditionally ate around the 1960s, before modern trends like fast food and packaged products took hold. The ideal Mediterranean diet emphasizes fish and shellfish, legumes (such as starchy beans and lentils), vegetables, fruits, whole grains, and monounsaturated fats (mainly from olive oil and nuts). It minimizes consumption of red meat and full-fat dairy products and incorporates moderate amounts of alcohol (particularly wine, with meals).

Columbia University researchers analyzed the diets of 1,875 older New Yorkers, and then, four years later, tested them for mild cognitive impairment, a sort of intermediate memory disorder that may progress to dementia. The investigators found that people whose diets most closely aligned with the Mediterranean style of eating were 28 percent less likely to develop mild cognitive impairment, compared with those whose diets were least similar to the Mediterranean model. If you use the grocery lists and meal plans outlined in my 4-Step Plan, you'll be eating more like our coastal European neighbors and reaping the benefits for your brain (and heart!).

## BONUS POINTS

- **Move your body.** Exercise is probably the single most effective action you can take to improve memory. Because your brain functions well only when it has a steady supply of oxygen, anything that improves bloodflow is good for your mind. Regular physical activity has been shown to decrease the risk of dementia and Alzheimer's disease by about half. Half! That's a huge benefit for doing any leisure activity you enjoy. And the best news is this: It's never too late to reap the rewards. In one fascinating study, adults in their midsixties who walked for 40 minutes just three days a week were able to increase the size of brain areas critical to memory formation—areas that typically shrink with age, leading to memory impairment. So take a walk after dinner, go bowling, do some gardening, ride your bicycle, sign up for tennis lessons, waltz around a golf course, or take advantage of equipment and group classes at your local gym. If you get 30 minutes of activity per day, you'll help turn back the clock on your brain for a lifetime of better memory.

- **Flex your mental muscle.** Memory is thought to be related to the number of brain cells (neurons) we have and the connections between those cells. For decades, scientists held fast to the belief that new brain cells could be formed only in childhood; it seemed that a neuron lost was gone forever. But in recent years, experiments have revealed that all mammals, including humans, can form new brain cells well into adulthood. These new cells can become integrated into the brain's vast network, forming more and more pathways that can encode and hold our memories. How can we increase the number of brain cells? The most documented and efficient way is by exercising your brain. "Use it or lose it" is certainly true, but so is "nourish and flourish." That is to say, the more active your brain, the better your memory will be. The trick is to keep your mind active and challenged. Learn new skills, such as playing a musical instrument, speaking a foreign language, or—best of all—cooking healthier meals. Reading; playing chess, bridge, or other games of strategy; starting a new hobby; or taking classes at a local college will also help keep your memory sharper longer. When tasks become too familiar, your brain goes into a less-active autopilot mode, so switch your daily activities up as much as possible to keep them from becoming old hat.

◆ **Be a social butterfly.** Listen up, chatterboxes! You can boost your brainpower by chasing the latest gossip! Interacting with others stimulates the mind, so being socially active can actually help keep your brain young. If you live alone, it's especially important to get active in your community or find other ways to expand your social network. Volunteer for local organizations, get a part-time job, attend religious services, join a knitting or book club, organize a weekly card game or poker night with friends, travel abroad or take day trips, or call long-distance friends and family regularly. The more social ties you maintain, the better.

◆ **Turn off the TV.** Zoning out in front of the television is the absolute opposite of challenging your brain. In 2005, researchers at the University of Washington in Seattle found that when very young children are exposed to television, they risk experiencing problems with thinking ability and memory years later. Adults who spend too much time watching TV miss out on beneficial brain-boosting activities. If you watch more than two hours of television a day, begin to cut down, and substitute a more challenging project to fill your valuable time.

◆ **Eat breakfast.** Decades of studies have demonstrated that children learn and remember more at school if they eat breakfast. The first meal of the day is just as important for you. If you tend to skip breakfast or make do with just a cup of coffee, listen up: Eating within 90 minutes of waking up will help jump-start your brain and improve your daily memory.

◆ **Don't smoke.** Just as smoking increases your risk of heart disease, it can also decrease bloodflow to the brain and do serious damage to your memory. As if all the other reasons for quitting weren't enough, add that to the list.

◆ **Give yourself a break.** Seek out ways to de-stress. Set aside a few minutes to meditate or just breathe deeply and relax. Try to simplify your life by taking on fewer projects and learning to say no to things you don't want to do. Exercise regularly, get enough sleep, and learn to go a little easier on yourself.

◆ **If you drink alcohol, do so in moderation.** Scientists are still actively exploring the complicated relationship between alcohol and cognitive health. We know for a fact that heavy alcohol use can impair mental function, contribute to memory loss, decrease brain volume, and increase the risk of dementia. And among older people who are already in the early stages of dementia, there's some evidence that alcohol may actually speed up the disease process. On the other hand, in healthy adults with normal cognition, moderate alcohol consumption may actually benefit brain health. The majority of studies show that alcohol in moderation is actually protective against age-related cognitive loss, Alzheimer's disease, and other forms of dementia. This may be because sensible alcohol use improves cardiovascular health, thereby enhancing bloodflow to the brain, or it may be because alcohol trains neurons to respond better to metabolic stress. There's some evidence that wine is more beneficial than other alcoholic beverages, perhaps due to its high antioxidant content. Health experts define moderate drinking as no more than two drinks per day for men and no more than one drink per day for women. If you are a healthy adult and currently enjoy a daily drink, there's no need to give up alcohol over long-term memory concerns, but (and you've heard this before) if you don't drink, please don't start.

## SUPPLEMENTS

Although I strongly believe that vitamins and minerals from food are your best defense against memory loss, if you want to consider supplements in addition to food fixes, start with a basic multivitamin. I've also included information on other supplements that have some scientific support and may be worth trying.

1. **A multivitamin.** At least one study found that people over age 65 who took a multivitamin every day for a year had significant improvements in short-term memory. Look for brands that offer 100 percent DV of most vitamins and minerals. Choose a formulation that contains at least 800 IU vitamin D. A handful of studies have associated low levels of vitamin D with faster cognitive decline, and a guaranteed daily dose from your multi helps ensure adequate intake.

2. **Huperzine A.** Although this chemical was originally made from a Chinese moss called *Huperzia serrata,* modern huperzine A formulations are either made from purified moss or synthesized in a laboratory. Huperzine A works by increasing the level of a brain chemical called acetylcholine and by protecting brain cells through its antioxidant properties. If you would like to try this supplement, I recommend taking 50 micrograms once or twice daily. Always check with your physician first. Notes and cautions: Huperzine A can decrease heart rate and therefore shouldn't be used by people with heart problems. Consult your doctor before taking huperzine A if you have a gastrointestinal or urinary obstruction, peptic ulcer disease, asthma, or chronic obstructive pulmonary disease. Because of its effects on acetylcholine, consult your doctor

before taking huperzine A if you are taking an anticholinergic medication (such as atropine, Cogentin, Akineton, or Artane) or a cholinergic medication or acetylcholinesterase inhibitor (such as Aricept, Razadyne, Exelon, Urecholine, Phospholine Iodide, Enlon, Reversol, Tensilon, Prostigmin, Antilirium, Mestinon, Anectine, Regonol, Quelicin, or Cognex).

3. **Ginseng.** For generations, people around the world have used this herb (also known as *Panax ginseng* or *Panax quinquefolius*) to improve memory. Study results are mixed—some show a benefit for certain types of memory and cognition, others don't. But some people I've worked with firmly believe that ginseng helps them stay sharp mentally. If you decide to try ginseng, look for an extract standardized to contain 4 to 7 percent ginsenosides. Take 200 milligrams daily for two weeks, followed by one week of "rest." If you feel it was helpful, continue the two-weeks-on/one-week-off prescription. Notes and cautions: Although side effects are very rare, talk with your doctor if you experience increased breast tenderness, postmenpausal vaginal bleeding, or menstrual abnormalities. Other possible side effects include insomnia, raised blood pressure and/or heart rate, and nervousness. Women who are pregnant or nursing should not take ginseng. Because of possible drug interactions, consult with your doctor before taking ginseng if you are taking an antidepressant, digoxin, insulin or oral diabetes medications or a blood-thinning medication such as warfarin (Coumadin).

4. **Phosphatidylserine (PS).** Although PS isn't widely known in the United States, it is very popular in Europe as a treatment both for dementia and for ordinary age-related memory loss. PS is a natural component of cell membranes— especially brain cells. Years ago, PS supplements were made from the PS found in cow brains. Of course, mad cow disease put an end to that. Now supplements are made mostly from soybeans. Nearly all the evidence showing that PS can improve memory was based on the cow-brain supplements. No one knows whether the current formulations from soy will work as well, but because most people can take PS with no problems, I sometimes suggest it for my clients who want to try everything possible to improve their memories. The usual dose for memory improvement is 100 milligrams once or twice a day. Opt for brands that combine PS with the omega-3 fatty acid DHA, as this formulation may be more effective than standard PS. Notes and cautions: PS is a mild blood thinner, so consult with your doctor before trying PS if you are currently taking regular doses of other blood-thinning drugs or supplements, including warfarin (Coumadin), aspirin, heparin, Trental, Plavix, Ticlid, garlic, or ginkgo.

For more information on foods that enhance memory, visit www.joybauer.com/memory.

# JOY'S 4-STEP PROGRAM
## FOR MEMORY

Follow this program if you feel that your memory has been "slipping" lately.

## Step 1 ... START WITH THE BASICS

These are the first things you should do to start improving your memory.

◆ See your primary care physician for a physical examination. Your doctor will check your blood pressure to make sure it is within the normal range (120/80 or less mm Hg). Blood tests may be done to check for high cholesterol, which could indicate the possibility of vascular disease.

◆ Quit smoking.

◆ Increase physical activity. Try to get up and move for 30 minutes every day.

◆ Lose belly fat. Measure your middle, and if your waist circumference is over 40 inches for men or 35 inches for women, make weight loss a top priority.

◆ Decrease stress. Relax. Be good to yourself.

◆ Try to get adequate amounts of sleep. Aim for seven to nine hours per night.

## Step 2 ... YOUR ULTIMATE GROCERY LIST

A nutrition plan is only as good as the foods you choose. This list contains foods with high levels of nutrients that might help improve memory, plus some healthy basics to help round out your daily menus. You don't have to purchase every item, but these foods should make up the bulk of what you eat each week. If you find yourself getting bored, try some unfamiliar foods from these groups—they may become new favorites.

## FRUIT

*All* fruits, but especially:

Apples (with skin)

Apricots

Berries (blackberries, blueberries, boysenberries, cranberries, elderberries, lingonberries, raspberries, strawberries)

Cherries

Currants

Grapefruit

Grapes (black, purple, red)

Lemons

Oranges (especially blood oranges)

Peaches

Plums

## VEGETABLES AND LEGUMES

*All* vegetables, but especially:

Arugula

Avocados

Beans, starchy (such as black, garbanzo, kidney, navy, pinto)

Beets (purple and red)

Bok choy

Broccoli

Broccoli raab

Brussels sprouts

Cabbage (all varieties)

Cauliflower

Celery

Chives

Collard greens

Dandelion greens

Eggplant

Green beans

Kale

Leeks

Lentils

Lettuce (especially darker lettuces)

Mustard greens

Onions (all varieties)

Peas, black-eyed and split

Peppers (all varieties)

Rhubarb

Soybeans (edamame)

Spinach

Swiss chard

Tomatoes (especially cherry tomatoes)

Turnip greens

Watercress (and other varieties of cress)

## SEAFOOD

*All* fish and shellfish, but especially:

Anchovies

Herring

Mackerel (not king)

Oysters, Pacific

Salmon, wild (fresh or canned)

Sardines

Trout (rainbow, wild)

## LEAN PROTEINS

Beef, lean

Chicken, ground (at least 90% lean)

Chicken, skinless

Eggs and egg substitutes

Pork tenderloin

Tempeh

Tofu

Turkey, ground (at least 90% lean)

Turkey, skinless

Turkey bacon

Turkey burgers, lean

Veggie burgers

## DAIRY

Cheese (fat-free, reduced-fat)

Cottage cheese (fat-free, 1%)

Milk (fat-free, 1%)

Milk alternatives (almond, rice, soy)

Yogurt (fat-free, low-fat)

## NUTS AND SEEDS (PREFERABLY UNSALTED)

Almonds and almond butter

Butternuts (white walnuts)

Cashews and cashew butter

Chia seeds

Flaxseed, ground

Hazelnuts

Macadamia nuts

Peanuts and peanut butter

Pecans

Pine nuts

Pistachios

Pumpkin seeds

Sunflower seeds and sunflower butter

Walnuts

## WHOLE GRAINS

Amaranth

Barley

Bread, whole grain (buns, crackers, English muffins, pitas, tortillas, wraps)

Bulgur

Cereal, whole grain

Millet

Oats

Pasta, whole grain

Quinoa

Rice (brown, wild)

Waffles, whole grain

Wheat germ

## MISCELLANEOUS

Canola oil

Cocoa powder, unsweetened

Coffee

Garlic

Guacamole

Herbs and spices (fresh, dried, ground)

Hot sauce

Hummus

Marinara sauce

Mayonnaise, reduced-fat

Mustard (all varieties)

Olive oil

Salad dressing, reduced-calorie

Salsa

Soft tub spread, trans-fat-free (reduced-fat or regular)

Tea (black, green, white)

Vinegar (all varieties)

# Step 3 . . . GOING ABOVE AND BEYOND

If you want to do everything you can for your memory, here are some additional things you might try.

- ◆ Take a daily multivitamin with 100 percent DV of most vitamins and minerals, along with at least 800 IU vitamin D.

- ◆ Although I can't personally recommend these supplements because of their potential for side effects in some people, some scientists believe that huperzine A, ginseng, and phosphatidylserine might help improve memory. Always talk with your doctor before trying these supplements.

- ◆ Increase mental challenges. Start doing a daily crossword puzzle, learn a musical instrument, or take classes at a local college—anything that makes you think.

- ◆ Be social. Engage with others wherever and whenever possible—at church, temple, a club, a gym, a community center, a friend's home, or any other place to meet and greet.

## KEEP YOUR BRAIN FIT

Community colleges, churches, and recreational centers offer a wide range of classes to challenge your mind. You can find something for just about any interest, at little or no cost. Looking for inspiration? Here are some classes I found listed around the country: CPR and First Aid Training; Interior Decorating; Flight Instruction; Television Production; Art of Bonsai Gardening; Secrets of Animal Training; Genealogy; Web Site Development; Flower Arranging; Scrapbooking; Acting for Beginners; Philosophy of Plato; Religions of the World; Creative Writing; Firefighting Tactics and Strategies; Surfing for Seniors; Principles of Tax Accounting; and—my personal favorite—Kitchen Chemistry.

# Step4 ... MEAL PLANS

These sample menus include the best memory foods, plus other nutrients related to vascular health.

Every day, choose one option for each of the three meals—breakfast, lunch, and dinner. Then, once or twice per day, choose from a variety of my suggested snacks. Approximate calories have been provided to help adjust for your personal weight-management goals. If you find yourself hungry (and if weight is not an issue), feel free to increase the portion sizes for meals and snacks. Beverage calories are not included.

## BREAKFAST OPTIONS

(300 TO 400 CALORIES)

### Oatmeal with Berries and Nuts

Prepare ½ cup dry oats with 1 cup water, fat-free milk, or soy milk and top with 1 cup mixed berries (fresh or frozen) and 1 tablespoon chopped walnuts (or other nuts).

### Yogurt Berry Pancakes with Applesauce

Enjoy 2 Blueberry Pancakes (page 296) with ½ cup nonfat yogurt and ½ cup blueberries.

### Whole Grain Cereal with Milk and Fresh Fruit

Mix 1 cup whole grain cereal with 1 cup milk (fat-free, 1%, or soy) and serve with 1 cup berries (fresh or frozen) or purple grapes (or 2 red or purple plums).

### Peanut Butter Toast with Fruit

Spread 2 slices whole grain toast with 2 level tablespoons peanut butter (or other nut butter) and serve with your choice of 1 orange, ½ pink grapefruit, or 1 cup berries or purple grapes.

### Scrambled Eggs with Tomatoes and Spinach

In a small skillet coated with oil spray, sauté chopped onion and tomatoes until softened. Scramble 1 whole egg with 2 or 3 egg whites and add to the skillet, along with 1 to 2 handfuls roughly chopped spinach. Stir occasionally until the eggs are cooked. Enjoy with a toasted whole grain English muffin, dry (or skip the muffin and have 1 cup mixed berries, purple grapes, or cherries).

## LUNCH OPTIONS

(400 TO 500 CALORIES)

### Grilled Chicken Pita with Tomato and Avocado

Layer 5 ounces chicken (or turkey), unlimited baby spinach leaves and tomato slices, 2 thin slices avocado, and optional mustard in a whole grain pita. Enjoy with 1 apple (or 1 peach or 2 red or purple plums).

### Spinach-Bean Salad with Fruit

Top a large bowl of fresh spinach leaves (or arugula or mesclun mix) with a variety of unlimited cut-up vegetables (beets, broccoli, red onions, and tomatoes are all great additions) and ¾ cup any beans (chickpeas, kidney beans, and shelled edamame are all great options). Toss with 2 teaspoons olive oil and unlimited vinegar or fresh lemon juice. Serve with 1 orange (or ½ grapefruit or 1 apple).

### Lentil Soup with Whole Grain Crackers

Enjoy 2 cups lentil soup (or hearty vegetable, split pea, or black bean soup) with 150 calories' worth of whole grain crackers (or 3 rice cakes).

### Salmon Salad Sandwich with Tomato and Onion

Layer salmon salad (5 to 6 ounces canned or fresh wild salmon mixed with 1 to 2 teaspoons reduced-fat mayonnaise, optional minced onion, and preferred seasonings), unlimited lettuce or baby spinach, tomato, and onion slices between 2 slices whole grain bread or in 1 whole grain pita.

### Spinach-Cheese Omelet with Salad

Cook 1 whole egg plus 2 or 3 egg whites in a heated pan coated with 1 teaspoon canola oil or oil spray. Add unlimited raw or cooked spinach and 1 ounce grated reduced-fat (part-skim) mozzarella cheese. When the bottom is cooked, gently flip over. Fold over and cook until the egg mixture is firm. Enjoy with a mixed green salad topped with 1 tablespoon chopped walnuts or slivered almonds, 2 teaspoons olive oil, and unlimited vinegar or fresh lemon juice.

## DINNER OPTIONS

(500 TO 600 CALORIES)

### Grilled Asian Salmon with Broccoli and Potato

Enjoy 1 serving Grilled Asian Salmon (page 297) with a plain baked sweet or white potato and unlimited steamed broccoli or cauliflower.

### Vegetarian Chili with Brown Rice and Steamed Spinach

Enjoy 2 cups vegetarian chili (homemade or store-bought) with 1 cup cooked brown rice (or quinoa or lentils) and unlimited spinach, kale, Swiss chard, or Brussels sprouts (steamed, roasted, or sautéed in oil spray).

### Turkey Burger with Vegetable Salad

Serve one 5-ounce lean turkey burger on a whole grain bun (or pita) with a mixed green salad loaded with lettuce (or baby spinach leaves), tomatoes, carrots, beets, onions, and peppers and tossed with 2 teaspoons olive oil and unlimited vinegar or fresh lemon juice. Or skip the bun and instead enjoy 1 cup seasoned beans (black, pinto, etc).

### Pasta with Turkey Meat Sauce and Vegetables

Toss 1 cup cooked whole grain pasta with turkey meat sauce (4 ounces sautéed lean ground turkey meat cooked with ¾ cup marinara sauce). Serve with unlimited cauliflower, kale, broccoli, broccoli raab, cabbage, Brussels sprouts, spinach, or bok choy (steamed, roasted, or sautéed in oil spray).

### Shrimp and Vegetable Stir-Fry over Brown Rice

Stir-fry 5 ounces shrimp (fresh or frozen) with unlimited strips of onion and bell peppers (red, green, or yellow) in 2 teaspoons olive oil and 2 to 3 teaspoons low-sodium soy sauce. Add additional veggies, if you like. Serve over ½ cup cooked brown or wild rice (or quinoa) and enjoy with a mixed green salad tossed with 1 teaspoon olive oil and unlimited vinegar or fresh lemon juice.

## SNACK OPTIONS

100 CALORIES OR LESS

- *Best Vegetable Snacks:* up to 2 cups raw or cooked veggies such as broccoli, cauliflower, green beans, Brussels sprouts, beets, or cherry tomatoes
- *Best Fruit Snacks:* 1 apple, peach, or orange (especially blood orange); 2 plums; ½ grapefruit; 4 apricots; 20 whole strawberries; 1 cup cherries, blueberries, blackberries, raspberries, boysenberries, sliced strawberries, or grapes (red, purple, or black)
- Celery sticks with 1 level tablespoon peanut butter (or other nut butter)
- 10 almonds
- 25 pistachios in the shell

100 TO 200 CALORIES

- 10 almonds (or 25 pistachios) plus 1 serving fruit (see Best Fruit Snacks)
- Whole nuts: 1 ounce (about ¼ cup) of your choice of almonds, cashews, pecans, walnuts, or peanuts
- ½ cup pistachios or sunflower seeds in the shell
- 1 cup fat-free plain yogurt mixed with ½ cup berries and 1 tablespoon chopped nuts
- Berry smoothie: In a blender, mix ½ cup fat-free milk (or soy milk), ½ cup fat-free yogurt, ¾ cup fresh or frozen berries, and 3 to 5 ice cubes
- ¼ cup hummus or guacamole with celery sticks and/or bell pepper strips
- 1 sliced apple with 1 level tablespoon peanut butter
- 1 slice whole grain toast (or 2 rice cakes) with 1 level tablespoon peanut butter (or other nut butter)
- ½ cup dry oats prepared with water and topped with ½ cup berries
- 1 cup boiled edamame (green soybeans in the pod)
- ½ small avocado drizzled with lime juice and lightly sprinkled with kosher salt
- 1 cup lentil or black bean soup

# BLUEBERRY PANCAKES

*Antioxidant-rich blueberries taste better than ever in this easy and delicious flapjack recipe. It's perfect for guests or a casual family breakfast.*

**MAKES 4 SERVINGS (2 PANCAKES EACH)**

1 large egg

1 cup fat-free plain yogurt

1 tablespoon canola oil

½ cup whole wheat flour

½ cup all-purpose flour

1 tablespoon sugar

1 teaspoon baking powder

½ teaspoon baking soda

¼ teaspoon ground cinnamon

Pinch of kosher salt

½ cup fresh or frozen blueberries

In a blender, combine the egg, yogurt, and oil. Blend until smooth. Transfer to a large bowl.

Sift together the flours, sugar, baking powder, baking soda, cinnamon, and salt. Sift into the yogurt mixture and blend well.

Spray a griddle with oil spray and heat over medium-high heat. In batches, using about ¼ cup of the batter for each pancake, ladle the batter onto the griddle. Sprinkle each with some blueberries and cook for about 30 seconds (or until bubbles form in the middle of the pancakes). Flip over and cook until golden.

**Per serving:** 213 calories, 9 g protein, 34 g carbohydrate, 5 g fat (1 g saturated), 55 mg cholesterol, 320 mg sodium, 3 g fiber

# GRILLED ASIAN SALMON

*This mouthwatering entrée is easy to make and bursting with flavor and brain-friendly omega-3 fats.*

**MAKES 4 SERVINGS**

4 wild salmon steaks, 6 ounces each

½ cup reduced-sodium soy sauce

¼ cup orange juice

2 tablespoons chopped garlic

2 teaspoons Dijon mustard

2 teaspoons tomato paste

Juice of ½ lemon

Place the salmon in a zip-top bag. Mix the soy sauce, orange juice, garlic, mustard, tomato paste, and lemon juice in a bowl. Pour the mixture into the bag with the salmon. Seal the bag, pressing out excess air. Refrigerate to marinate for 4 to 6 hours.

Heat an indoor or outdoor grill, or heat a large sauté pan over medium-high heat. Remove the salmon from the bag, reserving the marinade. Place the salmon on the grill or in the pan and cook for about 5 minutes on each side, or longer for well done. For extra flavor, lightly drizzle a few tablespoons of the marinade on the salmon during cooking. Discard the leftover marinade.

**Per serving:** 270 calories, 37 g protein, 2 g carbohydrate, 11 g fat (2 g saturated), 100 mg cholesterol, 400 mg sodium, 0 g fiber

# PART 5

# FEELING GOOD

# CHAPTER 13

# MOOD

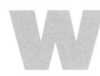hen Melissa came to see me with the goal of losing about 40 pounds, I quickly recognized how she got where she was, weightwise. She had the kind of unfortunate habits I see in so many of my clients: an erratic eating schedule, skipped meals, binges, and lots of ready-to-eat, grab-and-go foods. Constantly busy and overextended, Melissa often found herself feeling angry and resentful because she felt that there was no time she could call her own. Everyone and everything took priority—her kids, her husband, her boss, her friends, car pools, work—everyone got a slice of Melissa's time except Melissa.

One side effect of Melissa's hectic lifestyle was her chronic bad mood. Her day was ruined by things most of us would shrug off, like if the morning newspaper didn't arrive at the exact time she expected it, her kids were assigned an extra helping of homework, or the grocery store was out of her favorite brand of something. She complained about the amount of time her husband spent on the golf course, but she also complained about him hanging around the house and getting underfoot. She was irritated by coworkers and supervisors alike. She barked at the people she loved, sniped at the people she worked with, and hated herself for being so explosive. The other side of Melissa's personality was weepy—during our first meeting, she cried twice. That was my first clue that Melissa needed help with her moods as much as she needed to lose weight—and she couldn't have agreed with me more!

I did three things for Melissa: First, I put her on a schedule so she would eat meals more regularly to control her blood sugar and her moods. Second, I gave her a calorie-controlled program for weight loss, which would help raise her self-esteem. And third, I drew her a food "road map," which showed her the direction in which she needed to take her diet in order to get the right combination of foods, vitamins, and minerals specifically shown to help improve mood.

After the first week on her new food program, Melissa lost 4 pounds—just the boost she needed. Over the next several weeks, her weight loss was steady, if a bit less dramatic. The next time I saw her, Melissa had lost 20 pounds and was halfway to her weight-loss goal. She looked fantastic, but that wasn't the best part—Melissa felt better than she had in years. She was levelheaded and not as quick to react. As time went on, I saw Melissa morph from an uncertain, overbooked, overwrought slave to her emotions into a calm, beautiful, competent woman. She was slimmer. She ate better. And best of all, she was happy! She still had moments when she snapped or cried, but emotions didn't overwhelm her or rule her life. For the first time in a long time, Melissa didn't feel out of control.

Weight loss also bolstered Melissa's self-esteem and improved her moods. Mood-enhancing foods helped calm her inner turmoil. The covert part of this plan no doubt amplified its effectiveness: In order to diligently follow her weight-loss and mood program, Melissa needed to make time for herself, something she hadn't done in years. Like so many of us, Melissa rushed through her life, doing everything for other people but nothing for herself. If this sounds like you, hear this: It's critical for your physical health, your emotional well-being, and your moods that you learn to focus on your needs for at least some small portion of every day. I've found that taking time to shop for and prepare nutritious (and delicious!) meals can be the start of a new habit of caring for yourself. How much you pamper yourself after that is entirely up to you.

Over the years, I've worked with many clients who suffered with clinical depression and postpartum depression and, much more often, people like Melissa who struggled with chronic bad moods. As successful as I've been with this mood program, it is not a cure-all. Even if you follow the advice in this chapter to the letter, you won't be happy every minute of every day, and you will still sometimes lose your cool. That's life. But if you are feeling battered by your moods, this program should help you feel significantly better—perhaps even within the first week.

## WHAT AFFECTS MOOD?

If moods were merely psychological, if they were truly "all in your head," they wouldn't make us so miserable. Very few people would choose to remain in a pit of depression or keep their flash-point anger if they could simply change their state of mind. But we don't always have control over how our feelings affect our lives because, for many of us, mood is as physical as a broken bone.

Scientists believe that mood is caused by changes in the production or availability of brain chemicals called neurotransmitters. The three main neurotransmitters—norepinephrine, dopamine, and serotonin—work together to balance mood. If there is a decrease in one or all of these chemicals, we will feel differently, even if we don't know exactly why. Neurotransmitters are responsible for feelings of anger, anxiety, motivation, irritability, happiness, impulsiveness, and depression, and they can affect overall energy levels.

The reason you feel a particular way on a particular day is usually a complex combination of genetic susceptibility, life events and circumstances, and your body's general physical state. You may have noticed, for example, that your moods feel more intense at certain times of day or if you are feeling tired, ill, or stressed-out. Some women experience depression and irritability related to their monthly hormone fluctuations. (See Premenstrual Syndrome, page 348, for more on PMS.) And quite a few people are pushed over the emotional cliff by food-related issues, including what they eat, when they eat, and why they eat.

Nutrition-related mood problems have long- and short-term roots. Poor eating habits can, over time, lead to deficiencies in some of the vitamins, minerals, and other nutrients that contribute to good mood. For example, the neurotransmitters that regulate mood are built from amino acids, which are found in protein-rich foods. If you don't get enough of a variety of proteins in your diet, your brain chemistry will eventually suffer. Furthermore, the amino acid tryptophan can be converted in the brain to serotonin—a mood-calming neurotransmitter—only when adequate carbohydrate is present. Eating patterns can even affect your moods from hour to hour—the proverbial "midmorning slump"—and many cases of flaring irritability can be caused by a dip in blood sugar resulting from eating the wrong foods at the wrong time of day or from not eating often enough.

For most people, a mood is a temporary state—they feel it, react to it, and, after an hour or a day, forget about it. But sometimes a mood settles in and stays. Of all conditions seen in general medical practice, one of the most common is depression. Many people think of depression as extreme sadness, but that's just a partial description. Symptoms of depression also include feelings of hopelessness or helplessness, irritability, fatigue, sleeplessness, difficulty concentrating or making decisions, weight gain or weight loss, and loss of energy. Of course, depression is only one possible cause of these problems, but if you experience any or all of these symptoms for longer than two weeks, it is important to see a doctor. Bad moods that persist require medical attention—they can be signs of a serious medical problem, so you'll want to make sure you get checked out. And if you do receive a diagnosis of depression, your doctor may prescribe medication to help you feel markedly better.

## HOW FOOD AFFECTS MOOD

No matter where your moods come from or how long they last, eating the right foods can help you feel more energetic and less like you're riding an emotional roller coaster built for one. Here are some of the main guideposts on your mood-food road map.

### HIGH-QUALITY CARBOHYDRATES AND PROTEIN

There are two general categories of carbohydrates: high-quality and low-quality. High-quality carbs are full of vitamins, minerals, phytochemicals, and fiber. They are found primarily in plant foods, including whole grain products, oats, legumes, vegetables, fresh fruit, brown and wild rice, and potatoes. Low-quality carbs, on the other hand, have much less nutritional value. These less-than-stellar carbs include sugar itself, as well as candy, soda, syrup, jam and jelly, cakes, and most other foods that we typically think of as sweets or desserts. Refined starches—the "white" carbs—also fit into the low-quality carb category because your digestive system quickly breaks them down into simple sugars. Refined starches include white rice, white pasta, white bread, and anything else made with white flour, such as crackers, bagels, and sugary cereals.

Like all foods, carbohydrates affect body chemistry, and the type of carbs you eat makes a big difference in determining metabolism, energy, and overall well-being. All carbohydrates provide energy to the body in the form of glucose—the blood sugar that feeds our cells. When blood sugar is up, we feel good; when blood sugar goes down, mood can plunge, too. Ideally, we want to eat the types of foods that give us a steady level of energy so that we can go through the day feeling great from start to finish. The goal, then, is to find the right combination of foods that allows blood sugar levels to rise gently, stay even over a long period of time, and then fall off slowly.

**HIGH-QUALITY CARBS—NONSTARCHY VEGETABLES:** *artichokes, asparagus, beets, bok choy, broccoli, broccoli raab, Brussels sprouts, cabbage, carrots, cauliflower, celery, cucumber, dark leafy greens (collard, kale, mustard, Swiss chard, turnip), eggplant, fennel, green beans, lettuce (all varieties), mushrooms, okra, onions (all varieties), peppers (all varieties), pumpkin, radishes, rhubarb, snow peas, spaghetti squash, sugar snap peas, summer squash, tomatoes, water chestnuts, zucchini*

**HIGH-QUALITY CARBS—LENTILS AND BEANS:** *black-eyed peas, lentils, starchy beans (such as black, navy, pinto, garbanzo, kidney), split peas, soybeans (edamame)*

**HIGH-QUALITY CARBS—STARCHY VEGETABLES:** *corn, green peas, potatoes (sweet and white), winter squash (acorn, butternut)*

**HIGH-QUALITY CARBS—FRUIT:** *all fresh and frozen whole fruits (avoid dried fruit and fruit juice)*

**HIGH-QUALITY CARBS—WHOLE GRAINS:** *amaranth, barley, bulgur, millet, oats, quinoa, rice (brown and wild), whole grain breads, cereals, pastas*

All carbohydrates cause a rise in blood sugar that typically lasts about two hours before returning to baseline. With high-quality carbohydrates, blood sugar levels rise slowly and don't get very high. In addition, some of these high-quality carbs contain soluble fiber, a component of plant cell walls. Soluble fiber slows the absorption of glucose from food in the stomach, which also helps put a lid on blood sugar.

BEST FOODS FOR SOLUBLE FIBER: *psyllium seeds (ground), lima beans, starchy beans (such as black, navy, pinto, garbanzo, kidney), Brussels sprouts, oat bran, winter squash, parsnips, turnips, sweet potatoes, lentils, black-eyed peas, split peas, green peas, okra, eggplant, barley, oats, rice bran, guava, oranges, grapefruit, apples, peaches, plums, nectarines, pears, prunes, mangoes, strawberries, blackberries, raspberries, bananas, apricots, raisins, white potatoes, avocados, broccoli, carrots, green beans, spinach, cabbage, kale, wheat germ, ground flaxseed*

Low-quality carbs, on the other hand, cause an intense spike in blood sugar—it's quick and dramatic. These carbs trigger the highest highs, the Mount Everests of glucose levels. It is a long way down from the dizzying peak of surging blood sugar to your normal baseline. The steeper the drop, the worse you'll feel. That's why low-quality carbohydrates can lead to feeling irritable, depressed, sluggish, and foggy-headed. If you eat low-quality carbs regularly, your blood sugar won't have a chance to stabilize—and neither will your moods. That's why I recommend dramatically limiting sugary and refined foods in your diet.

To stay on an even keel all day, the majority of your meals and snacks should combine high-quality carbohydrates with protein. Protein is critical to moderating mood because it is the great stabilizer. It does not add to blood sugar but instead helps slow the absorption of carbohydrates from the blood. I recommend incorporating at least some protein into your meals whenever possible—breakfast, lunch, dinner, and snacks.

BEST FOODS FOR PROTEIN: *skinless chicken and turkey, fish and shellfish, pork tenderloin, lean beef, egg whites, yogurt (fat-free, low-fat), milk (fat-free, 1%), cheese (fat-free, reduced-fat), starchy beans (such as black, navy, pinto, garbanzo, kidney), lentils, split peas, tofu, tempeh, soybeans (edamame), soy milk, nuts and nut butters, seeds and seed butters*

## OMEGA-3 FATTY ACIDS

In our diet-conscious society, *fat* has become a synonym for *bad*. But some fat in the body and in your diet is necessary for good

## FAQS

**You say that protein is important for stabilizing blood sugar, but when I was on the Atkins diet, I felt terrible all the time. How come? Did I do something wrong?**

Protein is important, but it is just one part of the mood-balancing equation. Protein must be combined with high-quality carbohydrates for the best possible mood-regulating results. Because carbs provide the blood sugar to give us energy and are needed for the conversion of tryptophan to serotonin in the brain, people who severely restrict their carbohydrates may end up feeling more irritable than usual, an effect I call low-carb crabbiness. Mix moderate amounts of high-quality carbohydrates with protein and you'll inevitably feel better.

**I've been taking an antidepressant for about a year, and I feel like my mood is back to normal. Can I stop taking the medication if I commit to eating right and take omega-3 supplements?**

Please don't stop taking any medication without consulting your doctor. Clinical depression is a medical condition that should be taken seriously. Good nutrition can help, but it may not be enough for everyone. At the very least, it can make anyone feel healthier and stronger. But if you're determined to get off the antidepressants, I recommend that you follow my plan (while continuing your medication) for a couple of months. Then, together with your doctor, make the decision about whether tapering off the medication is a good idea for you.

health. For example, the type of polyunsaturated fat known as omega-3 fatty acids makes up part of the structure of our brain membranes, and they seem to help brain cells use neurotransmitters more efficiently. So it makes sense that omega-3s may help to regulate mood.

The relationship between depression and omega-3 fats is complex and not completely understood. Studies have shown that people who are clinically depressed have low blood levels of omega-3s, but their moods did not improve when they took omega-3 supplements. However, when depressed people took omega-3s along with antidepressants, the supplements helped reduce depressive symptoms better than the medication did alone. If you have been diagnosed with depression and would like to try a therapeutic dose of omega-3s as part of your treatment plan, see the Supplements section on page 309.

For people with milder problems—let's call them mood issues—I recommend going the food route (although you can certainly consider supplements if you can't get enough omega-3s through food). Although the research has been mixed, it's possible that foods rich in omega-3 fatty acids may help regulate brain function and level out everyday moods. Omega-3s are most abundant in fatty fish, so I recommend eating one or two meals containing fatty fish per week. (My Best Foods list includes only the fatty fish that have been shown to be low in mercury, PCBs, and dioxins.)

BEST FOODS FOR OMEGA-3 FATTY ACIDS: *wild salmon (fresh, canned), herring, mackerel (not king), sardines, anchovies, rainbow trout, Pacific oysters, chia seeds, ground flaxseed, walnuts, butternuts (white walnuts), seaweed, walnut oil, canola oil, flaxseed oil, soybeans (edamame)*

## VITAMIN D

In the past few years, research has suggested that vitamin D might help relieve mood disorders because it seems to increase levels of serotonin, one of the neurotransmitters responsible for mood. In particular, vitamin D seems to help the type of depression called seasonal affective disorder (SAD), or the winter blues. More than 10 million Americans are thought to suffer from SAD, experiencing anxiety, fatigue, and feelings of sadness for three to six months of the year. Scientists believe this is due to the shortened days and limited sunlight of winter. You see, our bodies can make plenty of vitamin D on their own from sunlight. Just 10 to 15 minutes of sun on the bare skin of the arms three or four times a week is enough to keep most of us healthy. The problem is that sunlight isn't always safe—too much causes skin damage and premature aging and may lead to skin cancer—and while using sunscreen protects your skin, it also prevents your body from making its own vitamin D. It becomes important, then, to get healthy amounts of vitamin D from the foods you eat and/or from supplements.

Scientists have discovered that people with SAD have normal blood levels of vitamin D in the summer, but their levels drop by as much as one-third in winter. No wonder they feel moody and tired! Those who took vitamin D supplements for a year had stable blood levels, and most experienced a significant improvement in their depression. If you would like to try supplements, see my guidelines for choosing a multivitamin on page 309. But everyone with minor depression and anxiety issues should strive to eat more foods rich in vitamin D to improve their mood profile.

> **BEST FOODS FOR VITAMIN D**: *wild salmon (fresh, canned), mackerel (not king), sardines, herring, milk (fat-free, 1%), soy milk, fortified yogurt (fat-free, low-fat), egg yolks, vitamin D–enhanced mushrooms\**
>
> *\*These mushrooms are treated with UV light, which dramatically increases their vitamin D content.*

## B VITAMINS: FOLATE AND B$_{12}$

Two B vitamins—folate and vitamin B$_{12}$—seem to be important for mood. Numerous studies have shown that low blood levels of these vitamins are linked to a higher risk of depression, particularly in older adults. Folate and vitamin B$_{12}$ are involved in the production and metabolism of neurotransmitters that help normalize mood. Although researchers don't understand exactly what role these vitamins play in brain function and mood regulation, it's scientifically plausible that low intake of these vitamins could contribute to mood problems. In addition, researchers have found that having higher B$_{12}$ levels seems to help depressed people respond better to treatment. Though questions still remain, these early results suggest that adding foods rich in these B vitamins may help people suffering from mood disorders or depression feel better faster.

If you are clinically depressed, it is important to continue to follow your doctor's treatment recommendations, but you should also go out of your way to eat foods rich in both folate and vitamin B$_{12}$. In addition, you may want to consider taking a multivitamin with appropriate amounts of these two vitamins as a backup, particularly if you're more than 50 years old (see the Supplements section, page 309).

BEST FOODS FOR FOLATE: *lentils, black-eyed peas, soybeans, oats, turnip greens, spinach, mustard greens, green peas, artichokes, okra, beets, parsnips, broccoli, broccoli raab, sunflower seeds, wheat germ, oranges and orange juice, Brussels sprouts, papayas, seaweed, berries (boysenberries, blackberries, strawberries), starchy beans (such as black, navy, pinto, garbanzo, kidney), cauliflower, Chinese cabbage, corn, whole grain bread, whole grain pasta*

BEST FOODS FOR VITAMIN B$_{12}$: *shellfish (clams, oysters, crab), wild salmon (fresh, canned), soy milk, trout (rainbow, wild), tuna (canned light), lean beef, veggie burgers, cottage cheese (fat-free, 1%), yogurt (fat-free, low-fat), milk (fat-free, 1%), eggs, cheese (fat-free, reduced-fat)*

## BONUS POINTS

- ◆ **Eat consistently throughout the day.** If your blood sugar flags, your energy will fade and your mood can take a nasty turn. You need to eat at least once every four to five hours in order to keep your brain well fueled and happy. Some people who are extremely sensitive to frequent blood sugar dips may need to eat every two to three hours to keep from feeling that postmeal letdown. To keep from gaining weight, make absolutely sure the meals and snacks are calorie controlled. And each meal and snack should contain a mix of high-quality carbohydrates and protein to best stabilize your blood sugar levels (see the meal plans, page 315, for examples).

- ◆ **Exercise.** Too many people underestimate the benefits of exercise. In addition to accomplishing your weight-loss or fitness goals, exercise can make you feel stronger, more confident, and more self-assured. That alone is enough to improve your overall mood. But exercise exerts other mood-enhancing effects, as well: It raises blood levels of endorphins, those natural body chemicals that scientists believe might induce feelings of well-being. Plus, exercise improves bloodflow, which means that your brain gets more oxygen, helping improve its function. Most studies that have looked at the effects of exercise on mood find that nearly any kind of exercise reduces anxiety, tension, stress, and feelings of depression. These amazing results are most powerful after several weeks of regular exercise, but research shows that mood can improve even on the first day of exercise.

  Researchers at the University of Texas Southwestern put people with mild to moderate depression on an exercise program—30 minutes three to five times per week for 12 weeks. The study participants who did a moderately intense workout on a treadmill or stationary bike reduced their depressive symptoms by nearly half, similar to what might be seen after starting antidepressant medications. Less-intense exercisers reduced their symptoms by 30 percent, and even those participants doing only stretching exercises reduced their symptoms by 29 percent.

For mood improvement, my recommendation is to engage in some sort of exercise at least five times per week for 30 minutes per session. The more intense your workout, the more your mood will improve, so do what you can. Happiness really could be just around the corner—as long as you walk or run there!

◆ **Make time for your personal life.** Feeling frazzled, crazed, overextended, and overworked is a sure way to end up angry, anxious, or depressed—or all three. As impossible as it may seem, your family and friends may be your best "vaccine" against the daily stresses and strains that can wear you down. But it's not enough just to have family and friends—you have to make time to relax with them and enjoy the simple pleasures they can bring. On the same note, you need to find a way to enjoy your work. If you're like most people, you probably spend a minimum of eight hours a day at your job. That's one-third of your day, five days a week, and that's not counting your commute. If you hate what you do, it will eventually affect your emotions. I understand that not everyone can just quit a job or change careers, but everyone can learn to enjoy some aspect of their work (or at least meditate for relaxation). Alternatively, psychological counselors can help you develop a new set of responses to stressful circumstances or "reframe" how you think about them so that you can learn to enjoy something that you once found intolerable. If you're retired, then your challenge becomes finding activities that are challenging and emotionally rewarding to fill your days.

## SUPPLEMENTS

If you are concerned about mood and want to consider supplements in addition to the food fixes, here are some that might be beneficial.

1. **A multivitamin.** I recommend a standard multivitamin. Look for a brand that contains 100 percent DV of folic acid (the supplemental form of folate), 100 percent DV of vitamin $B_{12}$, and at least 800 IU of vitamin D.

   Note: It is especially important for people over 50 years old to take a supplemental dose of vitamin $B_{12}$. That's because as we age, we become less efficient at absorbing the $B_{12}$ that's naturally found in food. However, the crystalline form of $B_{12}$ found in supplements and fortified foods is well absorbed at any age. If you're over 50, it's vital that you take a multivitamin with 100 percent DV of vitamin $B_{12}$ and/or go out of your way to eat cereals that are fortified with $B_{12}$.

2. **Fish oil.** If you find that you don't eat enough fatty fish to get your share of omega-3 fats, you can always take fish oil capsules. The two most potent types of omega-3 fatty acids found in fish oil supplements are DHA (docosahexaenoic acid) and EPA (eicosapentaenoic acid). Aim to take a daily dose of 1,000 milligrams of EPA and DHA combined. Because fish oil supplement companies balance these fatty acids differently, you'll need to read the label carefully and tally up the DHA plus EPA total. You typically have to take more than one pill to reach the 1,000-milligram amount.

Doses of omega-3s much greater than 1 gram per day are often used alone or in conjunction with prescription antidepressants to treat clinical depression. Dosages this high should not be self-prescribed; always talk with your doctor before taking them.

To prevent rancidity, always store bottles of fish oil supplements in the fridge. To lessen the chance of fishy burps or aftertaste, buy enteric-coated capsules, which are digested in the intestines instead of the stomach. Avoid getting omega-3 fats from cod liver oil because it may contain too much vitamin A.

3. **St. John's wort.** This herbal supplement, which seems to prolong the action of mood-stabilizing serotonin and other neurotransmitters in the brain, is a popular treatment for depression. A large 2008 research review reported that St. John's wort works nearly as well as antidepressant medications for mild or moderate depression and has fewer side effects. However, it is unclear whether St. John's wort is effective in people suffering from severe depression. Typical dosages for mild to moderate depression range from 500 to 1,200 milligrams of St. John's wort extract daily.

Just because St. John's wort is a natural herb doesn't necessarily mean it's safe. This is not a supplement to be taken casually—it is recommended only for people with documented depression because it has physiological effects that need to be monitored by a doctor. General side effects can include dry mouth, dizziness, fatigue, nausea, diarrhea, and sensitivity to sunlight. Like some prescription antidepressant medications, St. John's wort can have sexual side effects in some people, including an inability to become aroused or reach orgasm. It can also interact with many other medications and can weaken oral contraceptives, which means that there may be an unintended pregnancy. Please don't try St. John's wort on your own; if you suffer from mild to moderate depression and want to try it, talk with your doctor first.

4. **SAMe.** Another natural treatment for mild to moderate depression is SAMe (S-adenosylmethionine), an amino acid derivative. SAMe seems to work by increasing the availability of dopamine and norepinephrine in the brain. Studies have shown that most people can take SAMe for up to two years with few side effects and noticeable mood improvement. SAMe may be especially helpful for

individuals who don't respond to traditional antidepressant medications. A 2010 Harvard University study showed that people who took SAMe supplements along with a common prescription antidepressant experienced greater treatment results. Specifically, after six weeks, 26 percent of individuals taking SAMe in conjunction with their meds experienced a remission of symptoms, compared with only 12 percent in the group taking the prescription antidepressant on its own.

Still, it is important to talk with your doctor before taking SAMe to make sure that your depression is being adequately treated. The usual recommended dose for depression is 400 to 800 milligrams twice a day. Here's the big drawback: the cost! SAMe can run $150 per month—much more expensive than a prescription for an antidepressant medication that may be covered by insurance.

For more information on foods that can boost your mood, visit www.joybauer.com/mood.

# JOY'S 4-STEP PROGRAM
## FOR MOOD

Follow this program if you find yourself feeling irritable, depressed, anxious, or angry more often than you would like.

## Step 1 ... START WITH THE BASICS

These are the first things you should do to take control of your moods.

◆ See your doctor if you have signs of depression that last longer than two weeks, including sadness, hopelessness, difficulty concentrating, a change in weight, or a change in sleeping patterns.

◆ Limit your intake of sugary treats and refined foods.

◆ Eat a small meal or snack that includes protein every four to five hours to avoid huge swings in blood sugar.

## Step 2 ... YOUR ULTIMATE GROCERY LIST

A nutrition plan is only as good as the foods you choose. This list contains high levels of nutrients that contribute to mood, plus other overall healthy foods to help round out your grocery list. You don't have to purchase every item, but these foods should make up the bulk of what you eat during the week. If you find yourself getting bored, try some unfamiliar foods from these groups—they may become new favorites.

### FRUIT

*All* fruits, but especially:

Apples
Apricots
Bananas
Berries (blackberries, blueberries, boysenberries, raspberries, and strawberries)

Cantaloupe
Grapefruit
Guava
Mangoes
Nectarines
Oranges
Papayas

Peaches
Pears
Plums
Prunes
Raisins

## VEGETABLES AND LEGUMES

*All* vegetables, but especially:

Artichokes

Avocados

Beans, starchy (such as black, navy, garbanzo, kidney, and pinto)

Beets

Broccoli

Broccoli raab

Brussels sprouts

Cabbage

Carrots

Cauliflower

Corn

Eggplant

Dark leafy greens (such as collard, kale, mustard, Swiss chard, and turnip)

Lentils

Lima beans

Okra

Onions

Parsnips

Peas (black-eyed, green, and split)

Peppers, bell (green, red, and yellow)

Potatoes (sweet and white)

Soybeans (edamame)

Spinach

Tomatoes

Squash, summer

Squash, winter (acorn and butternut)

Zucchini

## SEAFOOD

*All* fish and shellfish, but especially:

Anchovies

Herring

Mackerel (not king)

Salmon, wild (fresh and canned)

Sardines (fresh and canned)

Shellfish (clams, crab, and oysters [especially Pacific])

Trout, rainbow

Tuna (canned light)

## LEAN PROTEINS

Beef, lean

Chicken, ground (at least 90% lean)

Chicken, skinless

Eggs and egg substitutes

Pork tenderloin

Tempeh

Tofu

Turkey, ground (at least 90% lean)

Turkey, skinless

Turkey bacon

Turkey burgers, lean

Veggie burgers

## NUTS AND SEEDS (PREFERABLY UNSALTED)

Almonds and almond butter

Butternuts (white walnuts)

Cashews and cashew butter

Chia seeds

Flaxseed, ground

Hazelnuts

Macadamia nuts

Peanuts and peanut butter

Pecans

Pine nuts

Pistachios

Pumpkin seeds

Soy nuts

Sunflower seeds and sunflower butter

Walnuts

## WHOLE GRAINS

Amaranth

Barley

Bread, whole grain (buns, crackers, English muffins, pitas, tortillas, and wraps)

Bulgur

Cereal, whole grain (at least 3 grams fiber; no more than 8 grams sugar per serving)

Millet

Oat bran

Oats

Pasta, whole grain

Quinoa

Rice (brown and wild)

Waffles, whole grain

Wheat berries

Wheat germ

## DAIRY

Cheese (fat-free or reduced-fat)

Cottage cheese (fat-free or 1%)

Cream cheese (fat-free or reduced-fat)

Milk (fat-free or 1%)

Sour cream (fat-free or reduced-fat)

Milk alternatives (almond, rice, and soy)

Yogurt (fat-free or low-fat)

## MISCELLANEOUS

Canola oil

Garlic

Herbs and spices (fresh, dried, and ground)

Hot sauce

Hummus

Marinara sauce

Mayonnaise, reduced-fat

Mustard (all varieties)

Olive oil

Salad dressing, reduced-calorie

Salsa

Soft tub spread, trans-fat-free (reduced-fat or regular)

Vinegar (all varieties)

# Step 3 . . . GOING ABOVE AND BEYOND

If you want to do everything you can to improve your mood, here are some additional things you might try.

◆ Consider taking a multivitamin to make certain you get the recommended amounts of most nutrients necessary for a good mood—specifically, a brand with 100 percent DV of folic acid and $B_{12}$ and at least 800 IU of vitamin D.

◆ Take a daily fish oil supplement (1,000 milligrams DHA and EPA combined) if you don't eat fatty fish and/or other omega-3-rich foods at least two times per week.

## GET MOVING FOR YOUR MOOD

We know that exercise can help improve mood, but if you're feeling depressed, just getting up off the couch can be a major achievement. Here are some tips for turning exercise into a happy habit.

- If the thought of a half hour of walking sucks your energy, then commit to walking for only 5 minutes. The first minutes are always the toughest. You'll usually find that if you can walk for 5 minutes, the next 25 minutes are no problem.

- Plan to exercise in the morning, so you have no chance to come up with excuses later in the day.

- Invest in an MP3 player so you can listen to—and be energized by—your favorite music while exercising.

- Remember, the couch isn't going anywhere—let it be your reward for activity instead of your excuse for avoidance.

◆ Add some sort of exercise to your weekly routine. Start with 30 minutes at least four times a week. As you become comfortable with your routine, increase the intensity and length of your workout.

◆ If you have been diagnosed with depression, ask your doctor if St. John's wort or SAMe might be a good treatment option for you.

◆ Schedule downtime to spend with family and friends as actively as you schedule your work responsibilities.

◆ Take up a relaxing hobby, such as meditation or yoga.

# Step 4 . . . MEAL PLANS

These sample menus include some of the best mood foods. All meals incorporate both high-quality carbohydrates and lean protein and are rich in omega-3 fats, vitamin D, folate, $B_{12}$, and soluble fiber. Every day, choose one option for each of the three meals—breakfast, lunch, and dinner. Then, once or twice per day, choose from my suggested snacks. Be sure to eat consistently throughout the day—every four to five hours—to avoid potential blood sugar dips.

Approximate calories have been provided to help adjust for your personal weight-management goals. If you find yourself hungry (and if weight is not an issue), feel free to increase the portion sizes for meals and snacks. Beverage calories are not included.

## BREAKFAST OPTIONS

(300 TO 400 CALORIES)

### Cereal with Nuts, Wheat Germ, and Fresh Fruit

Mix 1 cup whole grain cereal with 1 cup fat-free milk (or soy milk) and top with 1 tablespoon chopped walnuts and 1 tablespoon wheat germ. Enjoy with 1 orange (or ½ grapefruit).

### Breakfast Burrito

Scramble 1 whole egg with 2 egg whites on a griddle coated with oil spray. Mix with ¼ cup black beans and 2 tablespoons shredded reduced-fat cheese. Wrap in 1 whole grain tortilla (150 calories or less) and add optional onion, salsa, and/or hot sauce.

### Banana-Berry Cottage Cheese with Almonds

Mix 1 cup fat-free or 1% cottage cheese (or fat-free flavored yogurt) with ½ sliced banana, ½ cup chopped strawberries, and 1 tablespoon slivered almonds.

### Apple-Cinnamon Oatmeal

Microwave ½ cup dry oats with 1 cup fat-free milk for 1½ to 2 minutes, mix with 1 chopped apple, and microwave for an additional 30 seconds. Sprinkle with optional cinnamon plus 1 teaspoon sugar, honey, or sugar substitute.

### Scrambled Eggs, Tomato, and Spinach with Toast

Beat 1 whole egg with 2 egg whites. Cook in a hot skillet coated with oil spray, add unlimited chopped tomato and spinach, and serve with a toasted whole grain English muffin (or 2 slices whole wheat toast), dry or with 1 to 2 teaspoons soft tub, trans-fat-free spread.

### Waffles Topped with Yogurt and Berries

Toast 2 frozen whole grain waffles and top with 1 cup fat-free flavored yogurt and ½ cup berries (or ½ sliced banana).

### Hard-Cooked Eggs with Turkey Bacon and Fruit

Enjoy 2 hard-cooked eggs, 2 strips turkey bacon, and 1 orange (or ½ grapefruit).

## LUNCH OPTIONS

(400 TO 500 CALORIES)

### Wild Salmon Salad over Greens

Enjoy 1 serving Wild Salmon Salad (page 321), or drain and mash 6 ounces canned salmon and mix with 2 teaspoons reduced-fat mayonnaise and minced onion to taste. Serve over a bed of leafy greens with 100 calories' worth of whole grain crackers or a mini whole wheat pita.

### Turkey Sandwich with Baby Carrots

Layer 4 ounces sliced turkey (or grilled chicken), lettuce, sliced tomato, and onion, plus 1 optional slice reduced-fat cheese, between 2 slices whole grain bread or in a pita. Spread with mustard, 2 teaspoons reduced-fat mayonnaise, or hummus. Serve with a large handful of baby carrots.

### Spinach-Cheese Omelet with Vegetable Salad

Beat 1 whole egg with 2 or 3 egg whites and cook in a heated skillet coated with oil spray. When the bottom is cooked, gently flip over. Top with unlimited raw or cooked spinach and 1 ounce (¼ cup shredded) reduced-fat cheese. Fold the omelet over and cook until the egg mixture is firm and the cheese melts. Enjoy with mixed salad greens topped with sliced beets and 1 tablespoon toasted walnuts (or sunflower seeds), 2 teaspoons olive oil, and unlimited vinegar or fresh lemon juice (or 2 to 4 tablespoons reduced-calorie dressing).

### Baked Potato with Broccoli and Cheese

Top 1 baked potato with cooked chopped broccoli and 1 ounce (¼ cup shredded) melted reduced-fat cheese. Serve with 1 cup Vegetable Oatmeal Bisque (page 322) or any prepared vegetable soup.

### Grilled Chicken Vegetable Salad

Place 4 ounces grilled skinless chicken breast on a large bed of mixed greens and top with cherry tomatoes, sliced beets, chopped bell pepper (red, green, or yellow), artichoke hearts, and ½ cup chickpeas or black beans. Toss with 2 teaspoons olive oil and unlimited vinegar or fresh lemon juice (or 2 to 4 tablespoons reduced-calorie dressing).

### Yogurt with Fruit, Wheat Germ, and Nuts

Mix a 6-ounce container of fat-free vanilla yogurt with 1 chopped apple (or pear), ½ cup berries (or 2 tablespoons raisins), 2 tablespoons wheat germ, and 2 tablespoons chopped walnuts.

### Peanut Butter Toast with Lentil Soup

Spread 1 slice toasted whole grain bread with 1 level tablespoon peanut butter. Serve with 2 cups lentil soup (or any noncreamy bean soup).

## DINNER OPTIONS

(500 TO 600 CALORIES)

### Grilled Salmon with Brussels Sprouts and Brown Rice

Enjoy 5 ounces grilled salmon (or flounder, sole, or shrimp) with unlimited Brussels sprouts and ½ cup cooked brown rice tossed with 1 tablespoon slivered almonds.

### Pork Tenderloin with Black-Eyed Peas and Cauliflower

Enjoy 5 ounces baked, grilled, or broiled pork tenderloin with 1 cup cooked black-eyed peas and unlimited steamed or roasted cauliflower or green beans.

### Whole Wheat Pasta with Sea Bass and Pea Sauce

Enjoy 1 serving Whole Wheat Penne with Sea Bass and Pea Sauce (page 323) with a side salad of leafy greens, beets, carrots, and 1 tablespoon chopped walnuts tossed with 2 teaspoons olive oil and vinegar or fresh lemon juice (or 2 to 4 tablespoons reduced-calorie dressing).

### Vegetable Bisque with Grilled Chicken and Sautéed Spinach

Enjoy 2 cups Vegetable Oatmeal Bisque (page 322) or any prepared vegetable, lentil, or vegetable-barley soup with 5 ounces grilled chicken breast and unlimited spinach sautéed in 1 teaspoon olive oil and crushed garlic.

### Cheddar Burger over Greens

Top a 5-ounce turkey or veggie burger with 1 slice reduced-fat cheese, sliced tomato, and onion and serve on a bed of unlimited salad greens tossed with 2 tablespoons reduced-calorie vinaigrette. Enjoy with 1 cup boiled edamame (green soybeans in the pod).

### Chopped Chicken Salad with Apples and Walnuts

Enjoy 1 serving (page 321).

### Turkey Chili with Brown Rice and Salad

Top 2 cups Turkey Chili (page 363) with 2 tablespoons shredded reduced-fat Cheddar cheese and serve with ½ cup cooked brown rice or quinoa and a side salad of leafy greens (and optional peppers, carrots, beets, and artichokes) tossed with 1 teaspoon olive oil and unlimited vinegar or fresh lemon juice (or 2 tablespoons reduced-calorie dressing).

## SNACK OPTIONS

100 CALORIES OR LESS

- ◆ 1 level tablespoon peanut butter with celery sticks
- ◆ 6 ounces fat-free flavored or plain yogurt (100 calories or less)
- ◆ 10 almonds, unsalted
- ◆ 25 pistachios (in the shell)
- ◆ 8- to 12-ounce skim latte or cappuccino (choose decaf if caffeine makes you jittery or if you have PMS or insomnia)
- ◆ 1 handful baby carrots and 2 level tablespoons hummus
- ◆ 1 cup Vegetable Oatmeal Bisque (page 322)

100 TO 200 CALORIES

- ◆ 10 almonds (or 25 pistachios in the shell) and 1 apple
- ◆ ¼ cup walnuts (or almonds, pecans, cashews, or peanuts)
- ◆ ½ cup pistachios or sunflower seeds in the shell
- ◆ ½ cup fat-free or 1% cottage cheese mixed with 2 tablespoons wheat germ
- ◆ 1 slice whole grain toast with 1 level tablespoon nut butter (or 2 ounces turkey or chicken)

◆ 1 cup whole grain cereal with ¾ cup fat-free milk (or soy milk)

◆ 1 cup fat-free plain yogurt mixed with ½ cup berries and 1 tablespoon wheat germ

◆ ¾ cup chickpeas (garbanzo beans)

◆ Handful of baby carrots with ¼ cup hummus

◆ 1 sliced apple with 1 level tablespoon peanut butter (or other nut butter)

◆ 1 frozen banana with 1 cup fat-free milk (or soy milk). (For frozen banana, peel one banana, slice into ½-inch wheels, place in a small plastic bag, and freeze before serving.)

◆ Fruit smoothie: In a blender, mix ½ cup fat-free milk (or soy milk), ½ cup fat-free yogurt, ¾ cup fresh or frozen fruit (such as berries, banana, peach, or mango), and 3 to 5 ice cubes.

# WILD SALMON SALAD

*Everybody seems to have a favorite tuna salad recipe, but it is just as easy to create fabulous salads using canned salmon, which has much more omega-3 fatty acids. This recipe can also be made using leftover fresh salmon. Serve over a bed of lettuce or in a sandwich with whole wheat bread.*

**MAKES 3 SERVINGS (ABOUT 1 CUP EACH)**

1 can (6 ounces) wild salmon, well drained (remove skin)

1 can (19 ounces) chickpeas (garbanzo beans), rinsed and drained

½ cup chopped red onion

½ red bell pepper, chopped

2 tablespoons extra-virgin olive oil

2 tablespoons red wine vinegar

In a medium bowl, mash the salmon. Mix in the chickpeas, onion, and pepper. In a separate bowl, whisk together the oil and vinegar. Pour over the salmon mixture and stir thoroughly. Cover and refrigerate for up to 2 days.

> **Per serving:** 339 calories, 19 g protein, 33 g carbohydrate, 14 g fat (2 g saturated), 26 mg cholesterol, 60 mg sodium, 9 g fiber; plus 203 mg folate (51% DV), 2 mg vitamin $B_{12}$ (35% DV), and a hearty dose of omega-3s and vitamin D

# CHOPPED CHICKEN SALAD WITH APPLES AND WALNUTS

*This salad is delicious, and it provides generous amounts of protein, high-quality carbs, soluble fiber, and 75 percent of your daily requirement of folate.*

**MAKES 1 SERVING**

2 to 3 cups chopped lettuce (preferably romaine)

4 to 5 ounces cooked chicken breast, chopped

2 tablespoons canned chickpeas

½ medium Fuji or McIntosh apple (with skin), chopped

¼ cup chopped cucumber (with peel)

½ tomato, chopped

¼ avocado, chopped

1 stalk celery, chopped

2 scallions, finely chopped

1 tablespoon chopped walnuts

2 tablespoons reduced-calorie vinaigrette (raspberry vinaigrette works well)

Place the lettuce in a large bowl. Add the chicken, chickpeas, apple, cucumber, tomato, avocado, celery, scallions, and walnuts. Drizzle with the vinaigrette and toss to coat.

> **Per serving:** 460 calories, 42 g protein, 41 g carbohydrate, 16 g fat (2 g saturated), 95 mg cholesterol, 450 mg sodium, 11 g fiber; plus 300 mcg folate (75% DV)

# VEGETABLE OATMEAL BISQUE

*You're probably thinking that veggies and oatmeal are one strange combination! But I promise, this hearty soup is easy to make and one of my most favorite (and filling) low-calorie recipes. For less than 100 calories, you'll get plenty of high-quality carbohydrates, fiber, and folate. Plus, you'll have lots of leftovers for the next few days.*

**MAKES 10 SERVINGS (1 CUP EACH)**

1 bag (16 ounces) frozen broccoli florets

1 bag (16 ounces) frozen cauliflower florets

1 bag (16 ounces) fresh baby carrots

1 zucchini, peeled and chopped

½ chopped onion

6 cups reduced-sodium vegetable or chicken broth

1 cup old-fashioned oats (not quick-cooking)

Kosher salt

Ground black pepper

In a large pot over medium-high heat, combine the broccoli, cauliflower, carrots, zucchini, onion, and broth. Cover and bring to a boil. Reduce the heat and simmer, stirring occasionally, for 1 hour.

Add the oatmeal and mix thoroughly. Simmer, stirring occasionally, for 40 minutes longer. With an immersion blender or in a food processor or blender, puree the soup. Add salt and pepper to taste and serve.

**Per serving:** 86 calories, 6 g protein, 16 g carbohydrate, 0 g fat, 0 mg cholesterol, 386 mg sodium, 4 g fiber; plus 80 mg folate (20% DV)

# WHOLE WHEAT PENNE WITH SEA BASS AND PEA SAUCE

*This meal tastes as decadent as it sounds, but it is low in calories and simple to prepare. If you prefer, substitute shrimp, salmon, or halibut for the sea bass.*

**MAKES 8 SERVINGS (1½ TO 2 CUPS PER SERVING)**

1 package (16 ounces) whole wheat penne

4 tablespoons olive oil

½ onion, chopped

2 cups fresh or thawed frozen peas

2 cups low-sodium vegetable broth

Kosher salt

Ground black pepper

¾ pound sea bass, cut into ½" cubes

4 plum tomatoes, peeled, seeded, and diced

1 teaspoon chopped fresh parsley (optional)

Cook the pasta in a large pot of boiling water for 8 minutes, or until al dente. Drain and keep warm.

Meanwhile, heat 1 tablespoon of the oil in a saucepan over medium-low heat. Add the onion and cook for about 3 minutes, or until softened. Add the peas and broth and bring the mixture to boil. Simmer for 5 minutes. Using an immersion blender, puree the broth mixture in the saucepan until smooth. (If you don't have an immersion blender, transfer the broth mixture to a blender or food processor in two separate batches and puree. Return the puree to the saucepan.) Season with salt and pepper to taste and keep warm over very low heat.

Heat the remaining 3 tablespoons oil in a large skillet over moderate heat. Add the sea bass and sauté, stirring, for 2 minutes, or until almost cooked through. With a slotted spoon, transfer the sea bass to a bowl. Add the tomatoes to the skillet and cook for 5 minutes. Return the sea bass to the skillet and season with salt and pepper to taste. Add the cooked pasta and toss to coat.

To serve, ladle some of the warm pea sauce into each serving dish and mound some of the sea bass and pasta on top. Garnish with the parsley, if desired.

**Per serving:** 359 calories, 18 g protein, 51 g carbohydrate, 9 g fat (1 g saturated), 17 mg cholesterol, 520 mg sodium, 8 g fiber

# CHAPTER 14

# MIGRAINE HEADACHES

ne of my friends describes her migraines as pain storms that split her skull across her right temple, liquefying her brain until it feels like it's oozing out through her ears. The sound of a phone ringing is like a frying pan slamming the top of her head. Bright light is like a paintball gun filled with needles shot straight through her eyeballs. Once they strike, these intense, throbbing headaches last anywhere from a few hours to three days—and all she can do is take rescue medication, lie in a darkened room, and wait for the incapacitating pain to resolve.

About one in every ten Americans has had at least one migraine. Some experience an aura that presages the coming pain. An aura is typically some unusual visual experience, such as blind spots, distortion, jagged lines running through the visual field, sparkling or flashing lights, or enhanced color or depth perception. But some auras can cause a feeling of pins and needles in arms or legs, speech difficulties, excessive thirst, sleepiness, food cravings, or unexplained mood changes, particularly feelings of depression and irritability. More often, however, there is no warning before the pain sets in.

Migraine headaches usually start on one side but often spread and encompass the other hemisphere, too. During an episode, most migraine sufferers become extremely sensitive to light and sound, and some may feel nauseated or even vomit. Migraines can come just once or twice a year, several times each month, or much more frequently. My friend used to get migraines three times a week. Working with her doctor, she was able to find the right preventive medication and cut the frequency by half—but that still meant six migraines a month. Then, after identifying and eliminating food triggers from her diet, the number fell to one or two.

You're probably thinking, "That's great for her, but how much pain relief can I expect?" Unfortunately, no one can say with any certainty. Everyone has different triggers, so what worked for my friend may have no effect on you. However, there is bound to be something in this chapter that will help. I recommend that you try everything, keep what works, and never lose hope that you'll someday be able to avoid or control your migraines.

## WHAT AFFECTS MIGRAINE HEADACHES?

Migraines are a mystery. Scientists don't know precisely what causes them or what exactly happens in the body once a migraine is triggered. They believe that there is a genetic component and that the headaches are a result of abnormal functions in certain brain structures. Early research suggested that migraine headaches were caused solely by changes in the way blood vessels in the head dilated and constricted. Now scientists understand that blood vessels are just one element involved in the migraine process. We know from brain scans that during migraine headaches, there is increased bloodflow in the brain stem and the cerebral cortex. Inflammatory chemicals, such as substance P, and other substances are released; nerve centers are stimulated; and there are changes in levels of brain chemicals called neurotransmitters. In addition, new research hints that defects in cells' mitochondria—the "powerhouses" of cells responsible for producing energy to fuel your entire body—may play a role. The main lessons are that migraines are physiologically complex and that they absolutely are not "all in the mind" of the sufferer.

But for our purposes, the more important questions are: What sets off the headache in the first place? Can it be stopped? Migraines are triggered by specific factors, many of which are understood—but what triggers one person's headache may not affect you in the least. The most common triggers are:

**Foods.** Many everyday foods are big triggers. I provide a specific list on the next page.

*(continued on page 328)*

## FAQS

**I've figured out how to avoid my trigger foods at home, but eating out seems like a chore. Do you have any guidelines for foods to avoid or foods that are safe to eat in restaurants?**

It's safest to avoid the following: cheap buffets that leave food sitting and use suspect ingredients; Chinese food (due to soy sauce, tofu, and miso); and Mexican food (due to the assortment of dishes with cheese, sour cream, and avocado). Your safest bets are high-quality American, seafood, or Italian restaurants. My suggestions for relatively safe ordering include:

- Grilled chicken or fish (request no MSG or vinegar)

- Steamed or sautéed vegetables in olive oil and garlic with a plain baked sweet or white potato (or rice, preferably brown or wild)

- Pasta with broccoli and grilled chicken tossed in an olive oil–based sauce

- For dessert, a nonchocolate treat like strawberries with whipped cream, rice pudding, or herbal tea with plain biscotti

Keep in mind that these suggested meals are free of *all* migraine triggers. After keeping a migraine diary, you'll probably find that you are sensitive to only a handful of foods. Once you've identified your personal triggers, it will be much easier to order a wide variety of dishes in most ethnic restaurants.

## POSSIBLE TRIGGER FOODS: THE ANTIGROCERY LIST

I advise migraine sufferers to follow an elimination diet to help identify their personal food triggers. To start, eliminate every potential food trigger from your diet for at least one month. Note whether your migraines improve. Then add back one food at a time—try no more than one new food every two days. If you get a migraine within 24 hours of eating the added-back food, stop eating it again. (When you get through the whole list, you can always test it again if it is a particular favorite.)

For a printable version of this list, visit www.joybauer.com/migraines.

### Fruit

Apple juice and cider

Apples (red-skinned only)

Bananas

Citrus fruits (clementines, grapefruit, lemons, limes, oranges, pineapple, tangerines)

Citrus juice (grapefruit, lemonade, orange, pineapple, and other citrus blends)

Dried fruits (including apricots, dates, figs, prunes)

Grapes and grape juice

Papayas

Passion fruit

Pears (red-skinned only)

Plums (black-skinned only, purple, and red)

Raisins

Raspberries

### Vegetables

Avocados

Beans (specifically fava/broad, Italian/flat, lima, navy)

Canned tomato sauce

Canned vegetables

Eggplant

Lentils

Olives

Onions

Peas

Pickles

Relish

Sauerkraut

Snow peas

Tomatoes (in rare cases)

### Fish

*All* cured, smoked, canned, pickled, or aged fish

Anchovies (canned)

Caviar

Lox

Pickled herring

Sardines (canned)

### Meats

*All* aged, canned, cured, pickled, or smoked meats

Bacon (including beef, pork, and turkey)

Beef (all aged, canned, cured, pickled, or smoked)

Beef jerky

Bologna (all varieties)

Chicken (all canned, cured, pickled, or smoked)

Corned beef

Deli meats (cured or smoked)

Ham (aged, canned, cured, pickled, or smoked)

Hot dogs (all varieties)

Liver and liverwurst

Organ meats (such as kidneys or liver)

Pastrami

Pâté

Pepperoni

Pork (all aged, canned, cured, pickled, or smoked)

Salami

Sausages (including beef, chicken, soy, and turkey)

Turkey (all aged, canned, cured, pickled, or smoked)

Turkey jerky

## Soy

Miso

Products made with soy protein isolate (check labels!)

Soy sauce (including reduced-sodium)

Tempeh

Teriyaki sauce

Tofu

## Nuts and seeds

All nut butters

All nuts

## Dairy

Aged cheeses (including blue, Brie, Camembert, Cheddar, Gouda, Gruyère, mozzarella, Parmesan, provolone, Romano, Roquefort, Stilton, Swiss, and all other aged or "moldy" cheeses)

Buttermilk

Chocolate ice cream

Chocolate milk

Chocolate pudding

Foods prepared with cheese (check labels)

Sour cream

Yogurt

## Grains

Sourdough bread

Yeast bread and bread products, freshly baked

## Miscellaneous

Alcohol (especially beer, red wine, sherry, and vermouth)

Chocolate

Cocoa

Coffee

Diet beverages/products that use the artificial sweetener aspartame (also known as NutraSweet and Equal)

Processed foods that contain MSG, yeast extract, hydrolyzed or autolyzed yeast, hydrolyzed vegetable protein (HVP), hydrolyzed plant protein (HPP), sodium caseinate, and kombu extract

Caffeinated soft drinks (Coke, Mountain Dew, Pepsi, Red Bull, and others; check labels for caffeine)

Tea (black and green)

Vinegar (except distilled white vinegar)

**Stress.** When we are stressed, our bodies react physically—our muscles tense, our hormones become elevated, and migraines can be triggered.

**Hormonal changes.** Because estrogen and progesterone are such potent migraine triggers, women are nearly three times more likely than men to experience migraines. In fact, there is a subset of headaches known as menstrual migraines, which can occur one or two days before the start of a woman's period or during the first couple of days of her period. Women with hormone triggers can take comfort in knowing that many cases of menstrual migraines disappear entirely after menopause.

**Intense sensory stimuli.** Bright light, loud noises, and strong smells—such as cleaning chemicals, cigarette smoke, raw onions, and perfume—can trigger migraines.

**Physical exertion or abrupt lifestyle changes.** Jumping into an extreme exercise program can trigger migraines, as can changing sleep patterns, alternating work shifts, or anything else that breaks your body out of its normal rhythms. If you push yourself in a demanding job all week long, you'll be more likely to get a migraine when you finally slow down over the weekend. On the flip side, if you enjoy a weekend with a little too much fun, you may develop a Monday migraine.

**Environmental factors.** Some people get migraines when there are changes in the air—literally. Their headaches coincide with the arrival of thunderstorms, sudden changes in altitude or barometric pressure, windstorms, seasonal changes, or pollen levels. Others are sensitive to the switch to daylight savings time or travel across time zones.

**Medications.** Medications can have a wide range of side effects, so it is no surprise that some can trigger migraines. You need to be especially wary of antihistamines, decongestants, blood pressure medications, oral contraceptives, hormone replacement therapy, and prescription pain medications. Interestingly, migraines can also be triggered if you stop taking prescription or over-the-counter pain medications (such as aspirin, acetaminophen, or ibuprofen) that your body has become accustomed to. This phenomenon is called rebound.

Some neurologists believe that all those trigger factors can be additive. They theorize that everybody has a tolerance limit for triggers, and once that limit is exceeded, a migraine is in your near future. If you have extreme sensitivity, then a single mild trigger may be enough to cause a headache. But if you have a greater tolerance, it may take two or three triggers occurring in close succession to push you past that limit. So you may be just fine if you have to use strong-smelling cleaning products. But if you clean, and then a thunderstorm hits, that combination of triggers may be enough to send you over the top. That's why it is critical to try to eliminate as many potential "controllable" triggers from your life as possible.

# HOW FOOD AFFECTS MIGRAINE HEADACHES

The most important role food plays in migraines is as a trigger. Not all of the foods on my list will cause migraines in all sufferers, and some sufferers have no food sensitivities. In order to determine what your particular triggers are, I recommend keeping a migraine diary for at least three months (see page 331). If you discover that one of the foods listed here is a trigger for you, then you know that you should avoid that particular food if you want to remain pain free.

It's important to remember, however, that you and your migraines are unique; what causes headaches for someone else might be perfectly safe for you. I can't stress this enough: Don't automatically eliminate foods permanently without confirming that they are personal triggers. Many of the foods on this list contain healthful nutrients, and it would be a shame to cut nuts, cheese, or (gasp!) dark chocolate out of your diet if your headaches aren't affected by them.

## POSSIBLE TRIGGER FOODS TO BE AWARE OF . . .

◆ **Tyramine, phenylethylamine,** and other **amines.** Although many foods contain these amines in trace amounts, the following specific foods can often be powerful migraine triggers: chocolate (and anything made with cocoa), aged or fermented cheeses (including Cheddar, blue, Brie, and all hard cheeses and "moldy" cheeses), yogurt, sour cream, buttermilk, soy products (including tofu, tempeh, miso, soy sauce, teriyaki, and foods made with soy protein/isolate), all varieties of vinegar except white vinegar (including salad dressings and condiments made with vinegars other than white vinegar), sauerkraut, relish, pickles, olives, freshly baked yeast breads (commercial breads are fine), sourdough bread, organ meats (including liver, kidney, and pâtés), processed meats and fish (smoked, pickled, cured, aged, or canned), all nuts and nut butters, snow peas, beans (specifically broad/fava beans, Italian/flat beans, lima, navy), lentils, eggplant, avocados, onions (especially raw), citrus fruits and juices (pineapple, oranges, grapefruit, lemons, limes, tangerines, and clementines), bananas, raisins, figs, plums (red, purple, and black), papaya, passion fruit, and raspberries.

◆ **Leftovers.** Tyramine content increases over time, especially if food is improperly stored. Take extra care to avoid eating leftovers if you find that you're tyramine sensitive.

◆ **Alcohol.** Red wine, beer, sherry, and vermouth contain large amounts of tyramine and other naturally occurring compounds that are thought to precipitate migraines. In addition, all alcohol can cause dehydration, which can also trigger headaches. Clear liquors, like vodka and gin, are typically better tolerated.

◆ **Caffeine.** Caffeine is a double-edged sword for migraine sufferers. People with a sensitivity to caffeine can develop migraines after drinking coffee, black tea, green tea, cola, or other caffeinated beverages. If you're a steady coffee or tea drinker and you abruptly cut out caffeine (or you accidentally miss your cup o' joe one day), a painful withdrawal headache can result.

Paradoxically, caffeine can also be used to stop a migraine that is just beginning—that's why many over-the-counter migraine medications contain caffeine. German researchers reported that when people took a combination of 250 milligrams of aspirin, 200 milligrams of acetaminophen, and 50 milligrams of caffeine at the start of their migraines, they had better and faster pain relief than people who did not take the caffeine. But it gets even more complicated: If you start to rely on caffeine-containing pain relievers and use them nearly every day, you can induce what physicians refer to as a medication overuse, or "rebound," headache.

Bottom line: Migraine sufferers should limit their intake to no more than 200 milligrams of caffeine per day (that's equivalent to one to two 8-ounce cups of coffee or about four cups of tea) or give it up completely. If you need to cut back, taper down slowly over the course of several weeks. Finally, to minimize your risk of medication overuse headaches, don't use caffeine-containing pain meds more than two days per week. Keep in mind that chocolate, both milk and dark, also contains small amounts of caffeine, so if you find that chocolate is a trigger for you, you'll need to make use of a migraine diary (see opposite page) and some clever detective skills to determine whether the actual offender is chocolate or caffeine in general—or both.

◆ **MSG and MSG-like flavor enhancers.** Check labels carefully for foods that contain monosodium glutamate (MSG), a popular flavor enhancer, or other ingredients that have a similar chemical makeup: yeast extract, hydrolyzed or autolyzed yeast, hydrolyzed vegetable protein (HVP), hydrolyzed plant protein (HPP), sodium caseinate, and kombu extract.

◆ **Nitrites and nitrates.** These common preservatives are found in processed meats, including deli meats, pepperoni, bacon, hot dogs, sausages (including chicken, turkey, and soy sausages/bacon/hot dogs that list nitrites in their ingredients), bologna, pastrami, jerky (beef and turkey), corned beef, and all other beef/poultry/pork/wild game/fish that have been cured, smoked, pickled, canned, or preserved with nitrites or nitrates. Fortunately, there are some quality brands that offer nitrate-free versions of poultry sausages, deli meats, and turkey bacon. You can typically find these products at health food markets and some mainstream grocery stores.

◆ **Artificial sweeteners.** Some people report getting headaches after consuming products with artificial sweeteners, most commonly aspartame (also known as

## MIGRAINE DIARY

Some neurologists believe that becoming too obsessive about tracking migraine triggers can be stressful, and we all know that stress can trigger a migraine. But unless you keep a basic diary, it will be difficult to spot patterns. If you see a doctor, you'll be required to complete a diary, so starting now will put you one step ahead.

For each migraine episode, note on a regular calendar or in a journal:

- Date and day of the week

- The location and type of pain. For example, would you describe the pain as stabbing, throbbing, steady, dull, or sharp? Use whatever adjectives come to mind—there is no wrong answer.

- Intensity level, on a scale of 1 to 10, where 1 = mild pain and 10 = the worst pain you've ever felt

- Duration, in number of hours

- Any warning signs that the migraine was on its way

- Weather at the time the migraine started and any changes during the subsequent 12 hours

- Activities or stress level in the 24 hours prior to the migraine

- Foods eaten in the 24 hours prior to the migraine

- What you did to try to stop the migraine and whether those treatments were effective

- If you are a woman, where you are in your menstrual cycle

NutraSweet and Equal). Aside from being distributed in small packets, artificial sweeteners pop up all over the place—in diet beverages, light yogurts, sugar-free candies, and low-calorie desserts.

◆ **Tannins.** Tannins are bitter plant compounds that are found in high amounts in tea, red-skinned apples and pears, apple juice and cider, coffee, and red wine.

◆ **Sulfites.** This preservative is commonly found in wine (white and red), dried fruits (including prunes, figs, and apricots), and many processed foods.

## NUTRIENTS AND FOODS THAT MAY REDUCE MIGRAINE FREQUENCY

The list of potential trigger foods seems long, I know, but remember that it's just a list of possibilities. Most likely, when you're done systematically eliminating and then reintroducing these foods, you will find that there are just a few you need to avoid. Now for the good news: There are some nutrients you should try to consume more often.

## Liquids

Dehydration is a common migraine trigger. When everyone seems to be rushing from work to a meeting to the gym and back home again without much thought about food or drink, migraine sufferers need to stay hypervigilant about their liquid intake. While the latest government guidelines say that most people can allow thirst to guide how much they drink, migraine sufferers should aim to preempt thirst. Try to drink about nine 8-ounce cups of liquid a day if you're a woman or about thirteen 8-ounce cups a day if you're a man. Eight ounces is a lot less than you think! I ask my clients to fill their favorite drinking glass with water, then transfer the water to a liquid-measuring cup to see exactly how many ounces they drink each time they fill the glass. Please remember that water is the single best way to stay hydrated—it is inexpensive, calorie free, and efficient. The worst hydrating liquids are sodas, sugary fruit drinks, sweetened tea or coffee, and juices; all of these add too many calories to your daily diet (and in some instances are migraine triggers).

> BEST HYDRATING LIQUIDS: *water, herbal tea, decaffeinated coffee, decaffeinated tea, milk (fat-free, 1%), plain and naturally flavored seltzer and club soda*

## Omega-3 Fats and Olive Oil

Adding some healthy fats into your diet may help reduce inflammation, which is thought to contribute to the pain of migraines. Omega-3 fatty acids (found in large quantities in fatty fish) and monounsaturated fats (found in olive oil) have both been shown to reduce the frequency, duration, and severity of headaches. I recommend eating fresh wild salmon, which is high in omega-3s, at least two times per week and making other omega-3 foods a regular part of your diet. (My Best Foods list includes only the fatty fish that have been shown to be low in mercury, PCBs, and dioxins.) Try to use olive oil or canola oil instead of butter in your cooking whenever possible.

> BEST MIGRAINE-SAFE FOODS FOR OMEGA-3 FATTY ACIDS: *wild salmon (fresh only), rainbow trout, Pacific oysters, sardines (fresh only), chia seeds, ground flaxseed, flaxseed oil, walnut oil, canola oil*

## Riboflavin

Riboflavin—also called vitamin $B_2$—is involved with the body's production of energy at the cellular level. Some research suggests that people with migraines may have a genetic defect that makes it difficult for their cells to maintain energy reserves, and this lack of basic energy could trigger migraines. Many neurologists recommend that their migraine patients take riboflavin supplements along with their prescription medications. Although it is difficult to get enough riboflavin to prevent migraines from food sources alone, I recommend adding some additional riboflavin-rich foods to your diet. If you would like to try riboflavin supplements, I recommend a 400-milligram dose or a combination product that includes riboflavin and other potentially beneficial supplements. See the Supplements section, page 335, for more information.

BEST MIGRAINE-SAFE FOODS FOR RIBOFLAVIN: *fresh lean beef and lamb, venison, whole grain cereal, milk (fat-free, 1%), eggs, mushrooms, asparagus, kale, broccoli, spinach*

## Magnesium

Magnesium deficiency has been linked to migraines. Getting enough magnesium through diet or supplements may help prevent all kinds of migraines, but it seems to be particularly valuable for women who get menstrual migraines. Eating a diet high in magnesium is safe and will contribute to headache prevention. However, most studies showing that magnesium benefits migraines have used supplements, not food sources. By all means, go out of your way to include foods rich in magnesium, but if you would also like to try magnesium supplements, see the Supplements section, page 335, for more information.

BEST MIGRAINE-SAFE FOODS FOR MAGNESIUM: *pumpkin seeds, spinach, Swiss chard, amaranth, sunflower seeds, quinoa, sweet and white potatoes, millet, artichoke hearts (fresh or frozen only, not canned), brown rice, whole grain pasta, whole grains (see best varieties on grocery list), sesame seeds, wheat germ, flaxseed*

## BONUS POINTS

◆ **Eat regularly.** Anyone who skips a meal risks developing a headache, but migraine sufferers are particularly sensitive. Going several hours without eating alters levels of brain chemicals and causes low blood sugar, both of which may spark a migraine in susceptible individuals. In fact, skipping meals is one of the most well-documented triggers. Don't let a crazy schedule stop you from eating regularly—that means at least every five hours, but it's possible that you need to eat even more often than that. Look at it this way: If you don't take the time to eat lunch and then you get a migraine, you'll lose a lot more than your lunch hour nursing the headache. Carry small, healthy "emergency snacks," such as rice cakes, dry whole grain cereal, sunflower seeds, baby carrots, or green apples, with you at all times. If you find that plain nuts are not personal triggers for you, they also make a terrific portable snack.

♦ **Lose weight if you are overweight.** A study published in the journal *Neurology* found that being overweight was linked to greater frequency and severity of migraine headaches in adults. In addition, a 2010 study found that overweight teens were more likely to report getting migraines and headaches than their peers who maintained a normal weight. Scientists are just beginning to explore possible explanations, but the relationship makes sense. Fat creates inflammation, and inflammation contributes to migraines, so it's not a big leap to think that fat could make migraines worse.

♦ **Quit smoking.** Smoking increases inflammation and can trigger migraines, so quitting could be a quick way to get rid of pain. If you need a more potent reason, how about stroke? Smoking increases the risk of stroke, and some types of migraines (migraines with aura) can also increase the risk of stroke, even in people under age 50. Adding the two together can be disastrous.

♦ **Exercise gently but regularly.** Intense or unusual exercise can precipitate migraines, but regular exercise can reduce the frequency or severity of headaches by reducing tension. The trick is to warm up before exercising and, if you are new to physical activity, ease into it. Try walking, gentle cycling, or swimming to start.

♦ **Practice relaxation.** Because stress can trigger migraines, relaxation can help prevent them. Relaxation can be as simple as taking a bubble bath, listening to music, or spending an afternoon reading. But more structured relaxation programs are custom designed to put body and mind at ease. I recommend practicing yoga, progressive relaxation, or meditation for at least 30 minutes each day. Look for classes at your local community college or hospital wellness center.

♦ **Get enough sleep, without oversleeping.** In these overbusy, overscheduled times, it is so easy to sleep too little or develop an erratic sleep pattern. But if you suffer with migraines, you need to pay attention to your sleeping habits. Both lack of sleep and too much sleep can trigger migraines, so it is important that you make your sleep pattern as regular as possible, no matter how busy you are. Ideally, aim for seven to nine hours of quality sleep each night.

♦ **Consider physical therapy along with acupuncture, biofeedback, or massage.** There are a lot of different physical treatments that can help control or even prevent migraines. Research shows that physical therapy, when performed by a licensed physical therapist, is effective at treating migraines when paired with acupuncture, acupressure, biofeedback, or massage. Acupuncture is an ancient Asian therapy that involves the placement of hair-thin needles into the skin along energy pathways called meridians. The precise placement of needles reopens blocked energy meridians, thereby reducing pain. Acupressure follows the same principles as acupuncture but uses finger pressure, rather than needles, to activate pressure points. Biofeedback uses sensitive electronic measuring devices to teach the body how to control muscle tension, heart rate, and other "automatic" body processes that we usually think are not controllable. It is a way to help disrupt that chain of action and reaction that starts with stress and ends with a migraine. Massage is . . . well, absolutely relaxing and wonderful. Although more research is needed before a definitive case can be made for any of these treatments, they all look promising.

## SUPPLEMENTS

If you suffer from migraine headaches and want to consider supplements, research suggests that these supplements might be helpful.

1. **Magnesium.** Some studies have found that magnesium supplements are effective for headache prevention. The recommended dose is 400 milligrams daily. Magnesium is available as a single supplement or in widely available combination migraine supplements that also contain riboflavin and feverfew (more information below).

2. **Riboflavin.** When a group of migraine sufferers took 400 milligrams of riboflavin (vitamin $B_2$) daily for three months, 59 percent experienced at least a 50 percent reduction in migraine attacks. Riboflavin is available as a single supplement or in widely available combination migraine supplements that also contain magnesium and feverfew (more information below). One additional note, just to prevent an unexpected shock: At these dosages, riboflavin can turn urine a bright fluorescent yellow. It isn't dangerous, just colorful.

3. **Omega-3 fish oil.** If you can't get enough omega-3 fats through diet alone, try fish oil supplements. I recommend 1,000 milligrams from a combination of EPA (eicosapentaenoic acid) and DHA (docosahexaenoic acid), the two most beneficial types of omega-3 fats. Because the amount of EPA plus DHA per capsule varies widely among brands, you'll need to read the label and add up the individual milligrams yourself to determine how many pills it will take to reach 1,000 milligrams total of EPA and DHA. Store pills in the fridge to prevent the fish oils from going rancid. To avoid fishy burps and aftertaste, take with food, and choose enteric-coated varieties, which are designed to dissolve in the intestines instead of the stomach. Because fish oil acts as a blood thinner, do not take it if you have hemophilia or are already taking blood-thinning medications or aspirin.

4. **Coenzyme Q$_{10}$ (CoQ$_{10}$).** CoQ$_{10}$ is a vitaminlike substance that helps enzymes create energy at the cellular level. Without it, cells can't work properly. A handful of studies have shown that CoQ$_{10}$ reduces the frequency and severity of migraines. If you're looking to try CoQ$_{10}$, I recommend a daily dose of 100 to 200 milligrams. Although there are very few side effects from CoQ$_{10}$, some people may experience flulike symptoms, itching, rashes, heartburn, lack of appetite, or gastrointestinal distress. If you have liver disease, diabetes, or thyroid disease, talk with your doctor before trying CoQ$_{10}$.

5. **Feverfew.** Of all the herbs and botanicals touted for migraine relief, feverfew is one of the most studied. Feverfew is a traditional medicinal herb that shares the same family as marigolds and chrysanthemums, and it has been used for centuries to treat headaches. A few trials, but not all, have shown that feverfew reduces the frequency and severity of headaches in chronic migraine sufferers, presumably by relaxing blood vessels and decreasing inflammation to improve circulation in the brain. Although the evidence is by no means watertight, feverfew has limited side effects and may be worth trying. However, choosing a quality formulation is critical. A common dose is 100 to 125 milligrams of powdered feverfew leaves, standardized to 0.2 percent parthenolide, which is believed to be the active ingredient in feverfew. Feverfew is also found in combination with riboflavin and magnesium in supplements formulated specifically for migraine prevention. Women who are pregnant or trying to become pregnant and individuals taking blood thinners should not take feverfew due to undetermined safety in these populations.

6. **Combination migraine relief supplements.** MigreLief, a popular migraine supplement, is formulated with a combination of ingredients that may help ward off headaches: 360 milligrams of magnesium, 400 milligrams of riboflavin, and 100 milligrams of standardized feverfew. This product may cause diarrhea in some people, due to magnesium's laxative effects. Do not take MigreLief if you are using potassium-sparing diuretics, have renal failure, or are pregnant or nursing.

For more information on how food can help manage migraines, visit www.joybauer.com/migraines.

# JOY'S 4-STEP PROGRAM
## FOR MIGRAINE HEADACHES

Follow this program if you suffer from migraine headaches.

## Step 1 . . . START WITH THE BASICS

These are the first things you should do to try to reduce the frequency and intensity of your headaches.

◆ If you haven't been diagnosed, see your doctor. Many disorders—everything from a simple sinus infection to a brain tumor—can cause severe headaches. If you are diagnosed with migraines, ask if there are medications that might be helpful for preventing or stopping headaches.

◆ Begin keeping a migraine diary.

◆ Eliminate all potential migraine trigger foods from your diet for one month. Slowly reintroduce potential trigger foods one at a time at two-day intervals.

◆ Carry sunglasses at all times to shield your eyes from bright lights. Also, wear ear protection (or block your ears with cotton) in loud settings.

◆ Delegate chores that require chemical cleaners to someone else, or look for products that have less of a noxious odor, such as natural cleaners.

◆ Make your routine as regular as possible. Try your best to stick to regular eating and sleeping schedules, work habits, and exercise routines.

◆ If you smoke, quit.

# **Step 2** . . . YOUR ULTIMATE GROCERY LIST

Many foods on this list have high levels of nutrients that can help give you some relief from migraine headaches (foods rich in magnesium, riboflavin, and omega-3 fats). I have also included additional foods used as ingredients in the meal plans. All foods on this list are generally considered "safe" for migraine sufferers. Conduct a month-long elimination diet by eating ample foods from this list only. After one month, begin to introduce potential trigger foods one at a time at two-day intervals. This will help you determine a personal (shortened!) list of foods to avoid.

For a printable version of this list, visit www.joybauer.com/migraines.

## FRUIT

Apples (green and yellow only, not red-skinned)

Berries (blackberries, blueberries, and strawberries)

Cantaloupe

Cherries

Cranberries

Honeydew

Mangoes

Nectarines

Peaches

Pears (brown and green only, not red-skinned)

Watermelon

## VEGETABLES

Artichoke (fresh or frozen only, not canned)

Asparagus

Beets

Beans, starchy (black, cannellini, garbanzo, kidney, and white)

Bell peppers (all colors)

Broccoli

Broccoli raab

Brussels sprouts

Carrots

Cauliflower

Celery

Corn

Cucumbers

Dark leafy greens (such as collard, kale, mustard, Swiss chard, and turnip)

Lettuce (all varieties)

Mushrooms

Potatoes (sweet and white)

Pumpkin

Rhubarb

Spinach

Squash, summer

Squash, winter (acorn and butternut)

Turnips

Zucchini

## SEAFOOD

*All* fresh fish and shellfish, but especially:

Oysters, Pacific

Salmon, wild (fresh)

Sardines (fresh)

Trout, rainbow

## LEAN PROTEINS

Fresh beef (lean cuts)                 Eggs
Fresh chicken, skinless                Fresh turkey, skinless

## NUTS AND SEEDS

Chia seeds                             Pumpkin seeds
Flaxseed, ground                       Sunflower seeds and
                                       sunflower butter

## WHOLE GRAINS

Amaranth                    Millet                      Quinoa

Bulgur                      Oats                        Rice (brown and wild)

Cereal, whole grain         Pancake and waffle mix      Rice cakes, plain and
                            (preferably whole grain—        flavored (no MSG)
*Bread, whole grain (buns,      check labels to ensure no
    English muffins, pitas,     buttermilk)             Waffles, whole grain
    tortillas, and wraps)                               Wheat germ
                            Pasta, whole grain
Crackers, whole grain (no
    MSG)                     Popcorn, air-popped

*Note: Freshly baked yeast breads, such as homemade bread from a bakery or bread maker,
may be a trigger.

## DAIRY

Cheese, American            Cheese, ricotta (part-skim)   Cream cheese (fat-free or
                                                              reduced-fat)
Cheese, farmer's            Cottage cheese (fat-free or
                                1%)                       Milk (fat-free or 1%)

## MISCELLANEOUS

Canola oil                  Jelly and jam (blackberry,    Soft tub spread, trans-fat-
                                blueberry, strawberry, or     free (reduced-fat or
Coffee, decaffeinated           other acceptable fruits)      regular)

Flaxseed oil                Olive oil                     Tea, decaf or herbal

Garlic                      Seltzer, plain and naturally  Vinegar, distilled white only
                                flavored
Herbs and spices (fresh,
    dried, and ground)

# Step 3 . . . GOING ABOVE AND BEYOND

If you want to do everything you can to reduce the number and intensity of your migraines, here are some additional things you might try.

◆ Generally speaking, medical doctors are not big fans of supplements, but migraine supplements seem to be an exception. Discuss supplements with your doctor for help choosing the right one for you. Ask about riboflavin, magnesium, CoQ10, feverfew, and fish oil supplements.

◆ Start a low-intensity exercise program.

◆ If you are overweight, try to lose weight.

◆ Try to get seven to nine hours of quality sleep each night.

◆ Practice relaxation, in whatever form works best for you.

◆ Talk with your doctor about physical therapy, acupuncture, acupressure, and biofeedback.

# Step 4 . . . MEAL PLANS

These sample menus are free of foods known to trigger migraines and rich in omega-3 fats, riboflavin, and magnesium—nutrients that may be protective against migraine headaches. Most important, be sure to eat at regular intervals throughout the day.

Every day, choose one option for each of the three meals—breakfast, lunch, and dinner. Then, once or twice per day, choose from my suggested snacks. Approximate calories have been provided to help adjust for your personal weight-management goals. If you find yourself hungry (and if weight is not an issue), feel free to increase the portion sizes for meals and snacks. Beverage calories are not included.

## BREAKFAST OPTIONS

(300 TO 400 CALORIES)

### Egg Tortilla Wrap with Spinach, Mushrooms, and Peppers

Sauté a handful of spinach leaves, sliced mushrooms, and half a bell pepper (chopped) in 1 teaspoon olive or canola oil until soft. In a small mixing bowl, beat 1 whole egg with 2 egg whites and scramble in a heated pan coated with oil spray. Warm a whole grain tortilla (150 calories or less) in the microwave for 15 seconds (or wrap in foil and place in the oven for a few minutes). Place the scrambled eggs, spinach, mushrooms, and peppers in the center of the tortilla. Roll up!

### Cantaloupe Stuffed with Cottage Cheese and Wheat Germ

Fill ½ cantaloupe with 1 cup fat-free or 1% cottage cheese and top with 1 to 2 tablespoons wheat germ, ground flaxseed, or sunflower seeds.

### Whole Grain Cereal with Milk and Berries

Mix 1 cup whole grain cereal with 1 cup milk (skim or 1%) and top with 1 cup blueberries or strawberries.

### Rice Cakes with Peach Ricotta Cheese

Combine ½ cup part-skim ricotta cheese (or 1 cup fat-free or 1% cottage cheese) with 1 chopped fresh peach or nectarine. Spread over 3 rice cakes (or 1 sheet whole wheat matzo or 1 slice whole grain toast).

### Oatmeal with Berries and Seeds

Prepare ½ cup dry oats with ½ cup water and ½ cup fat-free milk. Top with ½ cup blueberries (or chopped strawberries or peaches) and 1 to 2 tablespoons ground flaxseed, sunflower seeds, or wheat germ. (If you like, add 1 or 2 teaspoons of sugar, honey, or jam to taste.)

## LUNCH OPTIONS

(400 TO 500 CALORIES)

### Grilled Chicken Salad with Cranberry Basil Vinaigrette

Top a large portion of mixed salad greens with 4 ounces cooked skinless chicken. Feel free to add chopped bell pepper (any color), broccoli, sliced mushrooms, cucumbers, beets, carrots, and/or celery. Toss with 2 tablespoons Cranberry Basil Vinaigrette (page 346).

### Turkey Burger over Greens with Baked Potato

Enjoy 5 ounces turkey burger (or extra-lean hamburger) on a bed of salad greens with a 1 baked sweet or white potato topped with optional 1 teaspoon soft tub, trans-fat-free spread.

### Spinach Omelet with Toast and Fresh Fruit

Beat 1 whole egg with 2 or 3 egg whites. Cook in a heated skillet coated with 1 teaspoon olive or canola oil. When the bottom is cooked, gently flip over. Top with unlimited fresh or cooked spinach. Fold the omelet over and cook until the egg mixture is firm. Enjoy with 1 slice whole wheat toast and ½ cantaloupe (or 1 green or yellow apple or 1 cup cherries).

### Chicken and Tri-Colored Pepper Wrap

Mix 5 ounces grilled chicken with unlimited red, yellow, and green peppers sautéed in 1 teaspoon olive or canola oil. Wrap in a whole grain tortilla (150 calories or less).

### Turkey Roll-Up with Baby Carrots and Fruit

Enjoy 1 Fresh Turkey Tortilla Roll-Up (page 345). Serve with unlimited baby carrots and ½ mango (or 1 peach or 1 cup blueberries, sliced strawberries, or blackberries).

## DINNER OPTIONS

(500 TO 600 CALORIES)

### Sirloin Steak with Sautéed Spinach and Baked Potato

Enjoy 5 ounces grilled sirloin steak (or other fresh lean beef) with unlimited spinach sautéed in 1 teaspoon olive oil and garlic and ½ baked sweet or white potato with optional 1 teaspoon soft tub, trans-fat-free spread.

### Grilled Salmon with Brown Rice and Broccoli

Enjoy 1 serving Easy! 3-Step Microwave Salmon (page 345) or 5 ounces grilled salmon with 1 teaspoon olive oil and seasonings. Serve with ½ cup cooked brown rice or quinoa and unlimited steamed broccoli or cauliflower.

### Rosemary Chicken with Sautéed Swiss Chard and Potato

Enjoy 5 ounces grilled Rosemary Chicken (page 347) with 1 serving (1 cup) Sautéed Swiss Chard (page 346) and 1 medium plain baked sweet or white potato.

## Whole Wheat Linguini with Vegetables

In a large pan, sauté minced garlic in 1 teaspoon olive oil. Add 1 cup broccoli florets, 1 cup sliced zucchini, and 1 cup cut asparagus spears and sauté until slightly soft. Add 1½ cups cooked whole wheat linguini or penne with 1 additional teaspoon olive oil and preferred herbs and seasonings. Thoroughly mix until the pasta is coated with the vegetables and oil. Season with kosher salt and freshly ground black pepper to taste.

## Baked Fish with Brown Rice and Asparagus

Season 6 ounces grilled or baked sole, trout, cod, halibut, or tilapia with 1 teaspoon olive oil and preferred seasonings. Serve with 1 cup cooked brown or wild rice, quinoa, or amaranth (or 1 plain baked sweet or white potato) and unlimited steamed asparagus, cauliflower, or kale.

## SNACK OPTIONS

100 CALORIES OR LESS

◆ *Best Vegetable Snacks:* up to 2 cups raw or cooked bell peppers, broccoli, cauliflower, asparagus, carrots, celery, cucumbers, or zucchini

◆ *Best Fruit Snacks:* 1 apple or pear (yellow, green, or brown only), peach, or nectarine; 1 cup blueberries, blackberries, sliced strawberries, or cherries; 1 cup cubed honeydew or watermelon; 20 whole strawberries; ½ mango; ½ cantaloupe

◆ 1 hard-cooked egg (or 4 egg whites)

◆ 1 rice cake or ½ sheet whole wheat matzo with 1 tablespoon fat-free or reduced-fat cream cheese

◆ Celery sticks with 2 to 3 tablespoons fat-free or reduced-fat cream cheese

◆ 2 rice cakes

◆ 3 cups air-popped popcorn sprinkled with optional cumin, chili powder, cinnamon, or other preferred seasonings

100 TO 200 CALORIES

◆ 1 slice whole wheat toast with 1 tablespoon strawberry jam (or ½ cup fat-free or 1% cottage cheese)

◆ 1 slice whole wheat toast (or 2 rice cakes) with 1 level tablespoon sunflower butter

◆ 1 hard-cooked egg (or 4 egg whites) plus 1 serving fruit (see Best Fruit Snacks list)

◆ ½ cup fat-free or 1% cottage cheese mixed with 1 cup berries or 1 chopped peach or nectarine

◆ ½ cup sunflower seeds in the shell

◆ 1 cup whole grain cereal with ½ cup fat-free milk

◆ 2 rice cakes, each topped with 1 tablespoon fat-free or reduced-fat cream cheese and 1 teaspoon strawberry jam

# EASY! 3-STEP MICROWAVE SALMON

*If you're looking for the easiest way to prepare salmon, you've found the perfect recipe: Dinner will be ready in less than 10 minutes. Plus, you'll receive a healthy dose of omega-3 fats, olive oil, and magnesium—three ingredients that have been shown to help fight migraines. If you serve it with green vegetables (such as asparagus, broccoli, or spinach), you'll also add riboflavin to the mix.*

**MAKES 2 SERVINGS**

2 wild salmon fillets (6 ounces each), ½" thick

1 tablespoon olive oil

2 cloves garlic, minced

¼ teaspoon kosher salt

Ground black pepper

Arrange the salmon fillets skin side down in a microwave-safe dish. Brush the oil evenly over the salmon and sprinkle with the garlic. Season with the salt and pepper to taste. Cover and microwave on high for 1 to 2 minutes, or until the edges are flaky and the fish is cooked through. Let stand for 1 to 2 minutes before serving.

> **Per serving:** 306 calories, 34 g protein, 1 g carbohydrate, 17 g fat (3 g saturated), 93 mg cholesterol, 219 mg sodium, 0 g fiber; plus 50 mg magnesium (13% DV)

# FRESH TURKEY TORTILLA ROLL-UP

*This safe-food wrap also provides a good amount of riboflavin and magnesium. For some extra flavor, try adding 1 to 2 tablespoons of my Cranberry Basil Vinaigrette (page 346).*

**MAKES 1**

4 large leaves romaine lettuce

1 whole grain tortilla wrap (150 calories or less)

¼ pound fresh sliced turkey breast (nitrate-free)

4 medium-thick slices red tomato

Layer the lettuce on the wrap. On one side of the wrap, arrange the turkey. (This makes the roll a little neater.) Top with the tomato and roll it up.

> **Per serving:** 275 calories, 38 g protein, 20 g carbohydrate, 4 g fat (1 g saturated), 94 mg cholesterol, 380 mg sodium, 6 g fiber; plus 50 mg magnesium (13% DV), 0.17 mg riboflavin (16% DV)

# CRANBERRY BASIL VINAIGRETTE

*Salad dressings are often filled with ingredients that could trigger a migraine—the wrong vinegars, MSG, citrus fruits, preservatives, and more. The next time you're craving a salad at home, try this dressing. It's a tasty, easy-to-make combination of safe ingredients. Be sure to whisk thoroughly before each use (the oil will separate) and store it in the fridge.*

**MAKES 13 SERVINGS (2 TABLESPOONS EACH)**

1 cup extra-virgin olive oil

¾ cup cranberry juice (100% juice)

¼ cup plus 1 tablespoon white distilled vinegar

¼ cup fresh basil, finely chopped

½ teaspoon kosher salt

½ teaspoon black pepper

In a medium mixing bowl, combine the oil, cranberry juice, vinegar, basil, salt, and pepper. Whisk thoroughly for a few minutes. Store leftovers in the fridge.

**Per serving:** 150 calories, 0 g protein, 1 g carbohydrate, 16 g fat (2 g saturated), 0 mg cholesterol, 45 mg sodium, 0 g fiber

# SAUTÉED SWISS CHARD

*This vegetable is naturally loaded with magnesium. Sauté it in olive oil and you'll get the added benefits of monounsaturated fat. If you'd like to save some calories, skip the oil. When steamed or microwaved, 1 cup of Swiss chard contains only 35 calories!*

**MAKES 4 SERVINGS (1 CUP EACH)**

2 tablespoons olive oil

2 cloves garlic, thinly sliced

2 pounds red or green Swiss chard, thinly sliced

Kosher salt

Ground black pepper

Warm the oil in a large nonstick skillet over high heat. Add the garlic and cook, stirring constantly, for 1 to 2 minutes. Add the Swiss chard and sprinkle with salt and pepper. Cook for 4 to 5 minutes, or until the Swiss chard is soft and reduced by half. Serve immediately.

**Per serving:** 106 calories, 4 g protein, 9 g carbohydrate, 7 g fat (1 g saturated), 0 mg cholesterol, 483 mg sodium, 4 g fiber; plus 185 mg magnesium (46% DV), 0.21 mg riboflavin (19% DV)

# Rosemary Chicken

*While you are following an elimination diet, it's important to have a scrumptious, staple chicken recipe that uses only trigger-free ingredients. This simple chicken dish is perfect. Serve with Sautéed Swiss Chard for a blast of magnesium.*

**MAKES 4 SERVINGS**

1 tablespoon olive oil

2 teaspoons fresh rosemary, minced

1 teaspoon paprika

1 teaspoon chili powder

1 teaspoon ground coriander (optional)

½ teaspoon freshly ground black pepper

4 skinless chicken cutlets, pounded to ⅛" thick (6 ounces each)

Kosher salt

Preheat a grill pan over medium-high heat or heat an outdoor grill.

In a small bowl, mix the oil, rosemary, paprika, chili powder, coriander (if using) and pepper. Rub the spice mixture over the chicken and season with salt.

Grill the chicken, turning once, for about 8 minutes, or until no longer pink and the juices run clear.

To bake the chicken in the oven, preheat the oven to 450°F. Line a baking sheet with foil and coat with oil spray. Place the chicken on the baking sheet and coat with oil spray. Bake, turning once halfway through cooking, for 6 to 7 minutes, or until no longer pink and the juices run clear.

**Per serving:** 227 calories, 40 g protein, 2 g carbohydrate, 6 g fat (1 g saturated), 98 mg cholesterol, 263 mg sodium, 1 g fiber

# CHAPTER 15

# PREMENSTRUAL SYNDROME

any years ago, I had a client, Michelle, come to see me specifically to address her problem with premenstrual syndrome (PMS). For about one week of the month, just before she got her period, Michelle would descend into a nightmare—turning into what she called her serial-killer self. During that time, she was prone to wildly changing and unpredictable moods, mostly rage with occasional bouts of weeping. She would cry at the soft look a father and his son exchanged on a fast-food commercial, scream at the cabbie who dared to stop at a yellow light when she was in a hurry, fume or cry at the office over things that normally rolled off her back, and, just once, she took her car, stomped on the accelerator, and rammed into the back of a car belonging to an ex-boyfriend's current lover. She hadn't dated the guy in over a year. It ended up costing her a small fortune in car repair bills, not to mention the increase in her premiums.

For Michelle, every month followed a predictable pattern: one week of being totally out of control, followed by two weeks spent begging forgiveness and writing letters of apology to all the people she had hurt or offended the previous week. By the time she came to see me, she was desperate.

PMS is estimated to affect about 40 percent of American women of childbearing age. Between 3 and 9 percent of women have a more extreme form of PMS called premenstrual dysphoric disorder (PMDD). PMS and PMDD cause physical and emotional symptoms, including irritability, sadness, mood swings, low self-esteem, difficulty concentrating, lack of energy, water retention and bloating, and breast tenderness, all of which are triggered by the normal hormonal changes associated with the menstrual cycle. These symptoms most typically begin the week before a woman is due to get her period, peak the day before the start of her period, and then disappear within a day after her period starts. The vast majority of women with PMS have symptoms for five to seven days, but some women can have symptoms that last two or even three weeks each month. PMDD, the form of the disorder Michelle probably had (although she hadn't had a formal diagnosis when I knew her) is casually defined as PMS so severe that it significantly decreases a woman's quality of life. PMS feels uncomfortable and unpleasant, but PMDD can turn social lives, work lives, families, and marriages upside down.

Whether you experience a little extra moodiness or car-crashing emotional breakdowns near your period, good nutrition can help alleviate some of your premenstrual symptoms. I worked with Michelle to level out her moods, and she saw great results. Once she felt that she was able to make it through a month without

## FAQS
**There are lots of herbal "cures" for PMS. Do they help?**

Herbal remedies come in and out of fashion just like hemlines. You may have heard that black cohosh, wild yam root, dong quai, and evening primrose oil can help relieve your symptoms. However, there's no good scientific evidence to support that any of these particular supplements relieve PMS symptoms. For information on supplements and herbal remedies that may be beneficial, see the Supplements section on page 353.

potentially litigious behavior, we decided that she might benefit from talking with a therapist. I haven't heard from Michelle in a long while, but the last time I saw her, she was calm, happy, and—in a testament to her self-control—still in possession of her driver's license.

## WHAT AFFECTS PMS?

No one knows exactly why some women experience symptoms and others do not. One leading theory is that some women have a greater sensitivity to the effects the female hormones estrogen and progesterone have on their serotonin levels. Serotonin is a brain chemical that plays a key role in mood regulation and sensitivity to pain, and research and clinical results seem to confirm that it significantly influences the onset of PMS. When women with the most severe premenstrual symptoms are treated with a serotonin-enhancing antidepressant (similar to Prozac), about 70 percent get substantial relief. What we do know is that for many women, PMS is an uncomfortable fact of life. If you are a woman of childbearing age experiencing mood issues, I recommend keeping a PMS diary. Keep track of your menstrual cycle and write down your primary moods, emotions, and unusual physical symptoms on a calendar each day. If your troubling moods or other symptoms occur primarily within the two weeks prior to the start of your period, you may have PMS (in addition to all the regular aggravations of life). However, if the days you experience irritability or depression are evenly spaced throughout the month, PMS probably isn't the culprit, and you may be experiencing another mood issue or disorder.

It is important to note all your physical symptoms in your PMS diary. For reasons that aren't exactly clear, symptoms of many diseases or disorders get worse premenstrually, a phenomenon known as premenstrual exacerbation. Depression and anxiety are prone to this exacerbation, as are migraines, epilepsy, asthma, allergies, diabetes, irritable bowel syndrome, and many autoimmune disorders. Though your symptoms may not be included on the list of general PMS symptoms I mentioned, they may well be related to your menstrual cycle if they are at their worst the week before your period. Talk with your doctor about the best prevention and treatment options for you.

## HOW FOOD AFFECTS PMS

Many women with PMS define their monthly nutrition needs in terms of their cravings for anything involving salt or chocolate. Though indulging in chocolate-dipped pretzels might seem like the perfect remedy, junk food won't provide lasting mood enhancement or reduce the bloat you're likely experiencing. There are many healthier options to help you get your symptoms under control.

### CALCIUM

Calcium deficiency and PMS share many symptoms, which led researchers to investigate whether they might be related. The results suggest that they very well might be. Studies have shown that women with PMS have lower blood levels of calcium around their time of ovulation, compared with women who don't experience PMS symptoms. And when PMS sufferers take 1,000 to 1,200 milligrams of calcium supplements daily, their mood and bloating improve after just a few months. Therefore, I consider calcium-rich foods an absolute must for women with PMS.

> **BEST FOODS FOR CALCIUM:** *yogurt (fat-free, low-fat), milk (fat-free, 1%), soy milk, cheese (fat-free, reduced-fat), tofu with calcium (check nutrition label), soybeans (edamame), frozen yogurt (fat-free, low-fat), low-fat ice cream, bok choy, kale, white beans, collard greens, broccoli, almonds and almond butter*

### VITAMIN D

Our bodies can't absorb or use calcium without vitamin D. That's why the two are so often mentioned together and why some high-calcium foods (such as milk) are often fortified with vitamin D. In addition, research suggests that vitamin D may act on its own to prevent PMS. In a study that followed more than 3,000 women for more than 10 years, women who ate a diet high in vitamin D reduced their risk of PMS by about 40 percent.

BEST FOODS FOR VITAMIN D: *wild salmon (fresh, canned), mackerel (not king), sardines, herring, milk (fat-free, 1%), soy milk, fortified yogurt (fat-free, low-fat), egg yolks, vitamin D-enhanced mushrooms\**

*\*These mushrooms are treated with UV light, which dramatically increases their vitamin D content.*

## MAGNESIUM

Just as was found with calcium, women with PMS seem to have lower blood levels of magnesium, compared with women who do not experience PMS symptoms. Women with PMS who took magnesium supplements had better mood and less water retention than women who did not get enough magnesium. It's possible that magnesium might help regulate the activity of serotonin. Magnesium-rich foods are second only to calcium-rich foods for improving your chances for symptom reduction.

BEST FOODS FOR MAGNESIUM: *pumpkin seeds, spinach, Swiss chard, amaranth, sunflower seeds, cashews, almonds, quinoa, tempeh, potatoes (sweet and white), soybeans (edamame), millet, starchy beans (such as black, navy, pinto, garbanzo, kidney), artichoke hearts, peanuts and peanut butter, brown rice, whole grain bread, sesame seeds, wheat germ, flaxseed*

## VITAMIN B$_6$

Your body can't make dopamine—one of the mood neurotransmitters—without vitamin B$_6$. Research studies into the effects of vitamin B$_6$ on PMS have been mixed—some show that taking supplements reduces irritability, depression, and breast tenderness, while others don't find any effect at all. There's no need to take a supplement (beyond what you're getting in your multivitamin, if you take one), but I highly recommend eating vitamin B$_6$-rich foods because they seem to have helped many of my clients with PMS.

BEST FOODS FOR VITAMIN B$_6$: *chickpeas (garbanzo beans), wild salmon (fresh, canned), lean beef, pork tenderloin, skinless chicken, potatoes (sweet, white), oats, bananas, pistachios, lentils, tomato paste, barley, rice (brown, wild), peppers, winter squash (acorn, butternut), broccoli, broccoli raab, carrots, Brussels sprouts, peanuts and peanut butter, eggs, shrimp, tofu, apricots, watermelon, avocados, strawberries, whole grain bread*

## MANGANESE

The minute quantities of manganese found in certain foods are all we need to stay healthy, so if you eat a relatively balanced diet, you're probably getting enough.

However, blood levels of manganese vary throughout the menstrual cycle, so it is not surprising that a deficiency of this mineral might be involved in PMS. A handful of studies have suggested that manganese, in combination with calcium, may reduce the irritability, depression, and tension associated with PMS. One study found that women who did not get enough manganese in their diets had more pain and worse moods premenstrually, so I encourage you to incorporate manganese-rich foods into your diet, specifically around the time of PMS.

BEST FOODS FOR MANGANESE: *pineapple, wheat germ, spinach, collard greens, pecans, amaranth, lima beans, pumpkin seeds, walnuts, oats, tempeh, quinoa, brown rice, flaxseed, raspberries, chickpeas (garbanzo beans), sunflower seeds, peanuts, tofu, soybeans (edamame), soy nuts, lentils*

## OTHER FOOD FIXES

◆ **Avoid salt and salty foods,** which can exacerbate the bloating and water retention already caused by PMS.

◆ **Avoid caffeine.** Some research suggests that the effects of caffeine are magnified premenstrually, leading to greater breast tenderness, more nervousness, and, potentially, more irritability. If you think you become more sensitive to caffeine around the time of your period, stick to decaffeinated coffee and naturally caffeine-free herbal teas.

◆ **Drink chamomile tea.** Chamomile tea may be particularly helpful premenstrually because it contains properties that relieve muscle spasms and may therefore help reduce the severity of menstrual cramps. In addition, chamomile seems to reduce tension that may lead to anxiety and irritability, and it is naturally caffeine free, making it an ideal choice to replace some of your favorite caffeinated beverages when your period is approaching.

## BONUS POINTS

◆ **Read Chapter 13: Mood (page 301).** All of the advice to exercise, eat regularly throughout the day, get the right mix of proteins and high-quality carbohydrates, and decrease stress applies to PMS, as well.

◆ **Get enough sleep.** Hormonal shifts can make some women lose sleep, which in turn may make them irritable. It is generally important to get enough sleep to level out moods. Premenstrually, sleep becomes crucial. Try your best to get seven to nine solid hours of z's per night. Many women even feel the need to nap during the premenstrual week, so if you can manage a few minutes of sleep in the middle of the day, indulge. It may make the difference between a good day and a day of snapping and tears.

## POWER THROUGH PMS WITH PUMPKIN SEEDS

When it comes to fighting PMS, pumpkin seeds have a lot to offer. A ¼-cup serving of roasted seed kernels provides 75 percent of the DV for magnesium and 85 percent of the DV for manganese. Both of these minerals have been shown to reduce PMS symptoms. Pumpkin seeds are also especially rich in iron, which can help replace iron-rich blood that's lost through monthly menstruation. Plus, they deliver a hearty dose of protein, fiber, zinc, and heart-healthy fat.

You can enjoy pumpkin seeds in two forms. Whole pumpkin seeds (like the ones you scrape out of your Halloween pumpkins) have a flat, white hull and are often sold roasted as a packaged snack food. You can eat them whole or crack open the shell first—like you would sunflower seeds—and eat just the kernel inside. You can also buy already shelled pumpkin seed kernels, which are small, flat, and dark green in color. Pumpkin seeds may also be labeled as pepitas on a package. ("Pepitas" usually refers to the hulled kernels, rather than the whole seeds.)

Whole pumpkin seeds are great for snacking, but the kernels are much more versatile. You can mix roasted pepitas into yogurt, cottage cheese, cereal, or oatmeal or make your own low-fat granola with pepitas in the mix. Sprinkle them on quick breads or muffins as a crunchy topper, or make pepita-crusted chicken or fish. Pepitas are also a terrific garnish for pureed soups like butternut squash. Try substituting pepitas and cilantro for pine nuts and basil in any classic pesto recipe to make a delicious Mexican variation.

## SUPPLEMENTS

If you experience PMS and want to consider supplements in addition to the food fixes, I have a few recommendations.

1.  **A multivitamin.** In order to ensure that you get all the nutrients important for mood and the physical symptoms of PMS, look for a multivitamin that contains 100 percent DV of manganese (2 milligrams), at least 25 percent DV of magnesium (100 milligrams or more), 100 percent DV of $B_6$, and at least 800 IU of vitamin $D_3$, all of which may help improve mood and reduce bloating. (The vitamin D is necessary to help the body absorb calcium.)

2.  **Calcium plus vitamin $D_3$ (and optional magnesium).** I always prefer that women get their calcium from food, but if you're not consistently consuming at least three daily servings of calcium-rich foods or beverages, you may want to consider taking a separate supplement. When buying supplements, remember that calcium is worthless without vitamin $D_3$, so make sure you're getting a total of at least 800 IU of vitamin $D_3$ through your multi and/or calcium supplement. Also consider choosing a brand with additional magnesium, especially if you're not regularly eating magnesium-rich foods. For more information

on the amount of calcium you should be taking in and various types of supplements, see page 233 in the Osteoporosis chapter.

3. **Chasteberry extract.** If the foods and nutritional supplements in this chapter aren't enough to calm your premenstrual symptoms, scientists have found that chasteberry extract may also help. Preliminary studies have found that this extract can help relieve mood swings, irritability, headaches, and breast tenderness in some women. Scientists believe that the benefits of chasteberry are due to flavonoids and other phytochemicals that seem to relieve stress and reduce inflammation. While the current research looks promising, it's still in the early stages, so we aren't yet able to draw firm conclusions about chasteberry for PMS. If you do decide to give chasteberry a try (with your physician's consent), the typical dosage is a 20-milligram tablet taken once or twice a day. *Important note:* If you experience headaches, gastrointestinal distress, or rashes from chasteberry extract, stop taking it. Chasteberry lowers prolactin levels, so it should not be used by women who are pregnant or nursing. Because of possible interactions, do not use chasteberry if you are also taking drugs or hormones that affect the pituitary gland, such as bromocriptine or a birth control pill.

For more information on food cures for PMS symptoms, visit www.joybauer.com/pms.

# JOY'S 4-STEP PROGRAM
## FOR PREMENSTRUAL SYNDROME

Follow this program if you are a woman who experiences moodiness, irritability, water retention, or any other symptoms of PMS at predictable times corresponding to your menstrual cycle.

## Step 1 ... START WITH THE BASICS

These are the first things you should do to take control of your PMS.

◆ Keep a mood diary to see whether your mood and physical symptoms are related to your menstrual cycle. If not, you probably don't have PMS.

◆ If your moods or physical symptoms are overly distressing or have caused problems in your life, see a doctor. There are prescription medications that can help you feel markedly better.

◆ Limit your intake of salty foods and caffeinated foods or beverages. Salt and caffeine can often aggravate premenstrual symptoms.

◆ Consider reading Chapter 13: Mood (page 301). Many of the recommendations there may also help PMS, particularly the information about getting sufficient exercise and leveling out your blood sugar.

## Step 2 ... YOUR ULTIMATE GROCERY LIST

A nutrition plan is only as good as the foods you choose. This list contains foods with high levels of nutrients that can help relieve PMS symptoms, including foods high in vitamin $B_6$, calcium, vitamin D, magnesium, and/or manganese. I've also added a variety of overall healthy foods to help round out your grocery list.

## FRUIT

*All* fruit, but especially:

Apricots

Bananas

Berries (especially raspberries and strawberries)

Pineapple

Watermelon

## VEGETABLES AND LEGUMES

*All* vegetables, but especially:

Artichokes

Avocados

Beans, starchy (such as black, garbanzo, kidney, navy, and pinto)

Bok choy

Broccoli

Broccoli raab

Brussels sprouts

Carrots

Collard greens

Kale

Lentils

Peppers, bell (green, red, and yellow)

Potatoes (sweet and white)

Soybeans (edamame)

Spinach

Squash, winter (acorn and butternut)

Swiss chard

## SEAFOOD

*All* fish and shellfish, but especially:

Herring

Mackerel (not king)

Salmon, wild (fresh and canned)

Sardines (fresh and canned)

Shrimp

## LEAN PROTEINS

Beef, lean

Chicken, ground (at least 90% lean)

Chicken, skinless

Eggs and egg substitutes

Pork tenderloin

Tempeh

Tofu

Turkey, ground (at least 90% lean)

Turkey, skinless

Turkey bacon

Turkey burgers, lean

Veggie burgers

## NUTS AND SEEDS (UNSALTED)

Almonds and almond butter

Butternuts (white walnuts)

Cashews and cashew butter

Flaxseed, ground

Hazelnuts

Macadamia nuts

Peanuts and peanut butter

Pecans

Pine nuts

Pistachios

Pumpkin seeds

Soy nuts

Sunflower seeds and sunflower butter

Walnuts

## WHOLE GRAINS

Amaranth

Barley

Bread, whole grain (buns, crackers, English muffins, pitas, tortillas, and wraps)

Bulgur

Cereal, whole grain

Millet

Oats

Pasta, whole grain

Quinoa

Rice (brown and wild)

Waffles, whole grain

Wheat germ

## DAIRY

Cheese (fat-free or reduced-fat)

Cottage cheese (fat-free or 1%)

Cream cheese (fat-free or reduced-fat)

Frozen yogurt

Ice cream, low-fat

Milk (fat-free or 1%)

Milk alternatives (almond, rice, and soy)

Ricotta cheese (part-skim)

Sour cream (fat-free or reduced-fat)

Yogurt (fat-free or low-fat)

## MISCELLANEOUS

Canola oil

Garlic

Herbs and spices (fresh, dried, and ground)

Hot sauce

Hummus

Marinara sauce

Mayonnaise, reduced-fat

Mustard (all varieties)

Olive oil

Salad dressing, reduced-calorie

Salsa

Soft tub spread, trans-fat-free (reduced-fat or regular)

Tea, chamomile

Vinegar (all varieties)

# Step 3 . . . GOING ABOVE AND BEYOND

If you want to do everything you can to reduce PMS symptoms, here are some additional things you might try.

◆ I strongly recommend taking a multivitamin with 100 percent DV of manganese, at least 25 percent DV of magnesium, 100 percent DV of vitamin $B_6$, and at least 800 IU of vitamin $D_3$.

◆ If you don't consistently eat at least three daily servings of calcium-rich foods, consider taking a separate calcium supplement with vitamin D. If you don't regularly consume magnesium-rich foods, buy a calcium supplement with added magnesium.

◆ Women with severe PMS symptoms may also want to try chasteberry extract. See the Supplements section, page 353, for more information.

◆ Aim for seven to nine hours of quality sleep per night.

## MAKE IT TO MENOPAUSE

I have good news and bad news when it comes to PMS. The good news is that it eventually ends. The bad news is that you'll have to go through menopause first, and women who are most bothered by the emotional symptoms of PMS may also have a rough time with menopause. In your forties, you may notice your PMS symptoms becoming erratic as your ovulation and periods become less predictable. If you experience more physical or emotional pain than usual as you head into your hot-flash years, talk with your doctor—there are lifestyle changes you can make and treatments you can pursue to help ease this transition.

# Step 4 . . . MEAL PLANS

The following meals are rich in nutrients that may ease PMS symptoms—calcium, vitamin D, magnesium, manganese, and vitamin $B_6$—and low in those foods that aggravate symptoms. Be sure to drink a lot of water with (and between) your meals. If you'd like, enjoy chamomile tea and calcium-rich drinks, such as fat-free, soy, and almond milks. (The calories for beverages are not included in the following sample days.)

Every day, choose one option for each of the three meals—breakfast, lunch, and dinner. Then, once or twice per day, choose from my suggested snacks. Approximate calories have been provided to help adjust for your personal weight-management goals. If you find yourself hungry (and if weight is not an issue), feel free to increase the portion sizes for meals and snacks.

## BREAKFAST OPTIONS

(300 TO 400 CALORIES)

### Whole Grain Cereal with Milk and Fruit

Mix 1 cup whole grain cereal with 1 cup milk (fat-free, 1%, or soy) and top with 1 cup raspberries (or enjoy with 1 cup pineapple on the side). Serve with chamomile tea.

### Oatmeal with Wheat Germ and Berries

Prepare ½ cup dry oats with 1 cup milk (fat-free, 1%, or soy) and top with 2 tablespoons wheat germ (or ground flaxseed) and ½ cup berries (sliced strawberries and/or raspberries). Sweeten with optional 1 teaspoon sugar, honey, maple syrup, or sugar substitute. Enjoy with chamomile tea.

### Broccoli-Cheese Egg-White Omelet with Toast

In a heated pan coated with oil spray, sauté 1 cup broccoli florets until soft. Beat 1 whole egg with 3 egg whites and pour around the broccoli. When the bottom is cooked, gently flip over. Top with 2 tablespoons shredded reduced-fat cheese. Fold the omelet over and cook until the cheese is melted and the egg mixture is firm. Season with ground black pepper and preferred salt-free seasonings. Enjoy with 1 slice whole grain bread (or 2 slices reduced-calorie bread, 50 calories or less per slice), toasted and topped with 1 to 2 teaspoons soft tub, trans-fat-free spread. Enjoy with chamomile tea.

### Strawberry-Banana Cottage Cheese with Sunflower Seeds

Mix 1 cup fat-free or 1% cottage cheese (or 6 ounces fat-free plain or flavored yogurt) with ½ sliced banana, ½ cup sliced strawberries, and 1 tablespoon sunflower seeds. Enjoy with chamomile tea.

### Peanut Butter Pita with Yogurt

Spread 1 whole wheat pita with 1 level tablespoon peanut or almond butter. Enjoy with 6 ounces fat-free plain or flavored yogurt and chamomile tea.

## LUNCH OPTIONS

(400 TO 500 CALORIES)

### Chicken-Spinach Sandwich with Broccoli

Layer 4 ounces grilled chicken breast and unlimited spinach leaves, tomato, and onion between 2 slices whole wheat bread (or in a pita). Add 1 optional tablespoon hummus, ketchup, barbecue sauce, or Dijon mustard. Serve with unlimited steamed broccoli or Swiss chard topped with 2 tablespoons grated Parmesan cheese.

### Veggie-Bean Burrito with Guacamole

Fill 1 whole grain tortilla (150 calories or less) with ½ cup black beans, unlimited steamed vegetables (preferably collard greens, Swiss chard, and/or chopped broccoli), 2 tablespoons shredded reduced-fat Cheddar cheese, and 2 tablespoons guacamole.

### Yogurt Fruit Fiesta

Mix a 6-ounce container of fat-free plain or vanilla yogurt (or 1 cup fat-free or 1% cottage cheese) with ½ cup pineapple, ½ chopped apple (or pear), and ½ sliced banana. Top with 2 tablespoons ground flaxseed and 2 tablespoons pumpkin or sunflower seeds.

### Turkey, Swiss, and Avocado Sandwich

Layer 4 ounces sliced turkey or chicken, 1 slice reduced-fat Swiss cheese, 2 slices avocado, and unlimited lettuce, tomato, and onion between 2 slices reduced-calorie whole wheat bread (50 calories or less per slice). Add 1 optional tablespoon of mustard, hummus, or reduced-fat mayonnaise. Enjoy with unlimited bell pepper strips (red, green, or yellow).

### Baked Potato with Broccoli and Cheese

Top 1 medium baked potato with unlimited cooked chopped broccoli, 1 ounce (¼ cup shredded) reduced-fat cheese (or ½ cup fat-free or 1% cottage cheese), and optional salsa. Enjoy with a large handful of baby carrots.

## DINNER OPTIONS

(500 TO 600 CALORIES)

### Turkey Chili with Brown Rice and Salad

Top 1 serving (2 cups) Turkey Chili (page 363) with 2 tablespoons shredded reduced-fat cheese. Serve with ½ cup cooked brown rice (or amaranth or quinoa) and a tossed salad of leafy greens and optional peppers, carrots, and artichokes tossed with 1 teaspoon olive oil and unlimited vinegar or fresh lemon juice (or 2 tablespoons reduced-calorie dressing).

### Grilled Salmon with Edamame and Greens

Enjoy 1 cup boiled edamame (green soybeans in the pod) with 5 ounces grilled wild salmon seasoned with 1 teaspoon olive oil, preferred herbs, and fresh lemon. Serve with unlimited steamed Swiss chard or spinach.

### Whole Wheat Penne with Chicken and Broccoli

Enjoy 1 serving Whole Wheat Penne with Chicken and Broccoli (page 364) with a side salad of leafy greens, tomatoes, peppers, and 1 tablespoon pumpkin seeds or chopped walnuts tossed with 1 teaspoon olive oil and unlimited vinegar or fresh lemon juice (or 2 tablespoons low-calorie dressing).

### Pork Tenderloin with Brussels Sprouts and Sweet Potato

Enjoy 5 ounces grilled, baked, or broiled lean pork tenderloin (or chicken breast) with unlimited steamed Brussels sprouts (or collard greens, spinach, broccoli, or kale) topped with optional 1 to 2 teaspoons soft tub, trans-fat-free spread and 1 medium plain baked sweet potato on the side.

### Sweet and Sour Tofu-Veggie Stir-Fry with Brown Rice

Enjoy 1 serving Sweet and Sour Tofu-Veggie Stir-Fry (page 245) with 1 cup cooked brown rice (or 1 medium baked sweet or white potato).

## SNACK OPTIONS

100 CALORIES OR LESS

- *Best Vegetable Snacks:* up to 2 cups raw or cooked broccoli, mushrooms, bell peppers, or carrots
- *Best Fruit Snacks:* 1 cup pineapple, raspberries, or sliced strawberries; 1 cup cubed watermelon; ½ banana; 4 apricots; 20 whole strawberries
- 1 string cheese (or 1 ounce any variety reduced-fat cheese)
- 1 cup fat-free milk
- Celery sticks with 1 level tablespoon almond or peanut butter
- 1 hard-cooked egg (or 4 hard-cooked egg whites)
- ½ cup fat-free or 1% cottage cheese

## 100 TO 200 CALORIES

- ◆ 6-ounce container of fat-free plain or flavored yogurt topped with 1 tablespoon pumpkin or sunflower seeds
- ◆ 10 raw almonds plus 1 serving fruit (see Best Fruit Snacks on page 361)
- ◆ ½ cup sunflower seeds or pistachios in the shell
- ◆ Whole nuts: 1 ounce (about ¼ cup) plain or toasted almonds, walnuts, pecans, peanuts, soy nuts, or cashews
- ◆ 1 level tablespoon almond or peanut butter on a mini whole wheat pita or 1 slice whole wheat bread
- ◆ Frozen banana: Peel one banana, slice into ½-inch wheels, place in a small plastic bag, and freeze before serving.
- ◆ ½ cup frozen yogurt or low-fat ice cream
- ◆ 1 cup low-fat hot cocoa with 1 serving fruit (see Best Fruit Snacks on page 361)
- ◆ 1 cup boiled edamame (green soybeans in the pod)
- ◆ Unlimited bell pepper strips (red, green, or yellow) with 2 heaping tablespoons guacamole or hummus
- ◆ ½ cup fat-free or 1% cottage cheese mixed with 1 cup raspberries (or sliced strawberries) and 1 tablespoon wheat germ
- ◆ 1 serving (2 cups) Tropical Mango-Citrus Smoothie (page 114)
- ◆ Berry smoothie: In a blender, mix ½ cup fat-free milk (or soy milk), ½ cup fat-free yogurt, ¾ cup fresh or frozen raspberries or 8 whole strawberries, and 3 to 5 ice cubes.

# Turkey Chili

*You won't miss the high-fat beef in this hearty, well-seasoned dish, which relies on extra-lean ground turkey and black beans for its thick, crowd-pleasing consistency. Plus, you'll receive a healthy dose of magnesium, manganese, and fiber. Freeze leftovers in a tightly covered container or store in the fridge for up to 3 days.*

**MAKES 8 SERVINGS (2 CUPS EACH)**

2 pounds ground turkey (at least 90% lean)

1 can (28 ounces) crushed tomatoes (preferably no-salt-added)

2 cups water

2 large onions, coarsely chopped

2 tablespoons chili powder

2 teaspoons garlic powder

1 teaspoon paprika

1 teaspoon black pepper

1 teaspoon cumin

1 teaspoon dried oregano

½ teaspoon ground red pepper (or more, if you prefer a spicier chili)

2 teaspoons whole wheat or all-purpose flour

2 cans (15 ounces each) black beans, rinsed and well drained

2 cups frozen corn kernels

Brown the turkey in a large pot over medium-high heat, stirring to break up the meat. Drain the fat. Add the tomatoes, water, onions, chili powder, garlic powder, paprika, black pepper, cumin, oregano, and red pepper. Mix thoroughly. Cover and simmer, stirring occasionally, for 25 to 30 minutes.

Stir in the flour and cook, stirring, for 2 minutes. Stir in the beans and corn and cook, uncovered and stirring occasionally, for 20 minutes.

**Per serving:** 269 calories, 34 g protein, 29 g carbohydrate, 2.5 g fat (1 g saturated), 45 mg cholesterol, 220 mg sodium, 8 g fiber; plus 59 mg magnesium (15% DV), 0.38 mg manganese (15% DV)

# Whole Wheat Penne with Chicken and Broccoli

*This low-cal, nutrient-rich pasta dish is a favorite dinner among all three of my kids (and believe me, that's a feat). Even better, one serving provides 30 percent of the DV for vitamin B$_6$, 43 percent of the DV for manganese, and 17 percent of the DV for magnesium. Plus, the cheese and broccoli supply a healthy hit of calcium. Enjoy it with a colorful tossed salad and you've got a nutritional powerhouse!*

**MAKES 8 SERVINGS (2 CUPS EACH)**

¼ cup extra-virgin olive oil

½ large onion, chopped

4 cloves garlic, minced

1 pound skinless, boneless chicken breast, cut into
　　1" cubes

8 cups broccoli florets

1 package whole wheat penne

½ teaspoon kosher salt

2 tablespoons grated Romano or Parmesan cheese

Ground black pepper

Bring a large pot of water to a rolling boil over high heat.

Meanwhile, heat the olive oil in a medium skillet over medium heat. Add the onion and garlic and cook, stirring, until translucent, being careful not to let the onion brown. Add the chicken and cook, stirring, until no longer pink throughout. Remove from the heat and set aside.

Once the water boils, add the broccoli and cook for about 4 minutes, or until firm yet tender. Using a slotted spoon or skimmer, transfer the broccoli to the skillet with the reserved chicken. Cook until the broccoli is soft.

Return the large pot of salted water to a boil and add the pasta. Cook for about 8 minutes, or until al dente. Drain the pasta, reserving 1 cup of pasta water. Add the pasta, reserved water, and salt to the broccoli mixture and toss to mix. Add the cheese and mix again. Serve immediately on individual dishes and season with black pepper to taste.

**Per serving:** 378 calories, 23 g protein, 51 g carbohydrate, 9 g fat (1.5 g saturated), 34 mg cholesterol, 231 mg sodium, 8 g fiber; plus 6 mg vitamin B$_6$ (30% DV), 1 mg manganese (43% DV), 65 mg magnesium (17% DV)

# CHAPTER 16

# INSOMNIA

Catherine is 47 and for most of her life has been what she calls a champion sleeper. Once, when Catherine was 12 years old, her younger sister got sick and passed out in the middle of the night. An ambulance came to the house, accompanied by two police cars and a fire engine. Even though neighbors heard the ruckus and came out on their lawns to see what was happening, Catherine, as you may have already guessed, slept through the entire incident. Thirty-five years later, her family members still tell the story with genuine astonishment that anyone could sleep so soundly.

Catherine lost her supersleeper status after complex shoulder surgery two years ago. For eight weeks after surgery, she had to spend her nights sitting bolt upright on the couch, and for another eight weeks after that, she could only lean back on a huge pile of pillows—no lying down. For those four months, the pain was so bad that she barely slept—three solid hours of sleep was a good night. Months later, after she was done with physical therapy, she could lie down flat on the bed, but she still didn't sleep well. She says that it felt as though her body had forgotten how to sleep. No matter what time she turned in, no matter how many hours she had been awake or how tired she was, she couldn't seem to sleep for longer than four hours. Even the smallest sound would awaken her, and then she was up for the rest of the night. She mourned the loss of her sleep as though she had lost a close friend.

Catherine's sister Joanna has a different problem. As a busy stay-at-home mom, Joanna had always managed to carve out time to relax in those precious hours between her daughters' bedtime and her own. Joanna stuck to her routine as the girls grew; the only problem was that their bedtime got later and later. Preserving those few hours of private time meant staying up until 2:00 a.m. In a way, it's not a problem for her; she has no trouble staying awake and no trouble falling asleep once she goes to bed. She gets up at 6:00 a.m. to get the girls off to school and then settles in for a two-hour nap at 9:00 a.m. Now Joanna has decided to resume her career, but she can't seem to break her night owl ways. She doesn't want to apply for jobs until she knows that she can maintain a "normal" schedule, but she has been unsuccessful so far. Now she's wondering if she might have to take shift work.

Catherine and Joanna's father, Harry, is in his eighties. His insomnia has gotten steadily worse over the past decade, and he blames it on getting older. He has no trouble falling asleep, but staying asleep is a problem. No matter what time he goes to bed, he always wakes up between 3:00 and 4:00 a.m. and can't get back to sleep. He stays wide awake until about noon, but then he feels exhausted. By evening, when friends and family can schedule time to get together, he's too tired to enjoy their company. He feels like he is missing half his life.

One family, three distinct sleep problems. Sadly, this family's problems are not unusual. Experts at the National Institutes of Health estimate that around 70 million Americans experience sleep problems, and about half of those problems can be considered chronic. Insomnia is more than frustrating—it can be downright dangerous. Excess sleepiness increases everyone's risk of injury from accidents. And lack of sleep can weaken the immune system, raising your chances of developing everything from a common cold to type 2 diabetes. Of course, long-term disease prospects are no help when you are lying in bed in the dark, wide awake, with no hope of sleep. It is hard not to feel like you are the only person on earth staring at the ceiling. It's lonely and depressing—and unnecessary. Nutrition has solutions for many different cases and types of insomnia.

## WHAT AFFECTS YOUR ABILITY TO SLEEP?

Insomnia has many different faces. It can mean difficulty falling asleep, frequent waking throughout the night, or waking up too early in the morning. (But just because you don't sleep much doesn't necessarily mean you have a problem. Many people feel that three or four hours of sleep each night are sufficient. They are happy to have more time in their day and do not have insomnia.)

Just about everyone has difficulty sleeping once in a while, particularly in times of stress, during travel, or if the room they're sleeping in is too hot, cold, noisy, or bright. These types of short-term insomnia are annoying and can certainly affect the way you function the next day, but they are often easily remedied.

Temporary insomnia can also be caused by certain medications, including bronchodilators, pseudoephedrine (found in some over-the-counter cold medicines), antipsychotic medications, beta-blockers, calcium channel blockers, most antidepressants, and many, many others. If your insomnia started within two weeks of beginning a new medication, talk with your doctor about whether there is a different medication or dose that might work better for you.

If insomnia occurs at least three nights a week for a month or longer, it is considered chronic. At this point, lack of sleep becomes more than just an annoyance—it can be life altering. Almost all cases of chronic insomnia can be traced to a medical condition, lifestyle habit, or psychological preoccupation. Let's take a closer look at all three.

## MEDICAL CONDITIONS

Conventional wisdom once had it that insomnia was age related and you could reasonably expect your sleep habits to change after age 60. That's no longer considered true. Although people do seem to have more difficulty sleeping as they get older, the underlying reason is usually medical. In other words, insomnia is not an inescapable companion of aging. For example, we know that sleep can worsen in people who have depression, gastroesophageal reflux disease (GERD), sleep apnea, restless legs syndrome, arthritis, kidney or heart disease, osteoporosis, cancer, or Parkinson's disease—most of which occur in older age. Those disorders can affect neuron function and cause pain, interfere with breathing, or trigger major muscle movements—all of which can lead to sleeplessness. It is important to have all new cases of insomnia checked out by a doctor to rule out the possibility of a physical disorder.

Remember Harry, Catherine and Joanna's dad, who thought that his ten-year problem with insomnia was due to old age? It turned out that he had Parkinson's disease. Three months after starting medication for the disorder, he was surprised to find that his insomnia had disappeared. Now, he regularly sleeps until 7:00 a.m. (or later!), and he has more energy later in the day. But really, curing Harry's insomnia was just a side benefit—he was finally getting help for a disease that had gone untreated for years.

## LIFESTYLE FACTORS

Everything that affects the rhythms of your life can affect your sleep pattern: the long work hours leading up to a deadline, a new exercise routine, a suddenly busy travel schedule. For example, when people retire,

**FAQS**

**When I drink coffee, I drink only decaf, but on the nights I have a cup, I notice I have a hard time falling asleep. My friend told me that even decaffeinated coffees and teas contain small amounts of caffeine. Is that true? Do I need to stop drinking hot beverages at night?**

The teeny-tiny amount of caffeine in decaffeinated drinks is so inconsequential (generally less than 5 milligrams per cup, compared with more than 100 milligrams in regular coffee) that it really shouldn't affect your sleep. There are a couple of reasons why your beverages might keep you awake. First, if you order decaf coffee at a restaurant, you may not be drinking real decaf. It is a sad fact that some restaurants accidentally serve full-caffeine coffee when they think they're serving decaf. Even the color of the pot or the label on the tureen may be misleading. If caffeine is a real problem for you, I recommend you avoid coffee altogether when you eat out. Instead, order decaffeinated or herbal tea, and examine the tag to confirm that you received what you asked for. Your sleeplessness could also be psychological—maybe you are worried about being kept awake, or you are revved up from your evening's activities. If there is any lingering doubt, switch to herbal tea, which naturally contains no caffeine.

## FAQS

**I've been waking up with cookie crumbs in my pajamas and a mess in my kitchen. I think I'm getting up and eating at night, but I don't remember any of it. Is this possible?**

Yes, it is possible, and it's more common than you might think. There are several different reasons why this happens. If you are on a very restrictive weight-loss diet, your body may be doing what comes naturally—seeking the food it desperately wants. If this sounds like you, I recommend eating one of my bedtime snacks to make sure that you don't get hungry in the middle of the night.

Or maybe you eat enough during the day but are "overly preoccupied" with food, even while you sleep. I've had some clients who were forced to put padlocks on the kitchen cabinets and notes around the house reminding them to "Wake up" and "Do not eat!" In this case, I also recommend that you see a psychologist or psychiatrist who specializes in this area. Many times, sleep eating is a sign of an eating disorder of some sort. It's always better to have these kinds of extreme behaviors checked out by a professional.

they may sleep later or feel less stress than they did when they (or their spouses) were still working. These changes help some people sleep better, but others develop insomnia. It may take a while for the new lifestyle to become routine and for new habits to assert themselves. Until then, sleeplessness can be a real problem.

Some lifestyle choices have an immediate effect on sleep. For example, caffeine and nicotine are common causes of insomnia because they can activate the brain. So if you need yet another good reason to quit smoking, do it to improve your sleep.

## PSYCHOLOGICAL FACTORS

Mental preoccupation can have devastating effects on sleep. We all know that worrying over a plague-ridden work project can wreck a night's sleep. Imagine if those feelings lasted for years. A friend of a friend, a lovely man who had been the comedian of his suburban neighborhood, lost his 10-year-old daughter to a car accident. He started down a spiral of insomnia that continues to this day, many years later. He is not clinically depressed, but he is chronically sad, and he just doesn't sleep.

I wish he would see a doctor. All of his friends and family are encouraging him to do so. If you have experienced long-term insomnia, I encourage you to speak with your primary care physician and/or consult with a sleep specialist, no matter what you think the cause is. Help is available.

## HOW FOOD AFFECTS SLEEP

Combating insomnia through nutrition is about eating the right combination of foods in the evening, and—perhaps even more important—knowing which foods to avoid.

## WHAT TO EAT FOR A GOOD NIGHT'S SLEEP

Among the best natural sedatives is tryptophan, an amino acid component of many plant and animal proteins. Tryptophan is one of the ingredients necessary for the body to make serotonin, the neurotransmitter best known for creating feelings of calm and making you sleepy. A 2005 study of people with chronic insomnia found that diet made a big difference. After three weeks, those who ate foods with high amounts of tryptophan in combination with carbohydrates or who took pharmaceutical-grade tryptophan supplements had improvements on all measures of sleep—and food sources worked just as well as the supplements.

The trick is to combine foods that have some tryptophan with foods containing ample carbohydrates. In order for insomnia-busting tryptophan to work, it has to make its way to the brain. When you eat carbs, they trigger the release of insulin, which transports competing amino acids into muscle tissue but leaves tryptophan alone, so it can make its way to the brain.

BEST LOW-PROTEIN/HIGH-CARB FOODS FOR SEROTONIN PRODUCTION:
*whole grain breads, crackers, and cereal; whole wheat pasta; brown and wild rice; oats; fruits, especially mangoes, bananas, grapes, papayas, oranges, grapefruit, and plums; vegetables, especially spinach, yams, sweet and white potatoes, corn, winter squash (acorn, butternut), green peas, broccoli, Brussels sprouts, kale, asparagus, cauliflower, sugar snap peas, pumpkin, celery, and beets; milk (fat-free, 1%), yogurt (fat-free, low-fat), frozen yogurt, low-fat ice cream*

## WHAT NOT TO EAT OR DRINK BEFORE BED
### Caffeine

It seems obvious, but you'd be surprised how many caffeine junkies come into my practice complaining of sleep problems! People with troubled sleep should avoid caffeinated drinks and foods—coffee, tea, many sodas, and chocolate—for several hours before bed. Caffeine is a natural chemical that activates the central nervous system, which means that it revs up nerves and thought processes. If you drink anything containing caffeine too close to bedtime, chances are it will keep you awake. Of course, what "too close" means varies from person to person. Sensitive people should stop drinking caffeine at least eight hours before bedtime (that means by 3:00 p.m. if you hit the sack at 11:00 p.m.). You can play with your particular timing, but don't experiment on a night when you're counting on getting a good night's rest.

### Alcohol

It's true that a drink (or two) can make you sleepy and may help you get to sleep. But after a few hours, alcohol can cause frequent awakenings and lighter, less restful sleep. I'm not saying you need to give up alcohol, but don't use it like a sleeping pill. And if you have insomnia, I strongly recommend giving up alcohol for a few weeks to see if your sleep problem resolves.

## Large Meals

Eating a huge dinner or even a large before-bedtime snack may make you feel drowsy, but the sleep won't necessarily take. When you lie down and try to sleep, there's a good chance you'll feel uncomfortably full, which can keep you awake. Even worse, you may develop heartburn or gas, which will only increase your discomfort. I recommend eating a dinner of no more than 600 calories (optimally, at least three hours before bed). The good news: All the dinner meal plans in this book weigh in at 600 calories or less.

## Liquids

The single best piece of advice I can give to someone who wakes up in the middle of the night to visit the bathroom is to not drink water or fluids within 90 minutes of bedtime. It takes that long for your body to process liquid of any type. If you must have something to drink—for example, to take a prescribed medication—take a small sip. If the medication requires a full glass of water, take it earlier in the evening, if possible.

## BONUS POINTS

- **Make the room you sleep in comfortable and peaceful.** If your bedroom is a place of distraction and chaos, it will be that much more difficult for you to fall asleep. Remove the alarm clock from sight; instead, put it under the bed or in a drawer. Adjust the room temperature for your comfort—for most people, that's between 65° and 70°F—and make sure you have comfortable pillows and enough blankets. Hang blackout curtains or wear an eye mask if you are easily awakened by light.

- **Add white noise.** For many people, noise that is steady and not easily identifiable is easier to tune out than the sound of snoring, the rumble of traffic, or the musical stylings of the amateur trumpet player who lives next door. For others, total silence is disturbing. White noise machines emit a steady whirring or purring sound, similar to the sound of wind rustling through leaves, which provides a welcome distraction for both these problems.

- **Practice good sleep habits.** Sleeping well is often about establishing the right habits. Our bodies can become programmed to respond to various cues in our environment—think of how the smell of your favorite dinner can make your mouth water or how Sunday night can throw some people into a panic at the thought of returning to work on Monday morning. It's the same way with sleep.

If your bed has become a place of tension from an extended bout of insomnia (or even just worrying about insomnia), then you have to work that much harder to associate your bed with sleep again. First, get a different perspective and a fresh start on new habits by making the bedroom less familiar: Move the furniture around, buy a new set of bedding, or repaint the walls. Second, try to stick with a regular schedule of going to bed and waking up, even on the weekends. That way, your body will learn to associate certain times of day with a particular part of your sleep rhythm. Third, avoid using the bedroom for anything except sleeping and sex—no reading, no television, and definitely no eating. Finally, don't let insomnia back into the bedroom. If you are unable to fall asleep within about 20 minutes of when your head hits the pillow, get up, go to another room, and do something relaxing. Return to bed only when you feel sleepy again.

- **Eliminate naps.** People with insomnia often resort to afternoon naps to catch up on their missed sleep, but that's a mistake. Napping encourages insomnia because you'll be less likely to be tired at bedtime if you sleep during the day. It can also become a counterproductive habit. Fight the urge, but if you must nap, don't sleep for more than 20 minutes. After a day or two, your body will learn that the proper time for sleep is when you lie down in bed at the end of a day.

- **Make a to-do list.** People tend to lie awake in bed, angst-ridden over all the things they need to get done. Before you go to bed each night, draft a list of everything you need to do the next day. Getting it down on paper helps get it out of your mind.

- **Relax.** You can't run a crazy life and expect to just unplug your mind when you slip into bed. Sleep requires relaxation of mind and body. Try to take 30 minutes at the end of each day to unwind: meditate, read, do yoga, take a hot shower or candlelit bath—anything that helps you put worries away for the next eight hours.

- **Exercise regularly, early in the day.** Some scientists believe that regular exercise may be the single best and safest method for improving sleep. Exercise forces the body to work harder than usual, which means that we generally need more sleep to recuperate from the physical exertion, and it also increases the body's production of endorphins and other hormones that lead to feelings of calm and well-being. However, if you are struggling with insomnia, don't exercise vigorously right before bedtime—you may ramp up your energy and have trouble falling asleep. Calming routines like stretching or yoga are fine anytime of day.

- **Don't rely on sleeping pills.** Only you and your doctor can determine if sleep medication is a good option for you. For occasional use, medications can be helpful, but they are not magic. It is always better to try to fix the underlying problem.

## SUPPLEMENTS

If you are plagued by insomnia and want to consider supplements, two have been studied scientifically and shown to have beneficial effects.

1. **Valerian.** This herb has been used as a sedative for hundreds of years. Like sleep medications known as benzodiazepines (which include Xanax, Valium, Librium, and Ativan), valerian seems to enhance the action of the neurotransmitter GABA (gamma-aminobutyric acid), which acts to calm us down and make us sleepy. Studies examining the effectiveness of valerian as a sleep aid have been mixed—some studies show no benefit, while others show improvements in certain measures of sleep quality. If you'd like to give valerian a shot, look for an extract standardized to contain 0.4 to 0.6 percent of valerenic acid. Take 400 to 900 milligrams per day, two hours before bedtime. Although valerian has been well researched for safety, it shouldn't be taken for longer than 30 days. Common side effects include headache, itchiness, dizziness, and gastrointestinal distress. You should not take valerian if you are pregnant or nursing or if you are also taking a prescription sedative. Although valerian has not been shown to have any significant interactions with medications, it is always best to talk with your doctor before beginning any herbal supplement.

2. **Melatonin.** This neurohormone has long been linked to sleep. Research shows that people with some forms of insomnia have lower-than-normal levels of melatonin. Reviews of the medical literature suggest that taking melatonin may help some people with insomnia—especially the elderly and so-called night owls who naturally have a hard time falling asleep before 2:00 a.m. Melatonin seems to be safe if taken for only a month or two. The most common side effects are nausea, headache, and dizziness. If you want to try melatonin, the recommended dosage is 3 to 5 milligrams per day taken 30 to 60 minutes prior to bedtime. (When buying supplements, remember that 1 milligram = 1,000 micrograms.) If you have trouble falling asleep, use an immediate-release form; if you have trouble staying asleep, use a sustained-release form. You may need to take it for several days before you see any results. If you don't see results after two weeks, chances are it won't work for you at all.

For more information on foods that promote restful sleep, visit www.joybauer.com/insomnia.

# JOY'S 4-STEP PROGRAM
## FOR INSOMNIA

Follow this program if you have trouble falling asleep or staying asleep for at least three nights a week two weeks in a row.

## Step 1 ... START WITH THE BASICS

These are the first things you should do to improve your chances of a good night's sleep.

- ◆ If you have had insomnia for a month or longer, see your doctor to rule out a medical cause.
- ◆ Stop drinking caffeinated beverages after 3:00 p.m. (or at least eight hours before bedtime).
- ◆ If you're struggling with fragmented sleep, avoid drinking alcohol.
- ◆ To avoid having to get up to use the bathroom in the middle of the night, don't drink any beverages within 90 minutes of going to bed.
- ◆ Avoid heavy dinners, especially within three hours of going to bed.

## Step 2 ... YOUR ULTIMATE GROCERY LIST

This list contains the types of foods that help promote sleep, including those with high-quality carbohydrates and tryptophan. Foods marked with an asterisk (*) are the best sleep-inducing foods.

### FRUIT

| | | |
|---|---|---|
| *All* fruits, but especially: | *Grapefruit | *Papayas |
| Apples | *Grapes | *Plums |
| *Bananas | Lemons | Watermelon |
| Berries | *Mangoes | |
| Cantaloupe | *Oranges | |

## VEGETABLES AND LEGUMES

*All* vegetables, but
   especially:

*Asparagus

*Beets

*Broccoli

*Brussels sprouts

Carrots

*Cauliflower

*Celery

*Corn

Cucumbers

*Dark leafy greens (such as
   beet, collard, dandelion,
   kale, mustard, Swiss
   chard, and turnip)

Lettuce

Onion

*Peas, green

Peppers, bell (green, red,
   and yellow)

*Potatoes (sweet and white)

*Pumpkin

*Spinach

*Squash, winter (acorn and
   butternut)

Sugar snap peas

Tomatoes

## LEAN PROTEINS

Beef, lean

Chicken, ground (at least
   90% lean)

Chicken, skinless

Eggs and egg substitutes

Pork tenderloin

Tempeh

Tofu

Turkey, ground (at least
   90% lean)

Turkey, skinless

Turkey bacon

Turkey burgers, lean

Veggie burgers

## NUTS AND SEEDS (PREFERABLY UNSALTED)

Almonds and almond butter

Butternuts (white walnuts)

Cashews and cashew butter

Hazelnuts

Macadamia nuts

Peanuts and peanut butter

Pecans

Pine nuts

Pistachios

Pumpkin seeds

Sesame seeds

Sunflower seeds and
   sunflower butter

Walnuts

## WHOLE GRAINS

*Bread, whole grain (buns,
   crackers, English muffins,
   pitas, tortillas, and wraps)

*Bulgur

*Cereals, whole grain

*Oats

*Pasta, whole grain

*Quinoa

*Rice (brown and wild)

*Waffles, whole grain

*Wheat germ

## DAIRY

Cheese (fat-free or reduced-fat)

Cottage cheese (fat-free or 1%)

*Frozen yogurt (avoid coffee and chocolate flavors if consuming in evening)

*Ice cream, low-fat (avoid coffee and chocolate flavors if consuming in evening)

*Milk (fat-free or 1%)

Milk alternatives (almond, rice, and soy)

Pudding, low-fat (avoid coffee and chocolate flavors if consuming in evening)

*Yogurt (fat-free or low-fat)

## MISCELLANEOUS

Canola oil

Garlic

Herbs and spices (fresh, dried, and ground)

Hot sauce

Hummus

Marinara sauce

Mayonnaise, reduced-fat

Mustard (all varieties)

Olive oil

Salad dressing, reduced-calorie

Salsa

Vinegar (all varieties)

* Best sleep-inducing foods

# Step3 ... GOING ABOVE AND BEYOND

For a dreamy night's sleep, here are some additional things you might try.

◆ Talk with your doctor about whether you are a good candidate for taking valerian or melatonin supplements.

◆ Restructure your evening schedule and habits to be more conducive to sleep. Take some quiet time to relax, try to turn in at the same time each night, and make the bedroom a place for sleep (and sex) only.

◆ Try a white noise machine to block out distracting ambient sounds.

◆ Make a to-do list before going to bed each night.

◆ Exercise regularly.

## LAVENDER POWER

Generations ago, people put lavender sprigs in the bedroom to encourage a good night's sleep. Now it seems there is science behind the practice. Some research suggests that aromatherapy with essence of lavender calms the nervous system, allowing us to relax and fall asleep more easily. There are many different ways to use lavender to treat insomnia. The most potent is to receive a massage with essential oil or use an aromatherapy diffuser. Alternatively, try aromatic bath oils, lotions, soaps, air sprays, and sachets that include lavender oil. You can find a wide variety of products at health food stores and bath and body shops. I'm pretty sure lavender won't solve all of your sleep issues, but there's certainly no downside—and you and your house will smell divine!

# **Step 4** . . . MEAL PLANS

These sample menus include foods that may help you sleep better. You'll notice that protein is generously spread out between breakfast and lunch and then dramatically reduced at dinner. That's because in order to maximize serotonin production and induce sleepiness, your dinner and bedtime snacks should optimally be low in protein and high in carbohydrates (with foods that contain some tryptophan).

Every day, choose one option for each of the three meals—breakfast, lunch, and dinner. Between lunch and dinner, you may have one small healthy snack of your choosing (consider fresh fruit or vegetables, a handful of nuts, or a nonfat yogurt). Then, before bed each night, choose one option from my suggested bedtime snacks (see page 379). Approximate calories have been provided to help adjust for your personal weight-management goals. If you find yourself hungry (and if weight is not an issue), feel free to increase the portion sizes for meals and snacks. Beverage calories are not included.

## BREAKFAST OPTIONS

(300 TO 400 CALORIES)

### Hard-Cooked Eggs with Turkey Bacon and Fruit

Enjoy 2 whole hard-cooked eggs and 2 hard-cooked egg whites with 2 strips turkey bacon and 1 cup berries (or ½ grapefruit or ¼ cantaloupe).

### Cottage Cheese with Cantaloupe and Almonds

Fill ½ cantaloupe with 1 cup fat-free or 1% cottage cheese (or fat-free flavored yogurt) and top with 1 tablespoon slivered almonds.

### Scrambled Eggs with Vegetables and English Muffin

Beat 1 whole egg with 3 egg whites. Cook scrambled eggs in a skillet coated with oil spray, adding your preferred vegetables (onion, red and green peppers, or tomato sautéed in oil spray). Enjoy with 1 dry toasted whole grain English muffin.

### Whole Grain Cereal with Milk and Breakfast Sausage

Mix 1 cup whole grain cereal with 1 cup fat-free milk and enjoy with 1 lean poultry or sausage (120 calories or less) or 2 slices Canadian bacon.

### Toast with Cream Cheese, Tomato, Onion, and Lox

Top 2 toasted slices whole wheat bread with 1 tablespoon reduced-fat cream cheese, sliced tomato and onion, and 1 to 2 ounces smoked salmon.

## LUNCH OPTIONS

(400 TO 500 CALORIES)

### Turkey and Cheese Sandwich with Crunchy Carrots and Peppers

Layer 4 or 5 ounces turkey (or lean roast beef or grilled chicken), lettuce, sliced tomato, and onion between 2 slices whole grain bread or in a pita. Add optional 1 slice reduced-fat cheese, mustard, and 2 teaspoons reduced-fat mayonnaise or hummus. Enjoy with a large handful of baby carrots and green or red pepper strips.

### Grilled Chicken-Vegetable Salad

Serve 5 ounces skinless grilled chicken breast on a large bed of leafy greens with ½ cup cherry tomatoes, unlimited sliced cucumbers, chopped carrots, chopped bell pepper (red, green, or yellow), and artichoke hearts. Toss with 2 teaspoons olive oil and unlimited vinegar or fresh lemon juice (or 2 to 4 tablespoons low-calorie dressing).

### Turkey Burger with Veggies

Enjoy a 5-ounce lean turkey burger on ½ whole grain bun (or in a 70-calorie pita pocket) with unlimited steamed vegetables (broccoli, cauliflower, or spinach) topped with optional 1 tablespoon grated Parmesan cheese.

### Vegetable Tuna Salad with Whole Grain Pita

Enjoy Veggie Tuna Salad (page 271) with a whole grain pita or 150 calories' worth of whole grain crackers plus ¼ cantaloupe (or 1 cup watermelon or mixed berries).

### Turkey Chili with Mixed Green Salad

Top 1 serving (2 cups) Turkey Chili (page 363) or 2 cups prepared turkey or vegetarian chili with 1 ounce (¼ cup) shredded reduced-fat cheese. Enjoy with a tossed salad (leafy greens and other preferred vegetables) with 1 teaspoon olive oil and unlimited vinegar or fresh lemon juice (or 2 to 4 tablespoons low-calorie dressing).

## DINNER OPTIONS

(500 TO 600 CALORIES)

### Pasta with Roasted Pumpkin and Salad

Enjoy 1 serving Angel Hair Pasta with Roasted Pumpkin, Sage, and Walnuts (page 381) with a leafy green salad tossed with 2 teaspoons olive oil and unlimited vinegar or fresh lemon juice (or 2 to 4 tablespoons low-calorie dressing).

### Parmesan Couscous and Ratatouille with Olives, Tomatoes, and Fresh Basil

Enjoy 1 serving (page 383).

### Apple-Cinnamon Oatmeal for Dinner

Prepare 1 cup dry oats with 1 cup fat-free milk and 1 cup water (microwave for 1½ to 2 minutes). Mix with 1 chopped apple and microwave for an additional 30 to 60 seconds. Sprinkle with optional cinnamon and 1 teaspoon sugar or honey (or sugar substitute).

### Sweet Potato–Cauliflower Mash with Warm Turkey Bacon–Spinach Salad

Enjoy 1 serving Sweet Potato–Cauliflower Mash (page 382) with Warm Turkey Bacon–Spinach Salad (page 380) and 1 plain toasted whole wheat pita or 2 servings Tangy Pita Chips (page 384).

### Baked Potato with Broccoli and Cheese

Top 1 baked white potato with unlimited cooked chopped broccoli and 1 ounce (¼ cup shredded or 1 slice) melted reduced-fat cheese. Serve with 2 servings (2 cups) Vegetable Oatmeal Bisque (page 322) or 2 cups of any prepared vegetable soup.

## BEDTIME SNACK OPTIONS

*(SEROTONIN-PRODUCING)*
100 CALORIES OR LESS

- ◆ *Best Vegetable Snacks:* up to 2 cups raw or cooked broccoli, Brussels sprouts, asparagus, cauliflower, sugar snap peas, celery
- ◆ *Best Fruit Snacks:* 1 cup grapes (plain or frozen), 1 orange, 1 plum, ½ grapefruit, ½ banana, ½ mango, ½ papaya
- ◆ Tangy Pita Chips (page 384) with salsa
- ◆ 1 cup fat-free milk
- ◆ 6 ounces fat-free flavored yogurt

100 TO 200 CALORIES

- ◆ Banana-Mango Parfait (page 385)
- ◆ Cinnamon Oatmeal: Prepare ½ cup dry oats with ½ cup fat-free milk and ½ cup water, and sprinkle with cinnamon and optional 1 teaspoon sugar or sugar substitute.
- ◆ Frozen banana: Peel one banana, slice into ½-inch wheels, place in a small plastic bag, and freeze before serving.

- 1 slice whole wheat toast topped with sliced tomato and 1 slice reduced-fat cheese

- 1 banana with 1 level teaspoon peanut butter

- 1 cup fat-free milk with 1 orange (or 1 cup grapes, 1 plum, ½ grapefruit, ½ banana, ½ mango, or ½ papaya)

- ½ cup frozen yogurt or low-fat ice cream (avoid coffee and chocolate flavors if consuming in the evening)

- 1 low-fat ice cream pop (avoid coffee and chocolate flavors if consuming in the evening)

- ½ cup low-fat pudding (avoid coffee and chocolate flavors if consuming in the evening)

- ¾ cup whole grain cereal with 1 cup fat-free milk

- ½ baked sweet or white potato with optional 1 tablespoon grated Parmesan cheese

- 4 cups light or air-popped popcorn with 1 to 2 tablespoons grated Parmesan cheese

# WARM TURKEY BACON–SPINACH SALAD

*This simple dish is a nice change from your typical "garden variety" salad and a great addition to any main entrée. The warm, flavorful dressing adds plenty of zing, and the walnuts provide delicious crunch.*

8 cups baby spinach

4 slices turkey bacon

1 tablespoon olive oil

1 small shallot, thinly sliced

¼ cup low-sodium chicken or vegetable broth, heated

2 tablespoons vinegar, sherry or balsamic

½ teaspoon Dijon mustard

2 tablespoons toasted walnuts

Kosher salt

Ground black pepper

Place the spinach in a large bowl or divide evenly between two large plates. In a medium skillet over medium-high heat, cook the turkey bacon for 3 to 4 minutes, or until crisp and browned. Crumble and sprinkle over the spinach. In the same skillet, heat the oil over medium-low heat. Add the shallot and cook, stirring, for 1 to 2 minutes, or until softened. Add the broth, vinegar, and mustard and cook, stirring, until the mixture forms a dressing. Immediately pour over the salad. Top with the walnuts. Season to taste with salt and pepper.

**Per serving:** 200 calories, 7 g protein, 4 g carbohydrate, 17 g fat (3 g saturated), 30 mg cholesterol, 450 mg sodium, 6 g fiber

# ANGEL HAIR PASTA WITH ROASTED PUMPKIN, SAGE, AND WALNUTS

*If you love pasta but you're tired of eating the same old spaghetti with tomato sauce, definitely try this recipe. The unique combination of roasted pumpkin, walnuts, and sage creates a colorful and delicious dish.*

**MAKES 3 SERVINGS (2 CUPS PER SERVING)**

1 pound fresh pumpkin (or butternut squash), cut into ½" cubes (about 2 cups)

Kosher salt

1 package (8 ounces) whole wheat angel hair pasta

1 tablespoon olive oil

¼ cup fresh sage leaves, finely sliced

2 tablespoons walnuts, chopped

½ cup fat-free ricotta cheese, at room temperature

½ cup low-sodium chicken or vegetable broth, heated

Ground black pepper

Preheat the oven to 425°F. Cover a large baking sheet with parchment paper or aluminum foil and coat with oil spray.

Arrange the pumpkin cubes on the prepared baking sheet in a single layer so they are not touching. Coat the pumpkin with oil spray and sprinkle with salt. Roast for 15 to 20 minutes, or until the pumpkin has softened and begins to take on a gold color.

Cook the pasta according to package instructions. Drain, reserving 1½ cups of the cooking water.

Coat a large skillet with oil spray. Add the oil and heat over high heat. Add the sage and cook, stirring, for 1 to 2 minutes, or until the sage turns dark green (but not brown) and becomes crispy. Reduce the heat to low and add the pumpkin, pasta, walnuts, ricotta, broth, and 1 cup of the reserved cooking water. Stir to coat the pasta. Season with additional salt and black pepper. If the pasta is too dry, add more of the cooking water. Serve immediately.

**Per serving:** 388 calories, 18 g protein, 60 g carbohydrate, 10 g fat (1 g saturated), 10 mg cholesterol, 200 mg sodium, 13 g fiber

# SWEET POTATO–CAULIFLOWER MASH

*My low-cal mashed potatoes were accidentally created one night when I didn't have enough sweet potatoes and used leftover cauliflower to beef up mashed sweet potatoes. Clearly, it was an accident meant to happen: only 122 calories in 1½ cups, yet loaded with nutrition and fiber. Enjoy the mash with any meal you prepare, or couple with the Warm Turkey Bacon–Spinach Salad on page 380.*

**MAKES 2 SERVINGS**

1 large sweet potato (½ pound), peeled and cubed

¼ head cauliflower, cut into florets (about 1 cup)

½ cup low-sodium chicken or vegetable broth, heated

2 tablespoons fat-free sour cream

1 clove garlic, minced

¼ teaspoon freshly grated nutmeg

Kosher salt

Ground black pepper

1 scallion, minced

Steam the sweet potato and cauliflower over 1" of water for 9 to 10 minutes, or until fork-tender. In a large bowl, mash the potato and cauliflower with the broth. Stir in the sour cream, garlic, and nutmeg. Season to taste with salt and black pepper. Garnish each serving with some of the scallion. Makes 3 cups.

**Per serving:** 122 calories, 4 g protein, 27 g carbohydrate, 0 g fat, 0 mg cholesterol, 236 mg sodium, 5 g fiber

# Parmesan Couscous and Ratatouille with Olives, Tomatoes, and Fresh Basil

*Although this flavorful Mediterranean dish may appear complicated, it's not. I prefer it without the olives, but my husband and son insist on them. Of course, in your kitchen, you're the boss!*

**MAKES 3 SERVINGS (1½ CUPS RATATOUILLE AND 1½ CUPS COUSCOUS PER SERVING)**

### Ratatouille

½ pound kale, stems trimmed, thinly sliced

Kosher salt

1 tablespoon olive oil

1 large yellow squash, cut into small cubes (about 2 cups)

2 medium tomatoes, diced

¼ cup kalamata or Niçoise olives (7 or 8 olives), pitted and chopped

Pinch of ground red pepper

¼ cup whole basil leaves, torn

### Couscous

1 cup whole wheat couscous

1 cup sugar snap peas, chopped

1¼ cups low-sodium chicken or vegetable broth, heated

½ cup grated Parmesan cheese

Kosher salt

Ground black pepper

**To make the ratatouille:** Heat a deep sauté pan over high heat. Add the kale, a sprinkle of salt, and ³/₄ cup water. Cook, stirring occasionally, for 13 to 15 minutes, or until softened. If the kale becomes too dry, add more water. Stir in the oil, squash, tomatoes, olives, and red pepper. Cook for 5 to 6 minutes, or until the squash is tender and the tomatoes lose their shape. Remove from the heat and stir in the basil. Set aside.

**To make the couscous:** In a medium bowl, mix the couscous and sugar snap peas. Pour the hot broth on top, stir once, and cover with plastic wrap or aluminum foil. Allow the couscous to rest for 5 to 6 minutes, or until all the water is absorbed and the couscous is soft and fluffy. Fold the cheese into the couscous and season with salt and black pepper.

**To serve:** Spoon the couscous onto a plate or bowl and serve the ratatouille on top.

> **Per serving:** 514 calories, 22 g protein, 88 g carbohydrate, 12 g fat (3 g saturated), 0 mg cholesterol, 561 mg sodium, 15 g fiber

# TANGY PITA CHIPS

*If you're looking for crunch, my tangy pita chips will hit the spot. In fact, if you're anything like me, make sure you prepare only one portion at a time—it's too easy to gobble down several servings. Enjoy with your favorite fresh or jarred salsa.*

**MAKES 1 SERVING**

1 small whole wheat pita

1 clove garlic, cut in half lengthwise

¼ teaspoon onion powder

⅛ teaspoon ground cumin

⅛ teaspoon paprika

⅛ teaspoon kosher salt

Pinch of ground red pepper

Pinch of ground black pepper

Preheat the oven or toaster oven to 350°F. Split the pita and rub the top of each half with the cut side of the garlic clove.

In a small bowl, combine the onion powder, cumin, paprika, salt, red pepper, and black pepper. Sprinkle the spice mixture over the 2 pita halves. Coat the pita with oil spray.

Toast directly on a wire rack for 8 to 9 minutes, or until the spices become fragrant and the pita is crispy. Eat whole or cut into wedges.

**Per serving:** 70 calories, 3.5 g protein, 16 g carbohydrate, 0 g fat, 0 mg cholesterol, 290 mg sodium, 3 g fiber

# BANANA-MANGO PARFAIT

*You'll love the rich, decadent flavor of this sleepy-time snack. And because it's made up of three fabulous ingredients—banana, mango, and calcium-rich ricotta cheese—your body gets a blast of nutrition before bed. I like it supercold, chilled for at least an hour before serving.*

**MAKES 3 SERVINGS**

1 ripe mango, peeled and cubed (or 1½ cups frozen mango cubes, thawed)

2 tablespoons sugar

1 cup fat-free ricotta cheese

¼ cup mint leaves, finely sliced, plus 3 whole sprigs for garnish

1 large banana, thinly sliced

Place the mango and sugar in a blender and puree until smooth. Transfer to a large bowl and stir in the ricotta and sliced mint.

Spoon 2 tablespoons of the ricotta mixture into each of 3 parfait glasses. Top with half of the banana slices and another layer of ricotta. Top with the remaining banana and then the remaining ricotta mixture.

Garnish each glass with a sprig of fresh mint. Serve immediately or chill for up to 4 hours.

**Per serving:** 164 calories, 8 g protein, 33 g carbohydrate, 0 g fat, 20 mg cholesterol, 201 mg sodium, 2 g fiber

# CHAPTER 17

# IRRITABLE BOWEL SYNDROME

rritable bowel syndrome (IBS) is common, affecting as many as 20 percent of Americans, and yet it is a mystery. No one knows exactly what causes it, and there is no way for a doctor to make a definitive diagnosis. There is no single trigger and no single set of identifying symptoms, which can come and go in a day or plague sufferers for months or years. So much uncertainty attached to very real physical discomfort makes coping with IBS frustrating in the extreme.

IBS is called a functional bowel disorder, not a disease, because it doesn't cause permanent damage, it doesn't progress to serious illness, and it can usually be controlled with diet and lifestyle changes. There's another reason to be hopeful if your case is a persistent one: People with chronic symptoms like yours have been successfully treated with new medications and are less disabled by the condition than ever before.

Many people confuse IBS with IBD, which stands for inflammatory bowel disease (talk about acronym confusion!). Although IBD and IBS both affect the intestines and can cause similar symptoms, they are very different conditions. IBD actually refers to a cluster of disorders, but the two major types are Crohn's disease and ulcerative colitis. Both are chronic conditions characterized by inflammation of the intestines, which results from the body's impaired immune response. Treatment for IBD may require powerful anti-inflammatory medications and sometimes even surgery. Unlike inflammatory bowel disease, IBS does not involve a dysfunctional inflammatory response, cause permanent damage to the intestines, or increase the risk of colon cancer and other intestinal disorders. Though IBS can certainly be painful and debilitating, it fortunately does not carry the same health risks as IBD.

## WHAT AFFECTS IBS?

The agony of IBS comes from the pain, discomfort, and embarrassing inconvenience of symptoms, which include diarrhea or constipation, cramping, bloating, excess gas, and mucus in the stool. To understand what happens in IBS, imagine a football stadium full of spectators doing "the wave." If everyone cooperates, you can see the forward progress of the wave as each section stands and then sits again—it's amazing to see so many bodies working in concert. Now imagine that you have some very nervous spectators . . . they see the wave coming at them, and they stand up too early, starting a secondary wave, so now there are two competing waves. The rhythm is disrupted. Or imagine that one group stands up for the wave but doesn't sit back down again. The wave is "stuck," unable to move forward until the disrupting group decides to sit back down again.

Our intestines are lined with muscles that contract and relax in waves (aha!) called peristalsis, which push the food you eat through your system. Along the way, nutrients are absorbed, and the residual is eventually eliminated in feces. In people with IBS, normal rhythmic waves are disrupted because the nervous system is not communicating effectively with the muscles that control the gut. Sometimes the bowel contracts too much or too forcefully, so food moves through the intestines too quickly, resulting in diarrhea.

Other times the intestinal muscles contract but don't relax again, or they contract very slowly, resulting in constipation. These crazy, out-of-sync muscle movements are behind the pain of IBS, much like muscle spasms in your legs cause the pain of a charley horse. We all have intestinal gas, but for people with IBS, it can become trapped inside, resulting in bloating and distention. Some of my clients with IBS have admitted to buying two wardrobes—an everyday wardrobe and another specifically for their bloated, symptomatic days. It makes perfect sense: Who wants to wear a snug pair of jeans or a fitted dress when you feel like the Pillsbury Doughboy? In addition, the intestinal nerves of people with IBS are highly sensitive, so even minor bloating can have them doubled over in pain.

An individual with IBS might experience just a few of these symptoms or all of them. Although most sufferers have either diarrhea-predominant IBS or constipation-predominant IBS, some people alternate between diarrhea and constipation. No matter what type of IBS you have, the underlying problem is that the rhythm of intestinal muscle contractions periodically gets messed up. There is no test for messed-up intestinal waves, however, and the symptoms of IBS are common to many other diseases, so arriving at a diagnosis of IBS is often lengthy and full of guesswork. Your doctor will want to rule out all other possible disorders, including Crohn's disease, ulcerative colitis, and celiac disease, through a physical examination, blood tests, ultrasound, x-ray of your bowels, and sigmoidoscopy or colonoscopy, in which a lighted flexible tube is inserted into your lower intestines to get an up close and personal look at your intestinal lining. If there are no other problems, it's IBS by default. Once you have a diagnosis, you and your doctor can get to work to find a treatment that works for you. IBS can be managed with appropriate diet and lifestyle changes and sometimes medications or behavioral therapy. It's important to remember that although IBS can be uncomfortable, and strictly speaking there is no "cure," it also won't progress into anything more serious.

We don't know exactly what disrupts the workings of the intestines in the first place, but we do know what can trigger flares of the disorder. Food is a biggie, and I'll address that in the next section. Aside from food and eating issues, another significant IBS trigger is stress.

Stress can trigger a flare of IBS, and it can make food-triggered IBS symptoms worse. That's why many health experts recommend that people suffering from IBS actively explore a variety of ways to de-stress—there might be a terrific way to relax that you just haven't tried yet. Some doctors even talk about an IBS personality, one that is noticeably tense and anxious. I've seen this in my own practice. The client that comes to mind is Amy, a kindergarten teacher. The first time I saw Amy, I was struck by her rigid body language—every move she made told me she was a very controlled person. Sitting or standing, her posture was perfect, and she held her arms close to her body and used minimal gestures. She spoke in a clipped, drill-sergeant sort of way. Everything Amy did, she did quickly. She was always on the go doing things for the kids in her class, running errands for her family, setting up the classroom, and gobbling down her food. Amy didn't sit down to eat. If she couldn't wolf down a meal in five minutes, it wasn't worth eating. The challenge with Amy was getting her to recognize her food triggers and also—perhaps more important—helping her to understand that her stressful, on-the-go lifestyle was only making her IBS worse.

On a very basic level, eating quickly is risky because you are more likely to swallow air, which can directly lead to bloating and distention. But stress can also stimulate spasms in the gastrointestinal tract—like feeling butterflies in your stomach when rumors about impending layoffs start flying around the water cooler. In people with IBS, those butterflies are on a rampage. Amy's IBS was certainly made worse by her tense, never-stop, full-of-stress lifestyle. Fortunately, we were able to get her symptoms under control in pretty short order. We identified her food triggers (starchy beans, raw vegetables, gum, and coffee), which eliminated most of her problems, but stress education was the biggest eye-opener for her. Amy had no idea how much her driven personality affected her bowels. Although she still has a way to go, it's easier for her to relax now that she doesn't have to worry about whether her diarrhea will strike unexpectedly, and she's made a determined effort to be more relaxed. Ironically, she's as driven about finding time to de-stress as she is about everything else, but she's on her way to achieving the type of balanced life that can keep her IBS symptoms to a minimum.

## FAQS

**I've read that I should take fiber supplements for my IBS. Are they helpful?**

Many experts recommend fiber supplements, but they are not always the best medicine. I say this because many of my clients have complained that they've become more bloated and gassy after taking them. And this goes for both types—soluble and insoluble fiber supplements. People with IBS are very sensitive to fiber, so adding a concentrated dose of fiber isn't always beneficial, especially if you go overboard on the amount. Personally, I tend to treat IBS by focusing on foods.

I start by asking my clients about their symptoms. If it's predominantly diarrhea, I'll have them take a rest from most fiber-rich foods. Then, ever so slowly, we start adding them back, focusing first on the soluble type, which can be easily dissolved in the gut. If a client complains of persistent constipation, I immediately incorporate foods rich in soluble fiber (along with some insoluble fiber) evenly sprinkled throughout the day. When my clients feel well enough, we add more. Since I've had much more success with food than supplements, I suggest you skip the pills and instead add fiber-rich foods (slowly!) along with lots of flat water (not carbonated, which will add gas) to your diet.

While I prefer dietary modifications as the first line of defense, if you still can't find relief, you can certainly experiment with fiber supplements. Just be cautious—start with a small amount of a soluble fiber supplement (such as psyllium, wheat dextrin, methylcellulose, or inulin) and see how you react. If the product appears to be beneficial, you can slowly work your way up to the recommended daily dose. And if one type of supplement doesn't work for you, consider trying another; individuals can respond differently to different forms of fiber. Make sure to follow directions, and take your supplements with plenty of water to minimize bloating and constipation. This is definitely a trial-and-error process!

## HOW FOOD AFFECTS IBS

A sensitive gut needs to be treated like a fussy baby: You have to put it on a regular feeding schedule, keep it calm, and protect it from potential irritants.

### IDENTIFYING TRIGGER FOODS

Identifying your particular trigger foods can be difficult. Even people without IBS will have a gastrointestinal reaction to certain foods once in a while. It just happens, and it's perfectly normal. But people with IBS have a heightened sensitivity to foods. They know the awful consequences of a trigger food, so they might eat a spicy bowl of chili, for example, have a reaction, and condemn chili to a list of foods to be avoided forever. But what if the reaction was really due to unusual stress, a

## COMMON IBS TRIGGER FOODS

The following foods are the most commonly reported IBS triggers. It's important to emphasize that these foods do not cause IBS, but they can aggravate the condition.

- Concentrated sources of fructose, sugar, and other sweeteners, such as agave, honey, maple syrup, fruit juice, dried fruit, jams, jellies, and fresh fruit naturally high in fructose (apples, pears, mangoes, Asian pears); also, beverages, candies, syrups, ketchups, and other condiments that contain high amounts of sugar, high-fructose corn syrup, or other sweeteners

- Sugar alcohols: all foods, gums, mints, and candies containing sorbitol, maltitol, mannitol, and isomalt; also, fresh fruits naturally high in sorbitol: apples, pears, apricots, peaches, plums, prunes, cherries, and nectarines

- Milk and dairy products, including buttermilk, yogurt, ice cream, frozen yogurt, cottage cheese, ricotta cheese, sour cream, whipped cream, sherbet, cream cheese, all cheeses, and cream; also, prepared foods that contain dairy (creamy soups and sauces, mashed potatoes, pudding, etc.)

- Cruciferous vegetables, particularly broccoli, cabbage, Brussels sprouts, and cauliflower

- Beans and lentils

- Onions (all varieties) and garlic

- Raw vegetables

mild case of food poisoning, or just one of those normal gut reactions? You might avoid a food forever for no good reason. By the time some clients come to see me, they're downright food phobic. They are so afraid of an attack of diarrhea, constipation, or horrific gas that they err on the side of caution—but too much caution can result in low blood sugar, weight loss, poor nutrition, and another kind of socially awkward situation: They can become afraid of eating with friends and going out for fear of an attack.

For people with extreme IBS, the simplest way to identify trigger foods is to follow an elimination diet—a meal plan that has you avoid all potential offending foods—for five to seven days. Then you slowly reintroduce those same foods, one by one. Along the way, you keep track of reactions to the foods you are reintroducing in a food diary. Depending upon your symptoms, my guidelines for an elimination diet vary slightly. Please note: Following an elimination diet can be very difficult. It's just a week, but you still need to be pretty committed to put up with

- Foods high in insoluble fiber: Some people are sensitive to foods that are very high in insoluble fiber—specifically, wheat bran, high-fiber breakfast cereals, specially formulated high-fiber breads, and whole wheat pasta. Other people are extremely sensitive and react to foods with moderate amounts of insoluble fiber, such as whole grain breads and crackers, wheat germ, popcorn, bulgur, quinoa, millet, amaranth, and whole nuts and seeds.

- Wheat-based products: Some people have difficulty digesting compounds in wheat and wheat flour (unrelated to insoluble fiber). Common foods include white and whole wheat breads, crackers, pasta, cereals, and baked goods.

- Caffeinated drinks, such as coffee, tea, and colas

- Alcohol

- Fatty foods, especially fried foods (such as french fries, onion rings, and fried fish and chicken), fatty meats (such as marbled steaks, sausages, hot dogs, salami, bologna, ribs, and fatty ground beef and burgers), and full-fat dairy (such as butter, full-fat cheeses, cream, and creamy sauces and soups)

- Condiments, including ketchup, pickle relish, soy sauce, chutney, and barbecue sauce

- Carbonated beverages (any drinks that fizz with little bubbles)

- Chewing gum (sugared and sugar free)

- Chocolate (sorry!)

such a limited selection of food. Then again, if you're currently suffering, it's better to put up with a week of discomfort than a lifetime of untreated, debilitating abdominal pain.

If you have severe diarrhea-predominant IBS, your elimination diet will avoid all trigger foods plus all fiber, including soluble fiber. (Instructions are provided in my 4-Step Program under Extreme Elimination Diet—No Fiber, page 404.)

If you have severe constipation-predominant IBS, your elimination diet will avoid all trigger foods but incorporate foods rich in soluble fiber and small amounts of insoluble fiber. (Those instructions are provided in my 4-Step Program under Elimination Diet with Added Fiber, page 408.) The addition of soluble fiber can help encourage your intestines to "wave" more effectively.

Whichever plan you follow, after about a week, you'll be ready to test some of the potential trigger foods. I recommend trying one new food every two to three days and carefully documenting what you eat and how you feel during the 24 hours afterward. Although this chapter provides all the instruction you need to do this on your own, it's a big job. If you try on your own and find it unmanageable, I encourage you to work with a registered dietitian who specializes in gastrointestinal issues.

As I said, these elimination plans are only for severe cases of IBS. If you're among the majority of people who experience less debilitating IBS, feel free to skip the elimination meal plan altogether and go straight to keeping an IBS journal. Your journal should list exactly what you eat, when you eat, and what symptoms you experience, as well as your emotional state for the day. Make a special note if you feel particularly tense, anxious, or stressed.

When you have an IBS attack, consult your diary to see which foods you ate in the previous 24 hours and start a list of your potential triggers. Keep eating normally, always noting which foods you ate in the 24 hours prior to an attack and adding new items to your potential trigger list. When a food already on your list precedes an attack, make a hatch mark next to it each time it comes up. After a few weeks, those marks should tell you which foods are most likely to trigger an episode. Narrow down your list to the three most likely triggers, and avoid those foods entirely for two weeks. Continue to keep your IBS journal, and repeat the process. Every once in a while, test your trigger foods again (one at a time) to make sure you're not avoiding them for no reason. Over time, you'll get a good handle on which foods you need to avoid to feel well and which you can eat safely. Note: If you find yourself with more than five main trigger foods, see a dietitian to make sure that the rest of your diet is making up for whatever nutrients you're missing by eliminating those foods.

For everyone fighting IBS, there are a few mealtime guidelines that can make your life easier.

1. Try to eat meals at approximately the same time each day to get your body used to a schedule.

2. Eat smaller, more frequent meals so you don't overload your gut at any one time.

3. Slow down. Sit, relax, and take time to thoroughly chew your food. Think of it as time invested in training your digestive system to behave.

## GOOD FOODS TO CHOOSE

The best foods for IBS health are those that are gentle on the digestive system and encourage "smooth passage" through the intestines. Thus, vegetables, fruits, and whole grains—it pains me to say—should be limited until your symptoms subside and you identify foods that are problematic for you. It's hard to believe I just said that! Truth be told, these healthful foods are a bit hard for the body to break down, but remember that I'm recommending you watch your intake only until you get a handle on your triggers. Even with diarrhea-predominant IBS, you should eventually be able to tolerate moderate amounts of all three groups, although you'll probably need to cook vegetables.

## Soluble Fiber

Fiber comes in two main varieties: soluble and insoluble. Soluble fiber dissolves in water and turns into a kind of gooey substance with a gummy consistency—think what happens to oatmeal after it sits in a pot of water for a time. Insoluble fiber is tougher. It doesn't dissolve, and it pretty much keeps its form.

Although insoluble fiber is generally healthy, it can be hard on the intestines of IBS sufferers. Insoluble fiber speeds food through the colon, something that many diarrhea-predominant IBS sufferers want to avoid. People with constipation-predominant IBS may want to experiment with how much insoluble fiber they can eat without experiencing too much gas and bloating.

Soluble fiber, on the other hand, promotes gentle regularity, regardless of the type of IBS you have. That's why you'll find plenty of soluble fiber integrated into my Elimination Diet with Added Fiber. (It doesn't, however, include soluble fiber–rich foods that also act as potential triggers, such as beans, lentils, broccoli, and cabbage.)

Most foods high in soluble fiber are considered safe for people with IBS. The trick is to eat a variety of foods in moderation, without eating too much of one particular food or too much food in general at one time. If you have diarrhea-predominant IBS, I recommend slowly adding more foods high in soluble fiber to your diet. If you experience too much bloating or pain, back off a little, wait a few days, and then add fiber again. The key is to eat just a little bit of extra fiber, building up to about six servings a day over the course of weeks, not days. However, for constipation-predominant IBS, you can be more aggressive, fiberwise. The Elimination Diet with Added Fiber (for constipation-predominant IBS) works in three to six (or more) daily portions of soluble fiber, depending upon the meals and snacks you choose. Of course, even then you'll want to moderate the portions and spread them throughout the day (as opposed to eating them all at one sitting) to avoid the risk of excess gas. Remember to drink plenty of water to help move things along.

My Elimination Diet with Added Fiber incorporates at least one serving of soluble fiber–rich food at each meal. If you have diarrhea-predominant IBS and you're ready to follow the less extreme Elimination Diet with Added Fiber, you may want to move more slowly: Start with a single serving for the entire day. All foods rich in fiber included in Your Ultimate Grocery List have an asterisk (*), so you'll know what to include and what to avoid. Everything is explained in the 4-Step Program, page 404.

## LACTOSE INTOLERANCE VERSUS IBS

Milk can sometimes trigger IBS, so you'll find dairy on the list of foods to initially avoid. But sensitivity to dairy foods is most commonly a sign of lactose intolerance. Lactose intolerance is not IBS. In fact, it's a completely different problem and one that's easily remedied.

What is lactose intolerance? Milk products contain a form of natural sugar called lactose. In order to digest lactose, our bodies produce a specific enzyme called lactase. For a variety of reasons, including genetics, digestive disorders, intestinal injury, and/or the natural aging process, some people end up with very low levels of lactase. Depending on how much of the offending food you eat and how much lactase enzyme your body can produce, symptoms can be mild or severe and include nausea, cramping, gas, bloating, and diarrhea. Sound familiar? The symptoms can be remarkably similar to IBS symptoms. So, how do you tell the difference?

If you suspect you're lactose intolerant, make dairy the first thing you test. Avoid milk and anything containing milk for three to five days (see the full dairy list under Common IBS Trigger Foods, page 390). If your symptoms disappear completely, you're most likely lactose intolerant. If you want a definitive diagnosis, you can ask your doctor about taking a hydrogen breath test. This simple test looks for a higher-than-normal amount of hydrogen in the breath, caused by the extra gases produced by the bacteria fermenting the undigested lactose in the intestines. Fortunately, many people with lactose intolerance can enjoy hard, aged cheeses (like Cheddar and Swiss), which have insignificant amounts of lactose, as well as lactose-reduced milk products, without any symptoms. You can also take lactase enzyme in a tablet or liquid form with your first bite or sip of a milk product to prevent digestive trouble.

If you test positive for lactose intolerance and avoid all milk products but *still* have gastrointestinal symptoms, it's possible that you have both lactose intolerance and IBS.

In addition, raw vegetables—whether rich in soluble *or* insoluble fiber—tend to be difficult for IBS sufferers to digest and can often trigger diarrhea, gas, and bloating. When you're ready to introduce vegetables into your diet, I strongly recommend that you stick to cooked vegetables.

IBS-FRIENDLY FOODS FOR SOLUBLE FIBER: *winter squash, parsnips, turnips, sweet and white potatoes, green peas, okra, eggplant, barley, oats, oranges, grapefruit, clementines, tangerines, strawberries, blackberries, raspberries, bananas, avocados, cooked carrots, cooked green beans, cooked spinach, cooked kale, cooked Swiss chard, ground flaxseed*

The following fruits are high in fructose and/or sorbitol and may be trigger foods for some people. If you find that you do not have a personal sensitivity to these foods, they are excellent sources of soluble fiber and should be regularly included in your diet: apples, peaches, plums, nectarines, pears, mangoes, apricots.

## LIQUIDS

All people with IBS should drink flat water regularly throughout the day. If constipation is your problem, water will help keep your stools moist so they pass more easily; the soluble fiber in your diet will help, too. If diarrhea is your problem, you'll need to replenish the water you lose through loose stools. Plain water and decaffeinated tea should be your first choices. Carbonated beverages are not advised because the gas from the carbonation can get trapped in your intestines, causing discomfort. You'll also want to avoid drinking caffeinated beverages and alcohol, which can stimulate the intestines and make symptoms worse, particularly if you have diarrhea-predominant IBS.

## BONUS POINTS

- ◆ **Rule out other disorders.** Don't assume that your symptoms are due to IBS unless your doctor has told you so. You need to get a thorough medical workup to rule out other, more serious conditions, including Crohn's disease, ulcerative colitis, celiac disease, and colorectal cancer. Even if you've had a diagnosis of IBS, be sure to go back to your doctor if your symptoms change or worsen.

- ◆ **Talk with your doctor about medications.** The first line of treatment for IBS is typically diet and lifestyle changes. But if you can't get your symptoms under control, and if the pain and other symptoms are affecting your life, ask your doctor about medications that have been approved for IBS. There are a variety of possible medications, including antispasmodics, antidiarrheals, and antidepressants. Yes, antidepressants—for your intestines, not your brain—because they seem to modulate intestinal pain and regulate gut function. Many antidepressants regulate the neurotransmitter serotonin, and (who knew?) 95 percent of serotonin is found in your gut, where it helps maintain smooth, regular contractions of the intestines. Some scientists believe that the intestines of people with IBS require more serotonin than they're getting for normal function. The theory is that antidepressants that make more serotonin available (the serotonin reuptake inhibitors—SSRIs— such as Prozac, Zoloft, or Paxil) will fix the problem. More research needs to be done before antidepressants are a first-line treatment, but if you've tried everything else, you may want to discuss this possibility with your physician.

- ◆ **Don't self-medicate without guidance.** You may be tempted to take control of IBS by stocking up on over-the-counter laxatives or antidiarrhea medication, but don't do so unless you get the go-ahead from your doctor. IBS is a chronic disorder, and over-the-counter medications are short-term solutions. Laxatives in particular can be hard on the intestines if used inappropriately. If you find yourself relying on over-the-counter meds, talk with your doctor to find a better solution.

◆ **Maintain healthy eating patterns.** Eat small meals regularly throughout the day. Try to eat at about the same time each day. Slow down your eating pace during mealtimes, and try to avoid on-the-run (or over-the-kitchen-sink) eating.

◆ **Put a lid on stress.** Stress is a complex problem. Although circumstances outside of our control can feel stressful, psychologists remind us that events don't create stress. Stress is of our own making, fueled by our own interpretation of events or thoughts about future outcomes. Those perceptions trigger a variety of physiologic responses, including changes in the way our gastrointestinal systems function. That's how the mind-body connection works: The things we think have very real effects on our bodies. But just as we create stress, we can also learn to control it by responding differently to life events. People with IBS can have extreme physical reactions to stress, so relaxation is especially important.

The first thing to try is deep breathing, which is breathing from the diaphragm instead of the chest. To get started, lie down on the floor on your back. Bend your knees and put your feet on the floor. Put one hand over your diaphragm, just under your ribs. Keeping your shoulders as flat as possible against the floor, take a deep breath. As you breathe in, focus on letting your diaphragm push your hand up, expanding your abdomen. Exhale naturally, and notice how your hand gently falls as the air leaves your lungs. (After you get the hang of this type of breathing, try it while standing or sitting up straight.) This type of deep breathing triggers a relaxation response in the body.

Along with deep breathing, you can bring in an arsenal of relaxation techniques, including massage, yoga, and meditation. Even taking quiet time for yourself—a half hour to read, take a bubble bath, garden, or just enjoy nature—may be enough to give your mind and body a much-needed break.

If stress has gotten out of control, you might want to consider a short course of counseling with a psychologist or psychiatrist to help you learn how to change the way you respond to the stressful events in your life. There are specific techniques that can help you experience life without tension, anxiety, or a feeling of being overwhelmed. In fact, researchers from Mount Sinai School of Medicine in New York found that people with IBS who were treated by both a gastroenterologist and a psychologist got better faster than those treated by just one type of specialist.

◆ **Make exercise a daily prescription.** Exercise is important for two main reasons. First, it is a great stress reliever. Dozens of studies have shown that no matter what the cause of your stress, no matter what symptoms your stress causes, regular moderate exercise can help make you feel better. Second, exercise is critically important for the proper functioning of the gastrointestinal system. If your body is sluggish, your gut may follow suit. If your body is fit and active, your gut will be healthier and better regulated. In a 2011 study, IBS sufferers who were counseled to exercise for 20 to 30 minutes three to five days a week saw dramatic improvements in abdominal pain, stool problems, and other IBS symptoms. If you don't already exercise, you may want to consider walking for 30 minutes a day, every day, at a moderate pace. But really, any daily activity will be helpful, so choose something you find fun.

## SUPPLEMENTS

If you suffer from IBS and want to consider supplements in addition to the food fixes, here's what I recommend.

1. **A multivitamin.** I recommend a multivitamin to ensure that you always get the basic nutrition you might otherwise miss if you're tiptoeing around a sensitive stomach. Unfortunately, many people with IBS find that vitamins upset the delicate balance of their digestive systems. Look for liquid or chewable multivitamins—any brand, even children's chewables, are great for adults with IBS. Read the label, and take the amount recommended for adults.

2. **Calcium and vitamin D$_3$.** If you avoid dairy because it triggers IBS symptoms, you may not get enough calcium in your diet for good health, so you may want to consider taking a separate calcium supplement. For more specific information on calcium supplements, including appropriate dosages (see page 233). Because too much calcium has been linked to an increased risk of prostate cancer, if you're male and have IBS, you should speak with your physician before taking calcium supplements. For women with IBS, I recommend brands that contain calcium citrate (instead of the more common calcium carbonate) because this form is easier on the stomach. Important note: Some calcium chews contain lactose, so if milk bothers your stomach, avoid the chews and instead buy the pill form. If you have trouble swallowing pills, use a pill crusher and mix them with natural applesauce to help them go down more easily.

3. **Probiotics.** Our intestines are full of bacteria and other microorganisms, but that's not necessarily bad. Some of the bacteria are there to keep us healthy. Some experts believe that people with IBS don't have enough of the "good" microorganisms, which is why their intestines seem to be out of balance. Probiotics are supplements that provide more of the good stuff, which can prevent the bad stuff from causing diarrhea or constipation. Current research suggests that a mix of probiotics may be more effective at alleviating IBS symptoms than a single bacterial strain. If you're interested in trying a probiotic to see if it reduces the pain, bloating, and flatulence associated with IBS, I advise choosing a probiotic blend that includes the strain *Bifidobacterium infantis.* One respected brand to consider is VSL#3; take ½ to 1 packet per day for IBS.

4. **Enteric-coated peppermint oil.** Peppermint naturally reduces gastrointestinal muscle spasms and cramping by relaxing the smooth muscles that line the intestines. There is good evidence that peppermint oil supplements are just as effective at relieving abdominal pain and other IBS symptoms as prescription smooth muscle relaxant medications (called anticholinergics). Studies have found that participants get some relief if they take capsules containing 0.2 to 0.4 milliliters (mL) of peppermint oil three times a day, 15 to 30 minutes before meals, for one to two weeks. Choose a brand that is enteric-coated, which means that the supplements are specially designed to bypass the stomach and dissolve only in the intestines, reducing the possibility of heartburn and stomach distress.

5. **Beano.** When we eat beans, we get gas. It's a fact of life. That's because we don't have enough of an enzyme called alpha-galactosidase, which breaks down certain components of complex carbohydrates. The bacteria naturally found in our intestines break down the undigested complex carbs, creating gas in the process. The product Beano contains alpha-galactosidase, so it helps break down more of the gas-producing foods. It works with beans, of course, but also with vegetables (including cruciferous vegetables like broccoli and cabbage) and whole grains. Follow the directions on the label for best results. If you struggle with gas, you may want to keep a bottle handy.

6. **Artichoke leaf extract.** Studies by researchers in the United Kingdom have shown that artichoke leaf extract (*Cynara scolymus*) can reduce IBS symptoms of pain and flatulence by more than 25 percent with just two months of use. About half of the IBS patients who claimed to have alternating constipation and diarrhea reported having "normal" bowel habits after treatment with the extract. The recommended dosage is 320 to 640 milligrams two or three times per day.

For more information on managing irritable bowel syndrome, visit www.joybauer.com/ibs.

# JOY'S 4-STEP PROGRAM
## FOR IRRITABLE BOWEL SYNDROME

Follow this program if you have been diagnosed with Irritable Bowel Syndrome.

## Step 1 ... START WITH THE BASICS

These are the first things you should do to take control of your IBS symptoms.

- ◆ If you haven't been officially diagnosed with IBS, see a doctor to rule out other possible causes of your discomfort.

- ◆ For severe diarrhea-predominant IBS, start the Extreme Elimination Diet—No Fiber on page 404.

- ◆ For severe constipation-predominant IBS (along with other persistent types that cause gas, cramping, or pain), start the regular Elimination Diet with Added Fiber on page 408.

- ◆ For less debilitating IBS, start an IBS diary to monitor your symptoms, diet, and stress levels and identify which factors trigger your IBS attacks.

- ◆ Eat all of your meals sitting down. Chew your food thoroughly. Make meals a leisurely experience, not a race.

- ◆ Remember, stress hurts. Make relaxation a priority.

- ◆ Exercise daily.

# Step2 . . . YOUR ULTIMATE GROCERY LIST

A food plan for IBS is more about avoiding your personal trigger foods than about specific nutrients that will help alleviate your symptoms. The foods on this list are considered generally "safe," avoiding all common triggers. Go easy on foods marked with an asterisk (*), especially if you have diarrhea-predominant IBS. These foods are rich in fiber, and although they can often help control IBS in the long run, they need to be slowly and cautiously introduced into your diet. (See Elimination Diet meal plans, pages 404 to 408.)

There are so many potential trigger foods that affect different people in different ways that my grocery list is, unfortunately, somewhat limited. This is where you come in. Take a few minutes to add healthful foods you know you can personally tolerate without a problem. For example, if you regularly eat apples, onions, beans, lentils, and yogurt without symptoms, add them to your personal grocery list. As you keep an IBS journal or follow an elimination diet, you'll identify many more safe and healthy foods. Use the allotted spaces below each food category for your personal notes.

For a printable version of this list, visit www.joybauer.com/ibs.

## FRUIT

All fresh and frozen, but be cautious with the following fruits, which are especially high in fructose and/or sorbitol: apples, apricots, Asian pears, cherries, mangoes, nectarines, peaches, pears, plums, and prunes and other dried fruits

Best choices (highest in soluble fiber) include:

*Bananas

*Blackberries

*Clementines

*Grapefruit

*Oranges

*Raspberries

*Strawberries

*Tangerines

## Personal Safe Items

_____

_____

_____

## VEGETABLES (COOKED VEGETABLES ARE TYPICALLY MUCH BETTER TOLERATED THAN RAW)

Be cautious with the following vegetables, which are common triggers: cruciferous vegetables, especially broccoli, Brussels sprouts, cabbage, and cauliflower; garlic; lentils, onions (all varieties); and starchy beans

Best choices (high in soluble fiber) include:
*Avocados
*Carrots
*Eggplant (peeled)
*Green beans
*Kale
*Okra
*Parsnips
*Peas, green
*Potatoes (sweet and white)
*Spinach
*Swiss chard
*Turnips
*Winter squash (acorn and butternut)

### Personal Safe Items

_____
_____
_____
_____

## SEAFOOD

_All_ fresh or frozen fish and shellfish

### Personal Safe Items

_____
_____
_____
_____

## LEAN PROTEINS

Beef, lean
Chicken, ground (at least 90% lean)
Chicken, skinless
Eggs and egg substitutes
Pork tenderloin
Tempeh
Tofu
Turkey, ground (at least 90% lean)
Turkey, skinless
Turkey bacon

### Personal Safe Items

_____
_____
_____

## NUTS AND SEEDS

Almond butter

*Almonds

*Butternuts (white walnuts)

Cashew butter

*Cashews

*Chia seeds

*Flaxseed, ground

*Hazelnuts

*Macadamia nuts

Peanut butter

*Peanuts

*Pecans

*Pine nuts

*Pistachios

*Psyllium seeds, ground

*Pumpkin seeds

Sunflower butter

*Sunflower seeds

*Walnuts

### Personal Safe Items

_____

_____

_____

## LOWER-FIBER GRAINS

Bread, white/refined (buns, crackers, English muffins, and pitas)

Breakfast cereals (less than 1 gram fiber per serving)

Cereal, puffed rice or hot cream of rice or wheat

Corn grits/polenta

Pasta, regular (white)

Rice (white and yellow)

Rice cakes

Tortillas (corn, rice, and white flour)

## HIGHER-FIBER GRAINS

*Amaranth

*Barley

*Buckwheat

*Bread, whole grain (buns, crackers, English muffins, and pitas)

*Bulgur

*Cereals, whole grain (if you're sensitive to large amounts of fiber, choose cereals with no more than 5 grams fiber per serving)

*Millet

*Oats

*Pasta, whole grain

*Quinoa

*Rice (brown and wild)

*Tortillas, whole wheat

### Personal Safe Items

_____

_____

_____

## DAIRY

Milk alternatives (almond, rice, soy)

### Personal Safe Items

_____

_____

_____


## MISCELLANEOUS (INCLUDING CONDIMENTS)

Canola oil                    Olive oil                     Vinegar (all varieties)

Herbs and spices (fresh,      Soft tub spread, trans-fat-free
  dried, and ground)            (reduced-fat or regular)

### Personal Safe Items

_____

_____

_____

*Foods rich in fiber that should be slowly introduced, especially if you have diarrhea-predominant IBS


# Step 3 . . . GOING ABOVE AND BEYOND

If you want to do everything you can to try to alleviate your IBS symptoms while still staying healthy, here are some additional things you might try.

- ◆ Consider taking a chewable or liquid multivitamin to ensure that you fill in any nutritional gaps caused by a limited diet.
- ◆ If you're a woman and your IBS symptoms are triggered by dairy products, consider taking a calcium citrate supplement that also includes vitamin $D_3$.
- ◆ Consider taking supplements to reduce your symptoms, such as probiotics, enteric-coated peppermint oil capsules, Beano, or artichoke leaf extract.
- ◆ If you can't get relief through dietary and lifestyle changes, talk with your doctor. There are new medications that can help you get control over your worst symptoms.

## PSYCHOLOGICAL THERAPIES FOR IBS

If nothing else helps relieve your IBS symptoms, you might want to try cognitive behavioral therapy or hypnotherapy. IBS is often intimately related to stress and anxiety, so learning techniques to better cope with emotions can help you manage your condition. Plenty of research shows that psychotherapy can provide substantial relief from IBS. Take some time to explore these treatment options.

# Step 4 . . . MEAL PLANS

For severe diarrhea-predominant IBS, follow the Extreme Elimination Diet—No Fiber, below.

For severe constipation-predominant IBS, follow the Elimination Diet with Added Fiber, page 408.

## Extreme Elimination Diet—No Fiber

*For severe diarrhea-predominant IBS (follow for five to seven days)*

This elimination diet is extreme and should not be followed for longer than one week. It's designed to help people who suffer from severe, persistent, diarrhea-predominant IBS determine which foods may be aggravating their condition. It avoids all common IBS trigger foods. This plan is very low in dietary fiber and is based on the few foods I've found that people with this type of IBS can tolerate best. Fiber (and nutrition) will be slowly increased as you introduce new foods.

If you're a candidate for this extreme plan, follow it for up to one week. Every day, choose one option for each of the three meals—breakfast, lunch, and dinner. Then, once or twice per day, choose from my suggested snacks. Eat slowly, and thoroughly chew your food. Approximate calories have been provided to help adjust for your personal weight-management goals. If you find yourself hungry (and if weight is not an issue), feel free to increase the portion sizes for meals and snacks. Stick with flat water as your beverage, and try to drink at least 8 cups throughout each day.

After following this plan for one week, you can start experimenting by adding new foods. You should add one new food every two or three days. (It's best to stick with one portion of a new food per day.) Keep an IBS diary, and write down everything you eat and everything you feel. Pay close attention to how you feel after eating each new food, which will help you determine whether that food can be permanently reintroduced into your diet. If any food bothers your stomach, stop eating it and add it to your list of problem foods. Move on to the next food category. You can always retest a problem food at a later date.

At the end of this tough assignment, you will have identified most of the foods that aggravate your IBS. Let's hope it's a short list. For the sake of good nutrition and food variety, here's my suggested order for reintroducing new foods.

1. Dairy (fat-free and reduced-fat milk, yogurt, cheese, etc.)

2. Sweet potatoes

3. Wheat products: Start with white versions of bread, crackers, and pasta. In the future, when symptoms subside, you can slowly test small amounts of whole wheat varieties.

4. Oats and barley

5. Brown and wild rice

6. Cooked vegetables (noncruciferous)

7. Fruit (without tough outer skins, at first)

8. Whole grains (whole wheat breads, cereals, pasta; popcorn; quinoa; millet; amaranth; etc.)

9. Whole nuts and seeds

10. Garlic and onion

11. Starchy beans and lentils

12. Cooked cruciferous vegetables

13. Raw vegetables

14. Ketchup, soy sauce, and other condiments (test one at a time)

15. Dried fruit and all-fruit jams

16. Chocolate

17. Fruit juice, sugar, and honey

18. Coffee or tea

19. Alcohol

## BREAKFAST OPTIONS

(300 TO 400 CALORIES)

### Hot Cereal with Banana Slices

Prepare 1½ cups cream of rice cereal with water and 1 tablespoon soft tub trans-fat-free spread. Enjoy with 1 sliced banana.

### Cold Cereal with Soy Milk

Enjoy 2 cups puffed rice cereal with soy milk (or rice or almond milk).

### Scrambled Eggs with Rice Cakes

Beat 2 whole eggs with 2 egg whites and scramble in a hot skillet coated with oil spray. Season eggs with preferred herbs. Enjoy with 2 rice cakes, each topped with 1 teaspoon soft tub, trans-fat-free spread.

## LUNCH OPTIONS

(400 TO 500 CALORIES)

### Grilled Chicken with Rice

Enjoy 5 ounces grilled chicken (or fish, shellfish, or lean beef) with 1 cup cooked white or yellow rice with preferred seasonings.

### Turkey Burger with Baked Potato

Serve a 5-ounce bunless turkey burger with 1 medium baked potato topped with 2 teaspoons soft tub trans-fat-free spread. Do not eat the potato skin.

### Turkey and Avocado on Rice Cakes

Divide 4 ounces sliced turkey (or chicken) over 2 plain rice cakes and top each with 1 thin slice avocado. Enjoy with 1 ounce of baked potato chips.

## DINNER OPTIONS

(500 TO 600 CALORIES)

### Salmon with Rice

Enjoy 1 serving of Easy! 3-Step Microwave Salmon (page 345, omit the garlic) or 5 ounces grilled salmon (or sole, haddock, cod, or tilapia) seasoned with 1 teaspoon olive oil and a pinch of kosher salt. Serve with 1 cup cooked white or yellow rice with preferred seasonings.

### Rosemary Chicken with Baked Potato

Enjoy 5 ounces Rosemary Chicken (page 347) with 1 medium baked potato topped with 1 tablespoon soft tub trans-fat-free spread. Do not eat the potato skin.

### Roast Turkey with Mashed Potatoes

Enjoy 6 ounces skinless roast turkey with 1 medium baked potato scooped and mashed with 1 tablespoon soft tub trans-fat-free spread (or 1 cup cooked white or yellow rice). Do not eat the potato skin.

## SNACK OPTIONS

100 CALORIES OR LESS

- 2 plain rice cakes
- 1 banana
- 1 hard-cooked egg (or 4 egg whites)
- 1 rice cake topped with 1 teaspoon nut butter
- 8 ounces soy, almond, or rice milk

100 TO 200 CALORIES

- 100 to 200 calories' worth of plain rice crackers
- 1 ounce baked potato chips
- ½ baked potato with 1 teaspoon soft tub, trans-fat-free spread (or 1 tablespoon guacamole); do not eat the potato skin.
- 2 rice cakes, each topped with 1 teaspoon nut butter
- 2 rice cakes, each topped with 1 tablespoon guacamole

## Elimination Diet with Added Fiber

*Follow this diet for severe constipation-predominant IBS and as a follow-up to the extreme elimination diet.*

This elimination diet is extreme and should not be followed long-term. It's designed to help people who suffer with persistent constipation-predominant IBS (and other debilitating types of IBS that cause gas, cramping, and pain) finally figure out which foods may be aggravating their condition. It avoids common IBS trigger foods and provides a moderate amount of dietary fiber, with a good amount specifically coming from soluble fiber sources. All foods rich in fiber are marked with an asterisk (*). If you're feeling gassy or uncomfortably distended, go easy on these foods. Your total fiber intake (and nutrition!) will slowly increase when you start introducing new foods.

If you're a candidate for this plan, follow it for one week. Every day, choose one option for each of the three meals—breakfast, lunch, and dinner. Then, once or twice per day, choose from my suggested snacks. Eat slowly, and thoroughly chew your food. Approximate calories have been provided to help adjust for your personal weight-management goals. If you find yourself hungry (and if weight is not an issue), feel free to increase the portion sizes for meals and snacks. Stick with flat water as your beverage, and try to drink at least 10 cups throughout each day.

After following this plan for one week, you're ready to add new foods. You should add one new food every two or three days. (It's best to stick with one portion of a new food per day.) Keep an IBS diary, and write down all the foods you eat, the amounts, and how they affect your constipation. Pay close attention to how you feel after eating each new food, and determine if that food can be permanently reintroduced back into your diet. If any food bothers your stomach, stop eating it and add it to your list of problem foods. Move on to the next category. You can always retest a problem food at a later date.

At the end of this tough assignment, you will hopefully have identified all (or most) of the foods that aggravate your IBS. Let's hope it's a short list. For the sake of good nutrition and food variety, here's my suggested order for reintroducing new foods.

1. Dairy (fat-free and reduced-fat milk, yogurt, cheese, etc.)

2. Wheat products (preferably whole wheat bread, pasta, cereal, and more) and other whole grains

3. Increased portions of daily cooked vegetables (noncruciferous)

4. More daily fruit

5. Whole nuts and seeds

6. Garlic and onion

7. Starchy beans and lentils

8. Cooked cruciferous vegetables

9. Raw vegetables

10. Ketchup, soy sauce, and other condiments (test one at a time)

11. Dried fruit and all-fruit jam

12. Fruit juice, sugar, and honey

13. Chocolate

14. Coffee or tea

15. Alcohol

## BREAKFAST OPTIONS

(300 TO 400 CALORIES)

### Oatmeal with Strawberries and Ground Flaxseed

Prepare ½ cup dry *oats with water and top with 1 cup sliced *strawberries and 2 tablespoons ground *flaxseed.

### Cold Cereal with Banana and Soy Milk

Mix 1½ cups puffed rice cereal with 1 cup soy milk (or almond or rice milk) and top with 1 sliced *banana (or 1 cup *berries) and 1 to 2 tablespoons ground *flaxseed.

### Banana Almond Muffin with Scrambled Eggs

Beat 2 whole eggs with 2 egg whites and preferred seasonings and scramble in a hot skillet coated with oil spray. Enjoy with 1 *Banana Almond Muffin (page 412) or 2 rice cakes, each topped with 1 teaspoon soft tub, trans-fat-free spread.

## LUNCH OPTIONS

(400 TO 500 CALORIES)

### Curried Chicken Salad with Sweet Green Peas and Rice Cakes

Enjoy 1 serving *Curried Chicken Salad with Sweet Green Peas (page 413) divided over 2 rice cakes. Serve with 1 *orange or ½ *grapefruit.

### Turkey and Avocado on Rice Cakes

Divide 5 ounces sliced turkey (or chicken) over 2 rice cakes and top each with 1 thin slice *avocado. Serve with 1 cup *berries (blackberries, raspberries, sliced strawberries) or 1 *orange.

### Turkey Burger with Sweet Potato

Top a 5-ounce bunless turkey burger with ½ cup mushrooms sautéed in oil spray. Serve with 1 plain medium baked *sweet potato or 1 serving *Whipped Cinnamon Sweet Potatoes (page 314).

## DINNER OPTIONS

(500 TO 600 CALORIES)

### Salmon with Green Peas and Rice

Enjoy 1 serving Easy! 3-Step Microwave Salmon (page 345; omit the garlic) or 5 ounces grilled salmon, sole, cod, haddock, or tilapia with 1 teaspoon olive oil and other preferred seasonings. Serve with ½ cup *green peas mixed with ½ cup cooked *brown or wild rice.

### Rosemary Chicken with Sautéed Spinach and Sweet Potato

Enjoy 5 ounces grilled Rosemary Chicken (page 347), 1 cup *spinach sautéed in 1 teaspoon olive oil with a pinch of kosher salt and pepper, and 1 plain medium baked *sweet potato or 1 serving *Whipped Cinnamon Sweet Potatoes (page 314).

### Roast Turkey with Cooked Carrots and Brown Rice

Enjoy 5 ounces roast turkey with 1 cup cooked *carrots and 1 cup cooked brown or wild rice (or 1 plain medium *sweet or *white potato topped with 1 tablespoon soft tub, trans-fat-free spread).

## SNACK OPTIONS

100 CALORIES OR LESS

◆ *IBS-friendly fruit rich in soluble fiber:* 1 banana or orange; 1 cup berries (sliced strawberries, blackberries, raspberries); ½ grapefruit; 2 tangerines or clementines; 20 whole strawberries

◆ 1 hard-cooked egg (or 4 egg whites)

◆ 1 rice cake topped with 1 teaspoon nut butter

## 100 TO 200 CALORIES

◆ 100 to 200 calories' worth of plain rice crackers

◆ 1 ounce baked potato chips

◆ ½ baked *sweet or *white potato with 1 teaspoon soft tub, trans-fat-free spread (or 1 tablespoon guacamole)

◆ 2 rice cakes, each topped with 1 teaspoon nut butter

◆ 2 rice cakes, each topped with 1 tablespoon guacamole

◆ 8 ounces soy, almond, or rice milk

◆ 1 *Banana Almond Muffin (page 412)

◆ ½ cup *oats prepared with water, topped with ½ cup *berries or ½ sliced *banana

◆ *Strawberry-Banana Smoothie: Combine 1 full cup strawberries (fresh or frozen), ½ medium banana, ¾ cup soy milk (or almond or rice milk), and 3 to 5 ice cubes in a blender and puree until smooth.

# Banana Almond Muffins

*A muffin works well as an on-the-go snack, or enjoy one fresh from the oven, with scrambled eggs for breakfast. For only 180 calories per muffin, you'll get great taste and 4 grams of IBS-friendly soluble fiber.*

**MAKES 12**

½ cup granulated white sugar (may substitute with sugar substitute)

½ cup soft tub, reduced-fat, trans-fat-free spread

2 egg whites

3 bananas, mashed (about 1½ cups)

¼ cup water

1 teaspoon almond extract

1 teaspoon vanilla extract

½ cup barley flour (or oat flour)

½ cup ground flaxseed

2 teaspoons baking powder

½ teaspoon baking soda

1 teaspoon ground cinnamon

Preheat the oven to 350°F. Line 12 cups of a muffin pan with paper liners.

In a large bowl, mix the sugar and soft tub spread. Add the egg whites, one at a time, mixing well after each addition. Stir in the banana, water, almond extract, and vanilla. Add the flour, flaxseed, baking powder, baking soda, and cinnamon. Stir until the flour is just combined, but do not overmix.

Fill each muffin cup half full with the batter. Bake for 13 to 16 minutes, or until the tops of the muffins are lightly browned and a toothpick comes out clean when inserted in the center. Turn the muffins out onto a wire rack to cool. Once cooled, the muffins can be stored in an airtight container at room temperature for up to 2 days or frozen for up to 1 month.

**Per muffin (based on using real sugar):** 180 calories, 4 g protein, 30 g carbohydrate, 5 g fat (0.5 g saturated), 0 mg cholesterol, 170 mg sodium, 4 g fiber

# Whipped Cinnamon Sweet Potatoes

*Sweet potatoes are nutritional gems! They provide a slew of vitamins and minerals, along with a hearty dose of soluble fiber—good news for IBS sufferers. This supersimple side dish is a nice variation on standard baked sweet potatoes.*

**MAKES 4 SERVINGS**

4 medium sweet potatoes

2 tablespoons soft tub, trans-fat-free, reduced-fat spread (or whipped butter)

2 tablespoons soy milk (or almond or rice milk)

½ to 1 teaspoon ground cinnamon

Kosher salt

Microwave the sweet potatoes on high for 15 minutes, or until fully cooked. Let the potatoes cool, then peel and place the flesh in a large mixing bowl. Add the spread, soy milk, and cinnamon and mash thoroughly. Season with salt to taste.

> **Per serving:** 198 calories, 3 g protein, 40 g carbohydrate, 3 g fat (0.5 g saturated), 0 mg cholesterol, 150 mg sodium, 6 g fiber

# Curried Chicken Salad with Sweet Green Peas

*Try this interesting twist on chicken salad—it's incredibly flavorful yet gentle on the stomach. And thanks to the addition of green peas, your system receives the perfect amount of soluble fiber. Bonus: Use last night's leftover cooked chicken and you'll have the salad ready in minutes.*

**MAKES 1 SERVING**

½ cup frozen green peas

5 ounces cooked chicken breast, shredded or chopped

1 tablespoon reduced-fat mayonnaise

1 teaspoon curry powder

Rinse the green peas in a colander under cold water until thawed. Mash the chicken breast and gently mix it with the mayo, curry powder, and peas.

> **Per serving:** 320 calories, 48 g protein, 11 g carbohydrate, 8 g fat (1.5 g saturated), 120 mg cholesterol, 310 mg sodium, 3 g fiber

# CHAPTER 18

# CELIAC DISEASE

eliac disease tends to take everyone by surprise—both those who receive the diagnosis and family doctors who are shocked when a physically robust patient's blood work comes back positive for the disease. A couple of decades ago, the stereotypical celiac patient was a pale, malnourished child, someone who wouldn't be out of place in a Charles Dickens novel eating gruel and wasting away in an orphanage. However, as screening tests become more sophisticated, we're learning that celiac disease is surprisingly common, affecting about one in every 100 people in the United States. According to a 2009 study, celiac disease is more than four times more prevalent today than it was in the 1950s. Researchers can't yet explain this dramatic rise in incidence.

Celiac disease can begin at any time in a person's life, and there is no consistent set of symptoms. Some people lose a tremendous amount of weight; others experience fatigue, joint pain, or seizures; and sometimes there are no symptoms at all and the disease is discovered quite by chance. In fact, people often learn they have celiac disease when their doctors investigate possible causes for unexplained anemia or nutrient deficiencies. One minute you feel fine and you're having blood drawn for tests during a routine physical examination, and the next you're facing nonnegotiable changes to your eating habits or the possibility of complications. If that scenario sounds familiar, you're actually lucky to have caught the disease. If celiac remains undiagnosed or untreated, it can lead to osteoporosis, reproductive problems, skin rashes, epilepsy, and even some cancers. The good news is that celiac disease is currently treated entirely with dietary changes, so feeling better is as simple as knowing which foods are toxic to your gut.

## WHAT AFFECTS CELIAC DISEASE?

Celiac disease (also called celiac sprue, nontropical sprue, and gluten-sensitive enteropathy) is genetic. All individuals who develop celiac are born with a genetic predisposition for the disease, but the age of onset can vary from infancy to old age. Some people are diagnosed at birth or during childhood, but in many people, the disease lies dormant until it is triggered later in life. No one knows exactly what causes celiac disease to become active, but experts believe that times of extreme emotional or physical stress—including surgery, a viral infection, pregnancy, or childbirth—can set the stage. Researchers are also beginning to explore whether changes in the types of bacteria living in your gut may be the spark that initiates adult-onset celiac.

It's important to remember that celiac disease is *not* a food allergy. Some people call it an allergy as a shorthand way to explain why those with a diagnosis need to avoid certain foods, but that description is both misleading and dangerous. Celiac disease is an autoimmune disorder, a category of diseases in which the body's immune system attacks itself. The immune system reacts to a protein called gluten, which is found in wheat, and related proteins found in rye and barley.

When even the smallest amount of gluten enters the digestive system, it sets in motion a cascade of inflammatory processes. The immune system begins to attack the body's own tissue, resulting in damage to the small intestine, which is not merely a smooth tube connecting the stomach to the colon. The inner lining of the small intestine is jam-packed with protruding ridges called villi, which absorb nutrients as food passes through. Celiac disease causes inflammation that damages and sometimes destroys the villi, which means they can't do their job, and the nutrients your body needs pass through your digestive system unabsorbed and are eliminated in waste. The outcome of this damage varies depending on the extent of the disease. In mild cases, there are no overt symptoms, but blood tests might reveal a deficiency in certain nutrients, especially folate, vitamin $B_{12}$, or iron (which can result in anemia). Over time, poor calcium and vitamin D absorption can lead to osteoporosis. In some people, celiac disease causes embarrassing and sometimes life-altering gastrointestinal symptoms, including gas, bloating, diarrhea or constipation, and weight loss. Other problems associated with celiac disease include nerve damage, migraines, seizures, infertility or miscarriages, joint pain, and even some cancers, including non-Hodgkin lymphoma and cancer of the esophagus or small intestine. The longer celiac goes untreated, the greater the risk of harm.

## HOW FOOD AFFECTS CELIAC DISEASE

There is no cure for celiac disease, and at present, the only treatment is to eliminate gluten from your diet. If you follow a gluten-free diet strictly, your villi will eventually heal, and, with the right foods, you can replenish stores of the nutrients you've been missing. In terms of limiting damage, nutritional treatment for celiac disease is all about which foods to avoid. However, because the list of forbidden foods is so extensive, it is also critically important that you pay attention to the vitamins and minerals that most people normally get from gluten-containing foods and be sure your diet is rich in other sources.

## AVOIDING FOODS THAT CONTAIN GLUTEN

If you have an allergy to cats or you know people who do, you've probably noticed that not every cat-allergy sufferer suffers in the same way. Some people start to sneeze if they are just in the same house with a cat, while others remain sneeze free until they bury their face in the animal's fur. That's not the case with celiac disease. Even the tiniest bit of gluten—the amount found in ⅛ teaspoon of wheat flour—can signal the body's immune system to respond with a full attack. The tricky part of celiac disease is that damage can occur without you noticing much in the way of symptoms. But the longer you eat foods containing gluten, the further the damage will progress until eventually, you become noticeably sick.

I wish the guidelines for avoiding gluten were as easy as telling you to stop eating wheat, barley, and rye flour. That's part of what you need to do, but it is much more complicated than that. There are many hidden sources of gluten, and beyond that, some naturally gluten-free products can be contaminated with gluten.

Here are lists of foods, ingredients, and additives to avoid. Study this list carefully and refer to it often. Eventually, you'll have the foods memorized.

## COMMON FOODS THAT CONTAIN GLUTEN

Barley (and anything with the word *barley* in it, such as barley malt)

Beer (all types)

Bleached flour

Blue cheese (sometimes made with bread mold)

Bran (also called wheat bran)

Bread flour

Bulgur

Cake flour

Communion wafers

Couscous

Cracker meal

Croutons

Durum

Farina

Farro

Flour (this usually means wheat flour)

Gluten, glutenin

Graham flour

Groats

Kamut

Malt (and anything with the word *malt* in it, such as rice malt, malt extract, or malt flavoring)

Malt beverages

Matzo

Oats and oat bran (see "The Oatmeal Question," page 426)

Orzo

Pasta (all varieties made with wheat, wheat starch, oats, barley, rye, or any ingredient on this list)

Rye (and anything with the word *rye* in it)

Seitan

Semolina

Soy sauce (check ingredients—it's often made with wheat)

Spelt

Suet

Tabbouleh

Teriyaki sauce

Triticale

Triticum

Unbleached flour

Vital gluten

Wheat (and anything with the word *wheat* in it, such as wheat grass, wheat berries, wheat germ, wheat starch; buckwheat is okay and is the only exception)

## LESS COMMON FOODS AND FOOD ADDITIVES THAT CONTAIN GLUTEN

Abyssinian hard (a wheat product)

Amp-isostearoyl hydrolyzed wheat

Brewer's yeast

Cereal binding

Cereal extract

Dextrimaltose

Dinkel

Disodium wheatgermamido Peg-2 sulfosuccinate

Edible starch

Einkorn

Emmer

Filler

Fu

Granary flour

Mir

Udon (wheat noodles)

Whole-meal flour

## FOODS AND FOOD ADDITIVES THAT *MAY* CONTAIN GLUTEN

If a favorite food contains one of the following ingredients, contact the company and ask questions. Depending on the manufacturing process, these suspect ingredients can sometimes be gluten free.

Artificial color

Artificial flavoring

Bouillon cubes

Brown rice syrup

Caramel color

Coloring

Dextrins

Dried fruit (may be dusted with wheat)

Flavored coffee

Flavored vinegar

Flavoring

Food starch

Glucose syrup

Gravy cubes

Ground spices (wheat is sometimes added to prevent clumping)

Hydrolyzed plant protein (HPP)

Hydrolyzed vegetable protein (HVP)

Maltodextrin

Maltose

Miso

Modified food starch

Modified starch

Monoglycerides and diglycerides

Monosodium glutamate (MSG)

Mustard powder (some brands contain gluten; check ingredients)

Natural flavoring

Processed cheese (check ingredients)

Processed meats (cold cuts, hot dogs, sausages, and canned meats that contain wheat, barley, rye, oats, gluten fillers, or stabilizers)

Rice malt

Rice syrup

Seasonings (including powdered flavorings and dustings on chips, nuts, popcorn, rice mixes, and rice cakes)

Smoke flavoring

Soba noodles

Starch

Stock/bouillon cubes

Surimi (imitation seafood)

Textured vegetable protein (TVP)

Vegetable starch

Vitamins

## TIPS FOR HEALTHY EATING WITH CELIAC DISEASE

◆ **Don't cheat.** I can't say this strongly enough. A minuscule amount of gluten can cause real damage to your small intestine. A single cookie, half a slice of bread, even a single cracker is toxic to your system.

# FAQS

## I just found out I have celiac disease, and it seems as though I have to spend hours at the grocery store reading labels. Does it ever get any easier?

Yes, it does get easier. You have a lot of new information to assimilate, but it's knowledge that will serve you forever. Most people with celiac disease need to see a registered dietitian only two or three times—after that, they understand exactly what they need to do to live a gluten-free life. I highly recommend consulting with a dietitian who specializes in celiac disease to get a handle on the details. Also, check out the natural foods aisle at your supermarket. Thanks to an increasing awareness of celiac disease, most mainstream grocery stores now offer a variety of gluten-free foods that are conveniently labeled. Specific health food stores, such as Whole Foods and Trader Joe's, have an even broader selection. If it's tough to find gluten-free products in your area, you can certainly shop online. The Gluten-Free Mall (www.glutenfreemall.com) offers a wide selection of gluten-free products, and Bob's Red Mill (www.bobsredmill.com), Arrowhead Mills (www.arrowheadmills.com), and Udi's (www.udisglutenfree.com) sell a variety of gluten-free grains, baking mixes, and/or breads. Even mainstream sites like Amazon now sell an abundance of gluten-free goods.

If you're struggling emotionally with the transition to a gluten-free lifestyle, you might find it helpful to talk with a psychologist or counselor. Some people need time to mourn the loss of their favorite foods or their vision of themselves as indestructible. One or two sessions with a professional can mean the difference between fighting the change and embarking on a journey of discovery. Read everything, join a celiac disease support group (in person or online), befriend your health care professionals, and don't be afraid to ask questions. In addition, there are many wonderful resources to help you and those you love with celiac disease, regardless of whether the disease was diagnosed last week or ten years ago. Visit my Web site at www.joybauer.com/celiac for printable lists of foods to avoid and include, gluten-free recipes, and more. In addition, here are a few more informative Web sites for people with celiac.

1. The National Foundation for Celiac Awareness (www.celiaccentral.org). This site offers a plethora of resources, including printable information on gluten-free foods, medications, and other topics, along with recipes and frequently asked questions that have been answered by registered dietitians.

2. The Celiac Disease Foundation (www.celiac.org). This is a great resource, especially as a launching point for people who have recently been diagnosed with celiac disease.

3. Celiac.com (www.celiac.com). The best feature on this site is the online forum with message boards where families affected by celiac disease can exchange information on gluten-free products and strategies for coping with the disease, among other subjects.

◆ **Don't cheat, part 2.** If you ever eat in a restaurant or at a friend's house, or if you cook with any jarred, canned, or packaged foods not labeled "gluten-free," you will inevitably ingest some gluten from time to time. There is really nothing you can do about it. I call this unintentional cheating because I know you don't mean to do it. Just don't expose your intestines to more toxic gluten by *consciously* cheating.

◆ **Whenever possible, choose packaged foods that are specifically labeled "gluten-free" ("GF").** Do not make the mistake of assuming that "wheat-free" or "yeast-free" means the same thing as "gluten-free." Read labels carefully, using the list of suspect ingredients as your guide. Fortunately, most supermarkets now carry a wide variety of gluten-free products, and many mainstream food companies have debuted gluten-free cereals, snacks, waffles, and other foods in the last few years.

## FAQS

### I have celiac disease. Will I have to follow a gluten-free diet for the rest of my life?

Maybe not forever—there are some exciting new therapies on the horizon. Immunotherapy is one of the most promising. With this treatment, people with celiac disease are exposed to small amounts of gluten in the form of injections under the skin. The hope is that with repeated injections, the immune system will gradually build up a tolerance to the offending gluten protein fragments, become desensitized, and no longer react when gluten is consumed as food. Immunotherapy is still in the early phases of testing in humans, so there's no consensus as yet on if and when it will be available to the public. That said, it's good to know there's a glimmer of hope for a "gluten-free"-free future!

◆ **Go easy on gluten-free baked goods.** Just like regular baked goods, gluten-free baked goods often contain unhealthy amounts of added fat and sugar. While gobbling down gluten-free muffins, cookies, and other sweet treats won't harm your intestines, it will pack on the pounds and drive up cholesterol.

◆ **Be a gluten sleuth.** Everything that goes in your mouth or touches your tongue needs to be screened for gluten. Read labels on vitamin supplements, toothpaste, mouthwash, cough medicine, and all over-the-counter medications. Talk with your pharmacist so that your prescription medications can be chosen with your special needs in mind (and look up gluten-free medicines at www.celiaccentral .org or www.celiac.com). Also, don't lick postage stamps or envelopes—the glue can contain gluten.

◆ **Avoid all uncertainties, including bulk bins and fried food in restaurants.** In other words, if you don't know, it's a no-go. Foods that are sold from bulk bins may contain gluten, no matter how they are marked. The problem is that you have no way of knowing what sort of food was in the bin before the food you are buying. You may think you're buying dried beans and dried beans alone, but you may also be getting dust from the bulgur wheat that was in the bin last week. The safest choice is to buy only packaged goods labeled "gluten-free" or foods with no suspect ingredients on the label. In restaurants, avoid fried foods. Even if the food itself doesn't contain gluten, the fry oil may have remnants of breading or other gluten-containing foods. Sauces, gravies, and other toppings may also contain gluten. You are safest if you eat pure, fresh, whole foods from sources you can trust. Foods that are generally considered safe for people with celiac disease are noted on the grocery list beginning on page 423.

♦ **Beware of contamination in your own home.** In nearly every jar of jam or tub of margarine are bread crumbs left behind by the last person to dip a knife or spoon into them. You have two choices: Either stock your own private pantry that other family members know is for your consumption alone, or make sure that everyone in the household uses only fresh, clean utensils to spoon out products.

## BONUS POINTS

♦ **Get regular screenings.** Experts recommend that all adults with celiac disease get annual blood screenings for ferritin (a measure of the amount of iron stored in the body), folate, vitamin $B_{12}$, and thyroid-stimulating hormone (TSH, a measure of how well the thyroid is working). In addition, you will probably be tested for calcium absorption, which is measured by a test called a 24-hour urine catch. This test is exactly what it sounds like—you urinate into a special container every time you use the bathroom during a 24-hour test period. These tests will allow you and your doctor to track how well your intestines have healed.

♦ **Ask your doctor if you should have a bone density scan.** Long-term malabsorption of calcium can lead to osteoporosis, the thinning and weakening of bones. But osteoporosis often goes unnoticed. If a scan shows your bones are strong, it will be one less thing for you to worry about, and you'll have a good baseline measure for future reference. If your bones show signs of thinning, you and your doctor can begin a treatment plan.

♦ **Urge family members to get tested.** Celiac disease is genetic, so first- and second-degree relatives should all be tested. People with autoimmune disorders, such as type 1 diabetes or Hashimoto's disease, also have an increased risk of celiac disease and should be tested.

♦ **If you are pregnant or recently had a baby:** Remember that your child may or may not have inherited celiac disease along with your soulful eyes. I highly encourage breastfeeding, which seems to offer some protection from celiac disease and other autoimmune disorders.

◆ **Take advantage of new technology.** Check out some of the gluten-free apps available for smartphones and tablets. The most popular ones offer extensive databases of foods that you can search for verified gluten-free products and restaurant menu options. Just another terrific example of how technology makes life easier!

## SUPPLEMENTS

If you have been diagnosed with celiac disease, I strongly advise you to consider taking the following supplements.

1. **A multivitamin.** Because a gluten-free diet is limited and may have some nutritional gaps, I recommend a good general multivitamin that provides about 100 percent DV of most vitamins and minerals and at least 800 IU of vitamin D.

2. **Calcium, plus vitamin D.** Because many people with celiac disease have experienced malabsorption of calcium over the years, I urge women with celiac to speak with their physicians about whether it's necessary to take a separate calcium supplement with vitamin $D_3$. Because too much calcium has been linked to an increased risk of prostate cancer, if you're male and have celiac, it's less likely that you'll be a candidate for calcium supplements, but speak with your physician. For more specific information on calcium supplements (including dosages and various forms), see page 233 in the Osteoporosis chapter.

## FAQS

**I'm thinking about going on a gluten-free diet to lose weight. Will eliminating gluten help me shed more pounds?**

No, not really. "Going gluten free" has become quite trendy, but the truth is, unless you have been diagnosed with celiac or have a gluten intolerance, cutting out gluten will not offer any health advantage or directly enhance your weight-loss efforts. However, when you eliminate gluten from your diet, you eliminate many of the starchy, high-cal foods that people tend to overeat, including bread, pasta, cookies, cakes, pastries, crackers, and other snack foods made with wheat flour. Ditching these foods can definitely help you save calories and drop a few pounds, but it's a wash if you're replacing them with their gluten-free counterparts. When it comes to losing weight, it's always a smart strategy to limit bread, pasta, and baked goods (especially the white, refined products), but there's no need to eliminate all traces of gluten or unnecessarily ban yourself from enjoying a slice of whole wheat toast or a bowl of vegetable-barley soup. Strictly following a gluten-free diet can be demanding and time-consuming, so unless you have a medical reason to avoid gluten, there's really no need to add that extra level of stress.

In summary, if you have not been diagnosed with celiac disease and are not gluten intolerant, there's no reason for you to cut gluten out of your diet—for weight loss or for any other purpose. For a rock-solid weight-loss plan to help you reach your goal, see Chapter 3 on page 17.

## FAQS

### What are your specific recommendations for staying gluten free while dining out?

Thanks to an increasing awareness of celiac disease, it's become much easier to identify gluten-free options while dining out. Many popular chain restaurants have special gluten-free menus available on request, and you should definitely make use of gluten-free Web sites and mobile apps when dining out to make the ordering process even easier. Of course, there's always a big risk of cross-contamination in restaurant kitchens, so be very, very clear with your ordering instructions, and strongly emphasize that your requests are related to a serious medical condition.

For restaurants that don't offer specific gluten-free options, here are a few basic suggestions that can be found in most restaurants.

**Appetizers:** Vegetable salad with olive oil and balsamic or red wine vinegar requested on the side, or sliced tomatoes and mozzarella. Avoid prepared vinaigrette dressings.

**Entrées:** Grilled, broiled, baked, or roasted skinless chicken or fish (seasoned with olive oil, salt, pepper, and lemon)

**Unlimited Vegetables:** Anything goes, steamed or sautéed in olive oil and garlic.

**Starches:** Plain baked sweet or white potato, plain brown or wild rice, polenta, corn grits, beans, or lentils. Take advantage if a restaurant offers quinoa, amaranth, or millet on the menu.

**Dessert:** Fresh fruit

3. **Additional supplements, as directed by a physician.** Once you are diagnosed with celiac, blood work will indicate which extra supplements you might need to take in order to avoid nutrient deficiencies. Additional supplements should be taken only if they're recommended by a doctor and only for as long as the doctor recommends—too much of a good thing can be harmful. For example, even though many people with newly diagnosed celiac disease have anemia, taking high doses of iron for prolonged periods can cause iron toxicity.

For more helpful information on maintaining your gluten-free lifestyle, visit www.joybauer.com/celiac.

# JOY'S 4-STEP PROGRAM
## FOR CELIAC DISEASE

Follow this program if you have celiac disease.

## Step 1 ... START WITH THE BASICS

These are the first things you should do to take control of celiac disease.

◆ Make sure you thoroughly understand what foods and additives to avoid. If you have any questions or problems following a gluten-free diet, make an appointment with a dietitian who specializes in celiac disease. He or she will answer every question in as much detail as you need.

◆ Review all of the products in your kitchen pantry, refrigerator, freezer, and bathroom medicine cabinet, including medications, toothpaste, and mouthwash. Read the ingredients on all food labels. Find ways to separate safe products from those that contain gluten.

◆ Don't cheat!

◆ Talk with your doctor about the value of screening for bone density, anemia, and other nutrient deficiencies.

◆ Consider taking a multivitamin. If you're a woman, also consider a separate calcium supplement containing vitamin $D_3$.

## Step 2 ... YOUR ULTIMATE GROCERY LIST

Controlling celiac disease is not so much about foods you should eat as foods you shouldn't eat. The foods on this list are considered to be generally safe for people with celiac. You'll need to carefully check labels on all foods marked with an asterisk (*) because ingredients can vary from brand to brand. Because most of the popular grains contain gluten, it is important to try new, safe whole grains. You'll also need to eat plenty of vegetables and fruits to make sure that you get a wide variety of naturally occurring vitamins, minerals, fiber, and antioxidants. Toward the end of the grocery list, I've listed additives and ingredients that are also thought to be safe.

For a printable version of this list, visit www.joybauer.com/celiac.

## FRUIT

*All* fresh fruits

*All* frozen whole fruits with no additives

## VEGETABLES AND LEGUMES

*All* fresh vegetables

*All* frozen vegetables with no additives, breading, or sauces

*Beans, canned

Beans, lentils, and peas, dried

Olives

Potatoes (all varieties)

*Pumpkin (100% canned puree)

## SEAFOOD

*All* fresh fish and shellfish

*All* frozen fish and shellfish with no additives or sauces

## LEAN PROTEINS

*All* fresh meats and poultry with no breading or additives

*All* frozen meats and poultry with no breading or additives

Eggs

Tofu

## NUTS AND SEEDS (PREFERABLY UNSALTED)

*All* natural nut butters

*All* nuts

*All* seeds (except barley and rye)

## GRAINS, CEREALS, PASTA, AND MORE

Amaranth

Arrowroot starch

Buckwheat

*Cereals, dry (puffed and flake varieties made with amaranth, buckwheat, corn, millet, rice, or soy)

*Cereals, hot (cream and flake varieties made with amaranth, buckwheat, cornmeal, hominy grits, quinoa, rice, or soy)

Corn bran

Corn chips, plain

Corn flour/cornmeal products

Crackers, gluten-free (such as brown rice, corn, and lentil)

Flour: amaranth, buckwheat, carob, chickpea, lentil, millet, potato, quinoa, rice, sago, sorghum, soy, tapioca, and teff

Grits (corn and soy)

Kasha (not the same as Kashi)

Masa

Millet

Pasta made from beans, brown rice, corn, lentils, peas, potato, quinoa, or soy

Polenta

*Popcorn (air-popped and gluten-free packaged varieties)

## GRAINS, CEREALS, PASTA, AND MORE *continued*

Potato chips, plain or
  *flavored

Quinoa

Ragi

Rice (preferably brown or
  wild)

Rice cakes, plain

*Soba, 100% buckwheat

Sorghum

*Soy crisps

*Tacos shells made with
  corn, hard and soft

Tapioca starch/flour

Teff

*Tortillas made with brown
  rice, corn, or soy

Tortilla chips, plain or
  *flavored

## DAIRY

*Cheese (preferably reduced-
  fat), not blue cheese

*Cottage cheese (preferably
  fat-free or 1%)

*Cream cheese (preferably
  reduced-fat)

*Ice cream (check labels;
  ingredients will vary from
  flavor to flavor)

Milk (preferably fat free or
  1%)

*Milk alternatives (almond,
  rice, soy)

*Sour cream (preferably
  fat-free or reduced-fat)

*Yogurt (preferably fat-free
  or low-fat)

## MISCELLANEOUS

*All* pure herbs (check
  ingredients of *herb
  mixes)

*All* pure spices (check
  ingredients of *spice
  mixes)

Apple cider vinegar

Baking chocolate

Baking powder

Baking soda

Canola oil

Cocoa powder

Coffee, ground and instant
  (check ingredients of
  *flavored coffees)

Cornstarch

Corn syrup

Cream of tartar

Garlic

Gelatin

Honey

*Hummus (check labels;
  ingredients will vary from
  flavor to flavor)

Jam and jelly

*Ketchup

Maple syrup

*Mayonnaise (preferably
  reduced-fat)

Molasses

*Mustard

Olive oil

Pickles

Relish

*Salsa

* Soft tub spread, trans-fat-
  free (reduced-fat and
  regular)

Sugar

Tea, black and green (check
  *flavored and herbal tea
  varieties)

Vanilla and other extracts

Vinegar (balsamic, red wine,
  and white)

Wine (red and white)

*The asterisk (*) indicates foods whose labels need to be carefully checked for gluten.

## SAFE (GLUTEN-FREE) ADDITIVES

| | | |
|---|---|---|
| Acacia gum | Aspic | Methylcellulose |
| Adipic acid | Astragalus gummifer | Microcrystallin cellulose |
| Agar | Benzoic acid | Pectin |
| Algae | BHA | Pepsin |
| Algin/alginate | BTA | Stearic acid |
| Allicin | Dextrose | Sulfites |
| Annatto | Ester gum | Tapioca starch/flour (not pudding) |
| Arabic gum | Fructose | |
| Arrowroot | Guar gum | Whey |
| Ascorbic acid | Locust bean gum | Xanthan gum |
| Aspartame | Malic acid | |

*The asterisk (*) indicates foods whose labels need to be carefully checked for gluten.

# Step 3 . . . GOING ABOVE AND BEYOND

There really is no "above and beyond" for people with celiac disease. The treatment is to stop eating gluten-containing foods and consider taking supplements to fill in any nutritional gaps. However, there are some things you can do to be helpful to others who may be at risk.

◆ Recommend that first- and second-degree relatives get tested for celiac.

◆ If you are pregnant or have a child, talk with the pediatrician so that he or she can be aware of your child's increased risk.

## THE OATMEAL QUESTION

Although oats are naturally gluten free, they can be contaminated with wheat during the growing, milling, or packaging processes. If you want to add oats to your diet, here are some guidelines.

■ Choose Bob's Red Mill certified gluten-free oats, which are grown on dedicated oat farms, processed in a gluten-free facility, and tested multiple times for gluten. You can also ask your doctor for another dedicated gluten-free brand recommendation.

■ Never order oats when you're at a restaurant, and don't buy prepared or packaged foods that contain oats.

# Step4 . . . MEAL PLANS

These sample menus include nutrient-rich foods that have proven generally safe for people with celiac disease.

Every day, choose one option for each of the three meals—breakfast, lunch, and dinner. Then, once or twice per day, choose from my suggested snacks. Approximate calories have been provided to help adjust for your personal weight-management goals. If you find yourself hungry (and if weight is not an issue), feel free to increase the portion sizes for meals and snacks. Beverage calories are not included.

You can also prepare some of the delicious recipes in my other chapters by simply substituting gluten-free ingredients when necessary. And always remember to check every ingredient listed on condiments, spreads, and other prepared food. Enjoy!

## BREAKFAST OPTIONS

(300 TO 400 CALORIES)

### Berry-Nut Yogurt Parfait

Spoon ⅓ cup fat-free yogurt into a parfait glass. Top with 2 heaping tablespoons berries and 1 tablespoon chopped nuts or seeds (walnuts, pecans, peanuts, slivered almonds, sunflower seeds, or ground flaxseed). Repeat the three layers (yogurt, berries, and then nuts) two times.

### Cold Cereal with Milk and Fruit

Mix 1 cup gluten-free cereal with 1 tablespoon ground flaxseed and 1 cup milk (fat-free, 1%, or soy/almond/rice). Enjoy with ½ sliced banana (or ½ grapefruit or 1 orange).

### Cantaloupe with Cottage Cheese and Sunflower Seeds

Fill ½ cantaloupe with 1 cup fat-free or 1% cottage cheese and sprinkle with 1 tablespoon sunflower seeds or chopped nuts (walnuts, pecans, almonds, peanuts, or cashews).

### Mexican Breakfast Spud

Split 1 medium baked potato and fill with scrambled eggs (beat 1 whole egg with 2 egg whites and cook in a hot skillet coated with oil spray). Season eggs with preferred herbs to taste and top with 2 heaping tablespoons salsa (check salsa ingredients).

### Apple Slices with Peanut Butter

Top 1 sliced apple (or banana) with 2 tablespoons peanut butter. Or toast 1 slice gluten-free bread, top with 1 level tablespoon peanut butter, and serve with 1 banana or apple.

### Scrambled Eggs with Broccoli and Cheese

Beat 1 whole egg with 2 egg whites and cook in a hot skillet coated with oil spray. When the eggs are almost cooked, add 1 cup cooked broccoli florets and 1 ounce (¼ cup) shredded reduced-fat cheese. Enjoy with ½ grapefruit (or ½ banana, ½ mango, or 1 orange).

### Tropical Mango-Citrus Smoothie with Rice Cakes and Cottage Cheese

Enjoy 1 serving (2 cups) Tropical Mango-Citrus Smoothie (page 114) with 2 plain rice cakes, each topped with sliced tomato and 1 heaping tablespoon fat-free or 1% cottage cheese.

### Apple Cinnamon Pancakes with Lemon Yogurt Topping

Enjoy 1 serving (page 433).

## LUNCH OPTIONS

(400 TO 500 CALORIES)

### Turkey Sandwich with Avocado

Layer 4 ounces fresh turkey (or chicken), 2 thin slices avocado, lettuce, tomato, and onion between 2 slices gluten-free bread (or on 2 or 3 rice cakes, or wrap in a gluten-free corn or brown rice tortilla). Spread with optional 1 tablespoon reduced-fat mayo, mustard, or hummus (check condiment ingredients). Enjoy with bell pepper strips and celery sticks.

### Grilled Chicken Salad with Apple and Walnuts

Mix 2 to 4 cups romaine lettuce and baby spinach leaves with unlimited preferred vegetables (chopped peppers, broccoli, sliced mushrooms, tomatoes, onions, cucumbers, carrots, or celery). Top with 4 ounces chopped skinless chicken and ½ chopped apple. Toss with 1 tablespoon chopped walnuts, plus 2 teaspoons olive oil and unlimited vinegar or fresh lemon juice. Season with a pinch of salt and pepper.

### Turkey Burger with Baked Potato

Top a 5-ounce turkey burger (or lean hamburger) with sliced tomato, onion, and 2 tablespoons ketchup (check ingredients). Enjoy with ½ plain baked sweet or white potato and optional 1 to 2 tablespoons reduced-fat sour cream (check ingredients).

### Tomato-Cheese Omelet with Toast and Veggies

Beat 1 whole egg with 2 or 3 egg whites. Cook in a heated skillet coated with oil spray. Add a few tablespoons chopped tomatoes and optional dried or fresh basil. When the bottom is cooked, gently flip over. Sprinkle with 1 ounce shredded reduced-fat cheese, fold the omelet in half, and continue cooking until the egg mixture firms and the cheese melts. Enjoy with 1 slice gluten-free bread, toasted and topped with optional 1 teaspoon soft tub, trans-fat-free spread and unlimited baby carrots or sugar snap peas.

### Lentil Soup with Rice Cakes

Enjoy 2 cups lentil or black bean soup (any gluten-free brand) with 2 rice cakes topped with sliced tomato and onion.

### Chicken Tortilla with Tri-Colored Peppers

Sauté red, yellow, and green pepper strips in 1 teaspoon olive or canola oil until soft. Season with a pinch of salt and ground black pepper. Layer 1 tortilla (any gluten-free brand, 150 calories or less) with large lettuce leaves, the sautéed peppers, and 4 ounces cooked skinless chicken. Fold in ends and roll tightly. Enjoy with unlimited preferred vegetables (sliced cucumbers, cherry tomatoes, celery, baby carrots, peppers, green beans, and sugar snap peas).

### Stuffed Baked Potato with Broccoli and Cheese

Split and fill 1 medium baked white potato with cooked chopped broccoli. Top with 1 ounce (¼ cup) shredded reduced-fat cheese (or ½ cup fat-free or 1% cottage cheese). Heat in a 350°F oven or microwave until the cheese is melted. Serve with a mixed green salad tossed with 1 teaspoon olive oil and unlimited vinegar or fresh lemon juice.

## DINNER OPTIONS

(500 TO 600 CALORIES)

### Poached Red Snapper with Fresh Herbs and Vidalia Sweet Potatoes

Poach 6 ounces red snapper fillet in ⅔ cup water with 2 tablespoons each fresh parsley, dill, thyme, and rosemary. (Or season any favorite fish with preferred seasonings and lightly brush with olive oil; grill or pan-roast on medium-high for about 3 minutes on each side, or until golden brown—cooking times will vary depending on the fish.) Serve with 1 cup steamed Brussels sprouts, Swiss chard, asparagus, sugar snap peas, or green beans and 1 serving Vidalia Sweet Potatoes (page 434) or 1 medium baked sweet or white potato with optional 1 teaspoon soft tub, trans-fat-free spread or 2 tablespoons reduced-fat sour cream (check ingredients).

### Turkey Tacos

Enjoy 3 Turkey Tacos (page 244; use hard or soft corn taco shells and check ingredients on seasoning packet) with optional salsa and hot sauce.

### Sirloin Steak with Sautéed Spinach and Potato

Enjoy 5 ounces grilled sirloin steak (or pork tenderloin, fish, or chicken) with unlimited sautéed spinach in 1 teaspoon olive oil and garlic and ½ baked potato with optional 1 teaspoon soft tub, trans-fat-free spread or 2 tablespoons reduced-fat sour cream (check ingredients).

### Rosemary Chicken with Swiss Chard and Brown Rice

Enjoy 5 ounces Rosemary Chicken (page 347), or coat skinless chicken breast with preferred safe seasonings and grill, roast, bake, or lightly pan-fry. Serve with 1 cup Sautéed Swiss Chard (page 346), and 1 cup cooked brown or wild rice (or amaranth, quinoa, or millet).

### Grilled Salmon with Edamame and Broccoli

Enjoy 1 cup boiled edamame (green soybeans in the pod) with 1 serving Easy 3-Step Microwave Salmon (page 345), or grill 5 ounces wild salmon with 1 teaspoon olive oil and preferred safe seasonings. Serve with unlimited steamed broccoli or cauliflower.

### Turkey Chili

Top 2 cups (1 serving) Turkey Chili (page 363; when recipe calls for 2 teaspoons flour, use chickpea flour) with 2 tablespoons shredded reduced-fat cheese. Serve with ½ cup cooked brown or wild rice (or amaranth or quinoa or ½ plain baked potato) and an optional side salad with lettuce, mushrooms, cucumbers, peppers, and onions tossed with 1 teaspoon olive oil and unlimited vinegar or fresh lemon juice.

### Grilled Rockefeller Oysters with Cajun Fish and Asparagus

Enjoy 1 serving Grilled Rockefeller Oysters (page 179; when recipe calls for flour, use chickpea flour) with 6 ounces baked fish (tilapia, black cod, shrimp, wild salmon, or trout) rubbed with Cajun spice or preferred safe seasonings and baked, broiled, or grilled. Serve with a green salad tossed with 1 teaspoon olive oil and fresh lemon juice or balsamic vinegar and unlimited steamed asparagus, broccoli, green beans, cauliflower, spinach, or other preferred vegetable.

## SNACK OPTIONS

100 CALORIES OR LESS

- ◆ *Best Vegetable Snacks:* up to 2 cups raw or cooked bell peppers (red, green, or yellow), broccoli, sugar snap peas, tomatoes, carrots, asparagus, cauliflower, or green beans
- ◆ *Best Fruit Snacks:* 1 apple, small banana, orange, pear, peach, tangerine, persimmon, or guava; 2 clementines, kiwifruit, or plums; ½ papaya, mango, grapefruit, or cantaloupe; 1 cup berries (all varieties), cherries, or grapes; 1 cup cubed watermelon, honeydew, or pineapple; ½ cup lychees; 20 whole strawberries
- ◆ 1 cup fat-free milk
- ◆ 1 string cheese or 1 ounce reduced-fat cheese
- ◆ 1 hard-cooked egg (or 4 egg whites)

◆ 1 rice cake with 1 level teaspoon natural peanut butter (or other nut butter)

◆ 1 level tablespoon natural peanut butter (or other nut butter) with celery sticks

◆ 10 almonds

## 100 TO 200 CALORIES

◆ 1 ounce potato chips, tortilla chips, soy crisps, or vegetable chips (check ingredients)

◆ Pumpkin pudding: Mix a 6-ounce container fat-free vanilla yogurt with ½ cup canned 100% pure pumpkin and optional cinnamon.

◆ ½ cup frozen yogurt or low-fat ice cream (any gluten-free brand)

◆ 1 Gluten-Free Gingerbread Muffin (page 435)

◆ 2 cups Tropical Mango-Citrus Smoothie (page 114)

◆ 2 cups Strawberry-Kiwi Smoothie (page 114)

◆ Everyday Fruit Smoothie: In a blender, mix ½ cup fat-free milk (or soy milk), ½ cup fat-free yogurt, ¾ cup fresh or frozen fruit (such as berries, banana, peaches, or mango), and 3 to 5 ice cubes.

◆ 1 ounce nuts (about ¼ cup each): soy nuts, almonds, walnuts, pecans, cashews, or peanuts

◆ ½ cup sunflower seeds or pistachios in their shells

◆ 1 cup boiled edamame (green soybeans in the pod)

◆ 1 cup baby carrots and/or pepper strips with ¼ cup hummus (check ingredients)

◆ ½ cup fat-free or 1% cottage cheese mixed with 2 tablespoons ground flaxseed (or 1 tablespoon chopped nuts)

◆ Sliced apple with 1 level tablespoon natural peanut butter (or other nut butter)

◆ 10 almonds plus 1 fruit (see Best Fruit Snacks on page 431)

# APPLE-CINNAMON PANCAKES WITH LEMON YOGURT TOPPING

*Nobody should have to live without pancakes! While testing this gluten-free version, ten "nonceliac" breakfast guests confirmed that scrumptious flapjacks do not need all-purpose wheat flour. Enjoy the pancakes, which include extra calcium and fiber.*

**MAKES 4 SERVINGS (3 PANCAKES AND ¼ CUP TOPPING EACH)**

**Topping**

1 cup fat-free plain yogurt

1 tablespoon grated lemon zest

1 tablespoon honey

1 teaspoon vanilla extract

1 teaspoon ground cinnamon

**Pancakes**

1 cup buckwheat flour

1 cup fat-free milk

1 egg white

¼ cup fat-free plain yogurt

1 tablespoon honey

2 teaspoons vanilla extract

1 teaspoon ground cinnamon

⅛ teaspoon ground nutmeg

½ teaspoon baking soda

1 cup diced apple

1 tablespoon canola oil

**To make the topping:** In a small bowl, whisk together the yogurt, lemon zest, honey, vanilla, and cinnamon. Set aside.

**To make the pancakes:** In a blender, combine the flour, milk, egg white, yogurt, honey, vanilla, cinnamon, nutmeg, and baking soda. Blend until smooth. Stir in the apple.

Spray a griddle or large frying pan with oil spray. Add the oil and heat over medium-high. When the oil is hot but not smoking, ladle about 2 tablespoons of the batter onto the griddle for each pancake. Cook for 2 to 3 minutes, or until small bubbles form around the edge. Flip the pancakes and cook for 2 to 3 minutes longer, or until the centers are cooked through. Serve immediately with the topping.

**Per serving:** 261 calories, 11 g protein, 45 g carbohydrate, 5 g fat (0 g saturated), 0 mg cholesterol, 260 mg sodium, 5 g fiber; plus 259 mg calcium (26% of DV)

# VIDALIA SWEET POTATOES

*When my producer at the Today show, Rainy Farrell, mentioned her delicious sweet potato dish, my mouth was watering! I knew it had to be included in the book. Her version was meant for the grill, but the weekend I got my hands on the recipe, it stormed nonstop and I was forced to create an indoor version. I hope you love it as much as I do.*

**MAKES 2 SERVINGS**

2 medium sweet potatoes (about 7 ounces each)

1 teaspoon garlic powder

Kosher salt

1 Vidalia onion, thinly sliced

4 teaspoons soft tub, reduced-fat, trans-fat-free spread

Preheat the oven to 400°F. Line a baking sheet with aluminum foil or parchment paper and set it aside.

Prick the potatoes several times with a fork. Microwave the potatoes on high for 5 to 6 minutes.

Make a large, lengthwise slit down the centers of the potatoes. Sprinkle each potato with ½ teaspoon of the garlic powder and season with salt. Press the onion inside and top with the spread.

Bake on the top rack of the oven for 9 to 10 minutes, or until the onion begins to brown and the potato is tender when pierced with a fork. Serve immediately.

**Per serving:** 264 calories, 4 g protein, 56 g carbohydrate, 3 g fat (0 g saturated), 0 mg cholesterol, 171 mg sodium, 9 g fiber

# GLUTEN-FREE GINGERBREAD MUFFINS

*Enjoy these warm gingerbread muffins as a late-afternoon snack, or serve for a relaxed Sunday-morning breakfast with low-fat cottage cheese or scrambled eggs. Muffins can be stored in an airtight container at room temperature for up to 2 days or frozen for up to 1 month.*

**MAKES 12**

½ cup honey

½ cup soft tub, reduced-fat, trans-fat-free spread

2 eggs whites

1 cup fat-free plain yogurt

1 tablespoon grated lemon zest

1 teaspoon vanilla extract

2 cups teff flour

2 teaspoons baking powder

½ teaspoon baking soda

½ teaspoon ground ginger

½ teaspoon ground cinnamon

½ teaspoon ground nutmeg

¼ teaspoon ground cloves

1 tablespoon crystallized ginger, chopped

Preheat the oven to 350°F. Line the cups of a 12-cup muffin pan with paper liners.

In a large bowl, mix the honey with the spread. Stir in the egg whites, yogurt, lemon zest, and vanilla. Add the teff flour, baking powder, baking soda, ground ginger, cinnamon, nutmeg, and cloves. Stir until the flour is just incorporated, but do not overmix. Fold in the crystallized ginger.

Fill each muffin liner three-fourths full with batter. Bake for 12 to 15 minutes, or until the tops of the muffins are lightly browned and a toothpick comes out clean when inserted in the center. Turn the muffins out onto a cooling rack.

*Tip: If you have trouble finding teff flour in your local health food store, you can order it online at www.bobsredmill.com or www.amazon.com.*

**Per muffin:** 200 calories, 5 g protein, 35 g carbohydrate, 4 g fat (0 g saturated), 0 mg cholesterol, 186 mg sodium, 4 g fiber

# CHAPTER 19

# CANCER PREVENTION

ancer prevention is the holy grail of medical research. Students in medical school dream of finding a cure, scientists hope their work will provide the foundation for the one true end of this disease, and patients and family members pray for a future without cancer. Until that grand discovery, we will have to count on the wisdom of our bodies.

Healthy immune systems work hard to spot and eliminate cancerous cellular mutations before the disease can begin its wild, uncontrolled growth. Prevention, then, is all about keeping ourselves as healthy as possible and eating the kinds of foods that have been shown to help protect us—right down to our cells.

## WHAT AFFECTS CANCER?

Cancer doesn't surface overnight. It is the end point of a process that spans years or even decades.

The process starts when normal body cells are damaged by a virus, radiation, toxic chemicals, inflammation, or randomly occurring errors in cells' DNA that accumulate as we age. Every time a cell is damaged, there is the possibility that its genetic structure may mutate. Cells can handle a certain number of mutations without serious consequences, but after a certain point, the mutations change the essential nature of cells, turning them from normal body cells into precancerous cells. This first stage of cancer development is called initiation. Precancerous cells can reside harmlessly in the body without ever progressing to full-fledged cancer, but sometimes they become activated. In this stage, called promotion, the cells begin to grow and multiply. The third stage of cancer development is called progression, when the cells multiply out of control and begin spreading.

The first step toward cancer prevention is avoiding the kinds of damage that cause mutations. Although scientists don't have all the answers regarding what turns a precancerous cell into a cancer cell, it is widely believed that the forces behind mutations also allow the promotion and progression of cancer. The primary cancer culprits are detailed below.

## SMOKING

Smoking has been estimated to cause about 30 percent of all cancers in the United States. You probably know that smoking is linked to the risk of lung cancer, but it also increases the risk of cancers of the mouth, throat, esophagus, stomach, pancreas, kidney, bladder, and cervix. Secondhand smoke increases the risk of cancer among people who live with smokers.

Tobacco smoke contains dozens of toxins capable of damaging cells. The delicate lining of the lungs is directly exposed to the smoke, but toxins move from the lungs to the bloodstream to cells throughout the body.

## ALCOHOL

Moderate drinking is defined as no more than two servings of alcohol per day for men and one serving per day for women. Excessive alcohol intake has been linked to an increased risk of cancer of the breast, mouth, throat, esophagus, colon, rectum, and liver. The association is especially strong for breast cancer—even one drink or less per day has been shown to increase a woman's risk. No one is really sure what makes alcohol so dangerous, but there are theories. Alcohol itself is toxic to cells, and so are some of the by-products created when it is metabolized. Alcohol also increases hormone levels, thus heightening the risk of hormone-related cancers like breast cancer. And because alcohol makes cells more vulnerable to other cancerous compounds, smokers who drink have a tremendously increased risk of mouth and throat cancers. And the more you drink and smoke, the greater the risk. Heavy drinkers who don't smoke have a risk of head and neck cancers that is 10 times higher than the risk for people who neither drink nor smoke. But if heavy drinkers also smoke, their risk jumps to about 150 times higher.

## RADIATION

It has been known for decades that radiation from excessive exposure to x-rays can cause cancer. The amount of radiation we get from medical x-rays is very small and is thought to contribute to only about 1 percent of cancer risk worldwide. Sunlight contains a form of radiation called ultraviolet rays, which penetrate skin cells and may cause mutations that can turn into skin cancer. Long-term, cumulative exposure to sunlight causes mainly basal cell and squamous cell carcinomas, which are types of cancer that can be disfiguring but are rarely lethal. Severe sunburns, usually in childhood, increase the risk of developing the more dangerous cancer, malignant melanoma, later in life.

## VIRUSES AND BACTERIA

Infection with some strains of the human papillomavirus (HPV) can lead to cervical cancer. Hepatitis B and C bacteria can lead to liver cancer, and the *Helicobacter pylori* bacterium, which causes stomach ulcers, increases the risk of developing stomach cancer. Some scientists believe that these infections represent just the tip of the cancer iceberg and that many more links between cancer, viruses, and bacteria are likely to surface.

Scientists don't fully understand why some infections lead to cancer. We know that viruses can insert copies of their own DNA into normal body cells, altering the genetic structure of the cell. Bacteria, on the other hand, can produce toxins that may damage body cells enough to promote cancer.

## OBESITY

After smoking, obesity is the largest risk factor for cancer. According to the National Cancer Institute, obesity contributes to the development of cancer of the colon, endometrium, kidney, esophagus, and breast (in postmenopausal women only). Gallbladder, ovarian, pancreatic, and certain types of prostate cancer may also be related, but the links are less consistent.

Since fat tissue produces and stores estrogen, postmenopausal women who are overweight can have up to twice the estrogen levels as lean women, potentially leading to the growth of estrogen-sensitive breast tumors. Other cancers may be due to the effects of high levels of insulin common among overweight people, the irritation of reflux disease, or inflammation caused by cytokines and related hormones produced in fat tissue.

## HORMONES

The longer women are exposed to high levels of estrogen, the greater their risk of developing breast cancer. Estrogen levels climb at puberty and remain generally high until menopause, so the risk is higher for women who begin menstruating early (before age 12) or who go into menopause later in life (older than age 55). In addition, anything that increases levels of estrogen is thought to also increase the risk of breast cancer—and that includes carrying excess body fat, drinking alcohol, and taking hormone replacement therapy after menopause. High estrogen exposure is also linked to endometrial and ovarian cancers.

## HOW FOOD AFFECTS CANCER

I've heard people say that they believe cancer is unavoidable—either you get it or you don't. It's true that we inherit a tendency to develop certain cancers, but scientists estimate that only about 5 percent of all cancers have a genetic origin. On the other hand, about 35 percent of cancers are related to nutritional factors. (To fill in the numbers, about 30 percent of cancers are thought to be related to tobacco use, and the remaining 30 percent are attributed to all remaining factors, including bacterial and viral infections, pollution, radiation, and occupational hazards.) Some foods can damage body cells, setting them up for precancerous changes, while other foods protect cells from damage. Cancer prevention depends on knowing the difference.

## FOODS TO LIMIT OR AVOID
### Processed and Red Meats

A growing body of evidence links high intake of processed meats (such as bacon, salami, and bologna) and red meat in general (beef, pork, and lamb) to an increased risk of colon and rectal cancer and possibly other cancers as well. The reasons are still being investigated, but many experts believe the high concentration of heme iron present in red meat plays a role. Heme iron is a type of highly absorbable iron found only in animal proteins. (Vegetables, legumes, fortified cereals, and other plant foods contain only nonheme iron, which doesn't appear to carry the same risks.) Heme iron may damage the cells that line the colon, making them more susceptible to cancerous growth. Processed meats are often made from red meat, and most contain chemical preservatives, such as nitrites and nitrates, which have been identified as possible cancer-causing agents. What's more, the processes of curing, smoking, or salting meat creates additional compounds with cancer-causing potential.

I advise avoiding or dramatically limiting your intake of processed meats, including pepperoni, salami, pastrami, hot dogs, bologna, ham, bacon, beef and pork sausages, and bratwurst. If you're a red meat lover, enjoy fresh, unprocessed beef, lamb, or pork (preferably lean cuts) no more than twice a week. In other words, go ahead and savor a good burger or steak once in a while, but don't make ground beef, pork chops, steaks, and beef roasts mealtime staples. Looking on the bright side, cutting more red meat out of your diet means you'll automatically make more room for healthful, waistline-friendly vegetarian proteins like lentils, starchy beans, and whole soy foods.

### Salty Foods

Salt is thought to increase the risk of stomach and esophageal cancers by damaging the lining of the throat and stomach. Too much damage can cause changes in DNA and increased cell growth. Also, salt allows *Helicobacter pylori* bacteria to thrive, which can increase the risk of stomach cancer. If you enjoy salty and pickled foods, eat them only in moderation. Limit your intake of salt itself, sauerkraut, pickles, all pickled vegetables and fish, salt-cured fish and meats, and, of course, all of those salty processed meats listed above.

## Meats Cooked at High Temperatures

Cooking meats at high temperatures produces chemicals called heterocyclic amines (HCAs), which have been linked to many cancers, including those of the colon, pancreas, bladder, prostate, and breast. The most HCAs are found in proteins (beef, pork, poultry, and fish) that have been fried, broiled, grilled, or barbecued— all cooking methods that typically use high temperatures. Roasting and baking produce fewer HCAs, and poaching, stewing, and boiling meat produce the least. There aren't any specific guidelines about the amount of HCAs that can be considered "safe" or "dangerous." I recommend limiting your intake of meat cooked at high heat, but there's no reason for paranoia. If you love a good grilled steak, feel free to indulge once in a while. Just be sure to trim away excess fat before grilling, and cut off charred or burnt parts before eating the meat. This goes for chicken, turkey, and seafood, too. To further reduce your risk of consuming harmful HCAs, marinate your meat before tossing it on the grill. Marinating meat in a flavorful liquid with plenty of herbs and spices has been shown to dramatically cut back on HCA formation, perhaps because the antioxidants in seasonings block the creation of HCAs. Also, small pieces of chicken, fish, and lean beef cook faster and spend less time on the grill, therefore producing fewer HCAs, so try cooking kebabs instead of large breasts and steaks whenever you can. In general, if you eat beef or other grilled meats more than three times per week, definitely consider cutting back.

## GOOD FOODS TO CHOOSE

Cancer is a disease of opportunity: If a rogue cell has a chance to mutate, it may become cancerous. Along with avoiding mutation triggers, cancer prevention depends on protecting our health and putting up roadblocks to stop precancerous cells from turning bad and running amok. Our best hope is to eat a wide variety of nutrient-dense plant foods, including vegetables, fruits, starchy beans, lentils, and whole grains. Please note that although scientists typically focus on certain nutrients in relation to particular types of cancer, there are probably many interactions among these healthy foods—and they may help prevent cancer in many areas of the body, not just the ones that are mentioned here. So the strongest cancer prevention plan is to eat a good mix of healthy plant foods, without focusing too strongly on any one nutrient.

### Antioxidant Vitamins (Vitamin C, Vitamin E, and Beta-Carotene)

Antioxidants are your body's version of a computer's antivirus software. Antioxidants circulate through your cells, repairing DNA that has been damaged by harmful, reactive oxygen molecules called free radicals in much the same way that an antivirus program combs a hard drive seeking out and restoring infected files. Left unchecked, damaged DNA may impair normal cell reproduction and growth and set in motion processes that can eventually result in cancer. For this reason,

## FAQS

### Can soy foods prevent breast or prostate cancer?

The jury is still out on that one, but the research is promising, particularly for women. Soy foods contain compounds called phytoestrogens, which are akin to very weak forms of estrogen. When eaten in foods (as opposed to supplements), the results are subtle but still potentially significant. Phytoestrogens can bind to estrogen receptors in the breasts and other tissues and in some ways provide a kinder, gentler substitute for natural, ovary-produced estrogen. In Asian women, who consume far more soy than American women do, a diet rich in soy foods has been linked to a lower risk of breast cancer and cancer recurrence. Current research indicates that soy may offer more cancer protection when it's consumed earlier in life, during childhood and the teen years. In men, phytoestrogens also act as estrogens—again, subtly—which may balance out testosterone levels. In terms of benefits for prostate health, the research is mixed. Some studies have shown that men who consume high-soy diets are less likely to develop prostate cancer, and others have shown no advantage. I do not recommend that men or women take soy, phytoestrogens, or isoflavones (a class of phytoestrogens) in supplemental form, since their effects are not fully understood. If you would like to add soy to your diet, skip supplements and highly processed soy foods. Instead try high quality, whole soy foods such as soybeans (edamame), tofu, tempeh, or soy milk. One caveat: If you are being treated for or have a history of breast cancer, speak with your doctor before incorporating soy foods into your diet. In many instances, consuming moderate amounts of whole soy foods is perfectly fine, but your doctor may advise you differently based on your personal medical history and treatment plan.

a diet that emphasizes antioxidant-rich foods like vegetables, fruits, and whole grains may be one of your best defenses against cancer. Note that the key word here is *foods*. Nearly two decades of disappointing research trials have taught us that you're far better off getting your antioxidants in their natural state, not in the isolated, purified forms found in supplements. Researchers have repeatedly tested high-dose antioxidant supplements to see if they reduce cancer rates, and time and time again, supplements have shown no benefit. (Sometimes they even have adverse health effects.) Some scientists believe that antioxidants work synergistically with other nutrients and compounds in foods, which may explain why stripping them out and plunking them into bottles doesn't seem to offer any cancer protection. The moral of the story: When it comes to fighting cancer, load up on antioxidants from healthy, delicious foods only.

Vitamin C is an antioxidant that helps prevent the formation of cancer-causing nitrogen compounds. Diets high in vitamin C have been linked to a reduced risk of cancers of the stomach, colon, esophagus, bladder, breast, and cervix. Again, these results have been found for vitamin C–rich foods, rather than supplements, which seem less reliable.

BEST FOODS FOR VITAMIN C: *guava, bell peppers (all colors), oranges and orange juice, grapefruit and grapefruit juice, strawberries, pineapple, kohlrabi, papayas, lemons and lemon juice, broccoli, kale, Brussels sprouts, kidney beans, kiwifruit, cantaloupe, cauliflower, cabbage (all varieties), mangoes, white potatoes, mustard greens, tomatoes, sugar snap peas, snow peas, clementines, rutabagas, turnip greens, raspberries, blackberries, watermelon, tangerines, okra, lychees, summer squash, persimmons*

Some research shows that eating a vitamin E–rich diet reduces the risk of stomach, colon, lung, liver, and other cancers, but, as with other antioxidants, vitamin E supplements have largely struck out. I recommend adding vitamin E—rich foods to your diet—they are safe and will help keep you and your cells healthy.

BEST FOODS FOR VITAMIN E: *almonds and almond butter, sunflower seeds and sunflower butter, wheat germ, hazelnuts, spinach, dandelion greens, Swiss chard, pine nuts, peanuts and peanut butter, turnip greens, beet greens, broccoli, canola oil, red bell pepper, collard greens, avocados, olive oil, mangoes*

Beta-carotene is a powerful antioxidant. Studies have shown that people who eat a diet high in beta-carotene—found primarily in orange and leafy green vegetables—have a reduced risk of cancer, particularly of the lung, colon, and stomach. (These results are for beta-carotene from food sources only. In one study, beta-carotene supplements actually increased the risk of lung cancer in smokers.) Among premenopausal women, one study found that eating a lot of vegetables that include beta-carotene, folate, vitamin C, and fiber reduced the risk of breast cancer by about half.

BEST FOODS FOR BETA CAROTENE: *sweet potatoes, carrots, kale, butternut squash, turnip greens, pumpkin, mustard greens, cantaloupe, red bell pepper, apricots, Chinese cabbage, spinach, lettuces (especially darker lettuces), collard greens, Swiss chard, watercress, grapefruit (pink, red), watermelon, cherries, mangoes, tomatoes, guava, asparagus, red cabbage*

## Vitamin D

Experts consider the United States to be in the middle of a vitamin D–deficiency epidemic. We just don't get enough. In previous generations, vitamin D deficiency wasn't a problem because people spent ample time in the great outdoors and took in large amounts of the primary source: sunlight. Our skin makes all the vitamin D we need when exposed to sunlight. But the world has changed. We now spend less time outside, and the protective ozone layer has eroded, so sunlight today contains more cancer-causing ultraviolet radiation than it did a few decades ago. Fortunately, most of us use sunscreen regularly to protect our skin—but unfortunately, sunscreen keeps our skin from using sunlight to produce vitamin D.

In some studies, low vitamin D levels have been linked to several cancers, including colon and breast. Scientists theorize that vitamin D may help block the development of blood vessels that feed growing tumors and help stop the proliferation of cancerous and precancerous cells. I recommend that, to cover your bases, you eat plenty of vitamin D–rich foods and choose vitamin D–fortified dairy products. Because few foods provide vitamin D, you should consider a daily multivitamin or separate supplement that provides 800 to 1,000 IU of vitamin $D_3$ (cholecalciferol, the most potent form).

BEST FOODS FOR VITAMIN D: *wild salmon (fresh, canned), mackerel (not king), sardines, herring, milk (fat-free, 1%), soy milk, fortified yogurt (fat-free, low-fat), egg yolks, vitamin D-enhanced mushrooms\**

*\*These mushrooms are treated with UV light, which dramatically increases their vitamin D content.*

## Omega-3 Fatty Acids

There is no consensus about the role of omega-3 fatty acids in cancer prevention. However, some research has shown that eating plenty of omega-3s in the form of fatty fish may reduce the incidence and progression of colon, breast, and prostate cancers. Researchers at Columbia University studied over 21,000 men and found that those who ate the most fish had a 37 percent reduced risk of colorectal cancer. It is believed that omega-3 fatty acids may help prevent cancer by inhibiting cancer cell proliferation and disrupting steps that are critical to tumor growth. Omega-3 fatty acids also help reduce inflammation, which means that they are likely to help reduce the possibility of cellular mutations. But even if omega-3s don't directly reduce the risk of cancer, they certainly help keep our bodies strong and healthy. Plus, fish and shellfish are terrific main course replacements for red meat, which may *increase* the risk of certain cancers. For all of these reasons, I highly recommend adding omega-3–rich foods to your diet. (My Best Foods list includes only the fatty fish that have been shown to be low in mercury, PCBs, and dioxins.)

**FAQS**

**I'm surprised not to see calcium on your list of recommended nutrients. What does the research say?**

There's good, solid evidence that eating calcium-rich foods, such as low-fat dairy products, protects against colon cancer. But scientists have also found that too much calcium—over 1,500 milligrams daily—may increase the risk of prostate cancer. So for men, I recommend consuming only two or three servings of dairy or other calcium–rich foods daily—and definitely not taking calcium supplements unless specifically directed by your physician. For women, I recommend getting 1,000 to 1,200 milligrams of daily calcium—preferably from food—to help keep bones strong and *perhaps* help prevent colon cancer.

BEST FOODS FOR OMEGA-3 FATTY ACIDS: *wild salmon (fresh, canned), herring, mackerel (not king), sardines, anchovies, trout (wild, rainbow), Pacific oysters, chia seeds, ground flaxseed, walnuts, butternuts (white walnuts), seaweed, walnut oil, canola oil, soybeans (edamame)*

## Phytonutrients

There's more to good nutrition than vitamins and minerals. All plant foods—grains, fruits, and vegetables—contain small amounts of phytonutrients: naturally occurring chemical compounds that are just as important as vitamins and minerals are for maintaining health. There are thousands of known phytonutrients, many of which have demonstrated the potential to protect us against cancer. Cruciferous vegetables, for example, contain phytonutrients known as glucosinolates, which help inhibit the metabolism of some carcinogens, may stop the proliferation of cancer cells, and cause the body to produce detoxification enzymes. Onions, garlic, and other members of the *Allium* family of vegetables are rich in sulfur compounds, such as allicin, that appear to have antitumor properties. Lycopene, an antioxidant found in concentrated amounts in cooked tomato products, may offer protection against prostate, lung, and stomach cancers.

Then there are the flavonoids, such as anthocyanins and quercetin, found in plant foods such as berries, onions, apples, and purple grapes. These powerful antioxidants seem to help reduce the type of inflammation associated with cancer progression. Ellagic acid is the latest phytonutrient to enter the scene, although it's been quietly hanging out in berries, nuts, and pomegranates for millennia. In laboratory and animal studies, ellagic acid has been shown to inhibit cancer cell growth and deactivate cancer-causing compounds.

Different fruits and vegetables contain various combinations of phytonutrients, so to ensure that you are getting as many different protective compounds as possible, I recommend eating nine servings of vegetables and fruits per day. Go for variety, rather than focusing on just one or two of your favorites.

BEST CRUCIFEROUS VEGETABLES: *broccoli, broccoli raab, Brussels sprouts, cabbage, cauliflower, collard greens, daikon, kale, kohlrabi, mustard greens, rutabagas, turnips, bok choy, arugula, horseradish, radishes, Swiss chard, wasabi (Japanese horseradish), watercress and cress*

BEST ALLIUM VEGETABLES: *onions, garlic, shallots, leeks, scallions, chives, ramps*

BEST FOODS FOR LYCOPENE: *tomatoes (and all tomato-based products including tomato sauce, paste, soup, and juice), watermelon, guava, pink grapefruit, red bell peppers*

BEST FOODS FOR QUERCETIN: *onions, kale, leeks, cherry tomatoes, broccoli, blueberries, black currants, elderberries, lingonberries, cocoa powder (unsweetened), apricots, apples with skin, grapes (red, purple, black), tomatoes, tea, green beans, lettuces, hot chile peppers, celery, chives, red cabbage, lemons, grapefruit*

BEST FOODS FOR ANTHOCYANINS: *blackberries, black currants, blueberries, eggplant, elderberries, raspberries, cherries, boysenberries, grapes (red, black, purple), strawberries, plums, cranberries, rhubarb, red onions, red apples, peaches, cabbage (red, purple), red beets, blood oranges*

BEST FOODS FOR ELLAGIC ACID: *raspberries, blackberries, strawberries, walnuts, pecans, cranberries, pomegranates, grapes (red, black, purple)*

## Tea

Tea contains compounds called catechins, which are thought to be able to stop the growth of cancer cells and help prevent cellular mutations that contribute to cancer development. In Japan, where tea is the preferred beverage, green tea consumption has been shown to reduce the risk of stomach cancer among women. In China, green tea drinkers were found to have a reduced risk of developing rectal and pancreatic cancers, compared with non-tea drinkers. Regular tea drinkers have also been shown to be at lower risk of colon, breast, ovarian, prostate, and lung cancers. After analyzing tea's chemical components, scientists have discovered that black, oolong, green, and white tea all seem to have value as cancer preventive agents, and each type seems to protect against different types of mutagens.

## Herbs and Spices

Herbs and spices have been used as folk medicines for thousands of years. These days, scientists are busy trying to determine which claims for cancer prevention are true and which are fairy tales. A few of the most promising herbs and spices are turmeric, rosemary, and ginger.

Turmeric is the yellow spice found in curry powder. Curcumin, the active ingredient in turmeric, functions as both an anti-inflammatory and an antioxidant, and it may help prevent cancer by interfering with aspects of cellular signaling. In laboratory animals, curcumin has been shown to help prevent cancer of the breast, colon, stomach, liver, and lung.

Rosemary is a wonderful, fragrant herb that is easy to grow and quite versatile when it comes to cooking. I use it in meat dishes, roasted vegetables, and savory baked goods. Rosemary contains the antioxidant compounds caffeic acid and rosmarinic acid. Laboratory studies have shown that rosmarinic acid can protect against cell damage and prevent DNA fragmentation.

Gingerroot has a pungent, spicy flavor that works well in both savory and sweet dishes. This one root contains more than 50 antioxidant and anti-inflammatory compounds, and some of these phytonutrients have been shown to suppress cancer cell and tumor growth in laboratory studies. Ginger isn't a miracle food, but it's certainly an incredibly healthy addition to a cancer-fighting diet. Try grating fresh gingerroot into stir-fries or hearty stews, steeping a few slices in hot water to make a delicious tea, or adding fresh or ground gingerroot to a healthy muffin or fruit crisp recipe.

## BONUS POINTS

- ◆ **If you smoke, quit.** Even the best nutrition can't override the toxic effects of smoking. If you can go cold turkey on your own, great. But there are other options, including nicotine replacement, hypnosis, support groups, and prescription medications. Talk with your doctor about a plan that makes sense for you.

- ◆ **Exercise regularly.** Cancer prevention requires a strong immune system, and your immune system gets a boost from regular physical activity. Studies have shown that moderate levels of exercise can reduce the risk of colon cancer by 50 percent and the risk of breast cancer among postmenopausal women by at least 20 percent. Regular exercise has also been strongly associated with lower rates of lung and endometrial cancers. I recommend working some form of activity into your schedule—for 30 to 60 minutes at least five days per week.

- ◆ **Be smart about sun exposure.** Protect your skin from radiation as much as you can. Cover up with extra clothing (especially sun-protective brands), wear a hat, use sunscreen, avoid spending time outdoors during the high-exposure times of 10:00 a.m. to 4:00 p.m., and don't tan—even tanning beds have been found to contribute to cancer.

- ◆ **Minimize your alcohol intake.** Moderate drinking has been shown to decrease the risk of heart disease, but alcohol also increases the risk of certain types of cancer. If you're a woman at risk of breast cancer, be extra selective when choosing times to drink.

- ◆ **Follow medical screening guidelines.** Some medical tests may help prevent cancer. For example, a fleshy growth in the colon (called a polyp) is usually harmless, but some may develop into cancer. Your doctor can check for polyps during a colonoscopy. Once polyps are snipped out, they cannot become cancerous. Other tests, such as mammograms and the blood test for prostate-specific antigen (PSA), help detect cancers when they are still small and more likely to respond to treatment. Your doctor will recommend which tests to get and how often, based on your family and personal medical history.

◆ **If you are a woman, do your hormone research.** Theories about the health effects of hormone replacement therapy are continually evolving. If you are currently taking or considering taking hormone replacement therapy, talk with your doctor about your personal symptoms and risk factors in order to make an informed decision.

◆ **Practice safe sex.** The human papillomavirus (HPV) can lead to cervical cancer, and infection with hepatitis C can lead to liver cancer. Both of these infections can be acquired through unsafe sexual practices, particularly with multiple partners. For more information about HPV vaccinations and other ways to protect yourself against these and other sexually transmitted diseases, speak with your physician, call your local Planned Parenthood, or visit the Web site of the nonprofit American Social Health Association at www .ashastd.org.

## SUPPLEMENTS

If you want to consider supplements in addition to food fixes, I recommend only a multivitamin. However, multivitamins don't appear to offer any protection against cancer, so if you already eat a healthy diet with a variety of vegetables, fruits, whole grains, and other foods, a daily multi is probably unnecessary. If you do choose to take one, look for a brand that includes 100 percent DV of most vitamins and minerals, without megadoses of any nutrient. Make sure your brand provides at least 800 IU of vitamin D in the most potent and beneficial form, $D_3$. Men and postmenopausal women should look for a formulation without iron.

Some supplement manufacturers hype special cancer-prevention formulas based on nutrient research. However, the absolute best source of those nutrients is from food, not pills. In some cases, high-dose supplements may even speed cancer development (or be contraindicated in cancer treatment). So for cancer prevention, focus on foods and leave the pills on the shelf.

For more food cures for cancer prevention, visit www.joybauer.com/cancer.

# JOY'S 4-STEP PROGRAM
## FOR CANCER PREVENTION

Follow this program if you have a family history of cancer or if you want to do everything possible to reduce your risk of developing cancer.

## Step 1 ... START WITH THE BASICS

These are the first things you should do to start preventing cancer.

- If you smoke, quit.
- Begin a regular program of exercise.
- Talk with your doctor about cancer screening.
- Be safe—in the sun and in bed.
- Drink alcohol sensibly, if at all.

## Step 2 ... YOUR ULTIMATE GROCERY LIST

A nutrition plan is only as good as the foods you choose. Everything on this list has high levels of nutrients that are thought to help prevent cancer.

### FRUIT

*All* fruit, but especially:

Apples (with skin)

Apricots

Berries (blackberries, blueberries, boysenberries, elderberries, lingonberries, raspberries, and strawberries)

Cantaloupe

Cherries

Clementines

Cranberries

Currants

Grapefruit

Grapes (black, purple, and red)

Guava

Kiwifruit

Lemons

Lychees

Mangoes

Oranges (especially blood oranges)

Papayas

Peaches

Persimmons

Pineapple

Plums

Pomegranates

Tangerines

Watermelon

## VEGETABLES AND LEGUMES

*All* vegetables, but
  especially:

Arugula

Asparagus

Avocados

Beans, starchy (such as
  black, garbanzo, kidney,
  navy, and pinto)

Beets (purple and red)

Bok choy

Broccoli

Broccoli raab

Brussels sprouts

Cabbage (all varieties)

Carrots

Cauliflower

Celery

Collard greens

Eggplant

Green beans

Kale

Kohlrabi

Leeks

Lentils

Lettuce (especially darker
  varieties)

Mustard greens

Okra

Onions (all varieties)

Peas, black-eyed

Peppers (all varieties)

Potatoes (sweet and white)

Pumpkin (fresh, 100% pure
  canned)

Radishes

Ramps

Rhubarb

Rutabagas

Scallions

Shallots

Snow peas

Soybeans (edamame)

Spinach

Squash, summer

Squash, winter (acorn,
  butternut)

Sugar snap peas

Swiss chard

Tomatoes (including juice,
  pasta sauce, and soup)

Turnip greens

Turnips

Watercress (and other
  varieties of cress)

Zucchini

## SEAFOOD

*All* fish and shellfish, but
  especially:

Anchovies

Herring

Mackerel (not king)

Oysters, Pacific

Salmon, wild (fresh or
  canned)

Sardines

Trout (rainbow, wild)

## LEAN PROTEINS

Chicken, ground (at least
  90% lean)

Chicken, skinless

Eggs and egg substitutes

Tempeh

Tofu

Turkey, ground (at least
  90% lean)

Turkey, skinless

Turkey burgers, lean

Veggie burgers

## NUTS AND SEEDS (PREFERABLY UNSALTED)

*All* nuts and seeds, but
  especially:

Almonds and almond butter

Butternuts (white walnuts)

Chia seeds

Flaxseed (ground)

Hazelnuts

Peanuts and peanut butter

Pine nuts

Sunflower seeds and
  sunflower butter

Walnuts

## WHOLE GRAINS

Amaranth

Barley

Bread, whole grain (buns,
  crackers, English muffins,
  pitas, tortillas, and wraps)

Bulgur

Cereal, whole grain

Millet

Oats

Pasta, whole grain

Quinoa

Rice (brown and wild)

Waffles, whole grain

Wheat germ

## DAIRY

Cheese (fat-free or reduced-fat)

Cottage cheese (fat-free or 1%)

Milk (fat-free or 1%)

Milk alternatives (almond, rice, and soy)

## MISCELLANEOUS

Canola oil

Cocoa powder, unsweetened

Curry powder

Garlic

Ginger

Guacamole

Herbs and spices (fresh,
  dried, and ground)

Horseradish, prepared

Hot sauce

Hummus

Marinara sauce

Mayonnaise, reduced-fat

Mustard (all varieties)

Olive oil

Rosemary, fresh

Salad dressing, reduced-
  calorie

Salsa

Soft tub spread, trans-fat-
  free (reduced-fat or
  regular)

Tea (black, green, and
  white)

Turmeric (curcumin) spice

Vinegar (all varieties)

Wasabi

# Step3 . . . GOING ABOVE AND BEYOND

If you want to do everything you can to prevent cancer, here are some additional things you might try.

- ◆ Consider taking a multivitamin. Select a brand that provides at least 800 to 1,000 IU of vitamin D in the form of $D_3$.

- ◆ Avoid or strictly limit your intake of processed meats, and eat red meat no more than twice a week.

- ◆ Cut down on salty, pickled, cured, and smoked foods.

- ◆ Avoid frying, grilling, and broiling meats as much as possible. Cook at lower temperatures to avoid creating heterocyclic amines (HCAs).

## SNACK ON BERRIES

Of all the fruits and vegetables studied, berries rank among the most likely to reduce cancer risk. Every year, we learn more and more about the benefits of these nutrition powerhouse fruits. Studies have shown that laboratory animals fed black raspberries have a 60 percent reduction in tumors of the esophagus and an 80 percent reduction in colon tumors. An antioxidant called pterostilbene, found in high quantities in blueberries, also has cancer-fighting properties. Cranberries contain a whole drugstore's worth of cancer-fighting natural chemicals (such as polyphenolic extracts, flavonols, proanthocyanidin oligomers, and triterpenoids) that may give it the potential to prevent the growth of tumors in the breast, colon, prostate, and lung. So the next time you want a sweet treat, skip the cookies and feast on berries.

# Step4 . . . MEAL PLANS

These sample menus include foods that have been shown to be protective against cancer, specifically those foods containing antioxidants, vitamin D, omega-3 fats, and a variety of phytonutrients.

Every day, choose one option for each of the three meals—breakfast, lunch, and dinner. Then, once or twice each day, choose from my suggested snacks. Approximate calories have been provided to help adjust for your personal weight-management goals. If you find yourself hungry (and if weight is not an issue), feel free to increase the portion sizes for meals and snacks. Beverage calories are not included. If you enjoy drinking tea, incorporate a cup or two each day. Rotate between white, green, and black tea if you like all three.

## BREAKFAST OPTIONS

(300 TO 400 CALORIES)

### Fiesta Vegetable Omelet with Toast

Sauté ½ cup chopped onion, ½ cup sliced mushrooms, and ½ cup chopped bell pepper in a heated pan coated with oil spray until soft. Beat 1 whole egg plus 3 egg whites and add to the vegetables. Add preferred seasonings. When the bottom is cooked, gently flip and cook other side. Fold one side over the other. Serve with 1 slice whole wheat bread (or 2 slices reduced-calorie bread), toasted and topped with 1 teaspoon soft tub, trans-fat-free spread.

### Whole Grain Cereal with Milk and Fruit

Mix 1 cup whole grain cereal with 1 cup milk (fat-free, 1%, or soy/almond/rice) and top with 2 tablespoons wheat germ and 1 cup berries (or enjoy 1 apple or orange on the side).

### Cottage Cheese with Berries and Flaxseed

Mix 1 cup fat-free or 1% cottage cheese with 1 cup berries or sliced strawberries and 2 tablespoons ground flaxseed (or chopped nuts). You can substitute 1 cup fat-free plain or flavored yogurt for the cottage cheese.

### Breakfast Burrito with Vegetables

Sauté ½ cup chopped onion; ½ cup bell pepper strips; and 1 cup spinach, kale, or Swiss chard in oil spray until soft. Beat 1 whole egg and 2 egg whites and pour over the sautéed vegetables. Add preferred seasonings and cook, stirring, until the eggs are cooked through. Wrap in a whole grain tortilla (150 calories or less) and serve with optional salsa and/or hot sauce.

### Vanilla Pumpkin Breakfast Pudding

Mix 1 cup fat-free vanilla yogurt with ½ cup canned plain 100% pumpkin puree and optional ground cinnamon, and top with 2 tablespoons chopped walnuts and 1 to 2 tablespoons wheat germ (or ground flaxseed).

### Oatmeal with Chopped Fruit and Nuts

Prepare ½ cup dry oats with water, and top with 2 tablespoons chopped nuts (walnuts, almonds, pecans, etc.) and 1 chopped peach (or plum or apple). Sweeten with optional 1 to 2 teaspoons sugar, honey, or sugar substitute.

### Citrus Smooth-See

Enjoy 1 serving (page 272).

## LUNCH OPTIONS

(400 TO 500 CALORIES)

### Turkey Avocado Sandwich

Layer 4 ounces sliced turkey (or chicken), 2 or 3 thin slices avocado, lettuce, tomato, and onion between 2 slices whole grain bread. Spread with optional mustard and 2 teaspoons reduced-fat mayonnaise or hummus. Enjoy with unlimited red, green, or yellow bell pepper strips.

### Edamame with Wild Salmon Dijonnaise

Enjoy 1 cup boiled edamame (green soybeans in the pod) with 5 ounces canned salmon, drained, mashed, and mixed with 1 tablespoon reduced-fat mayonnaise, 1 to 2 teaspoons Dijon mustard, and minced onion and black pepper to taste. Serve on a large bed of leafy greens (such as spinach, romaine, or arugula) tossed with 1 teaspoon olive oil and unlimited vinegar (or 2 tablespoons reduced-calorie dressing).

### Grilled Chicken Pepper Wrap

Cut 5 ounces cooked chicken into strips and mix with unlimited chopped onion and red, green, or yellow bell pepper strips sautéed in oil spray or 1 teaspoon olive or canola oil. Wrap in a whole grain tortilla (150 calories or less). Enjoy with baby carrots and sliced cucumber or 1 serving gazpacho (Judy's Gazpacho, page 463, or prepared).

### Super Health Salad

Choose 4 ounces of one of the following proteins: canned sardines, canned light tuna in water, canned or fresh wild salmon, chicken, turkey, shrimp, crab, tofu, or preferred fish. Serve on a large bed of leafy greens (such as spinach, romaine, or arugula) mixed with chopped bell pepper, cherry tomatoes, sliced mushrooms, chopped cucumbers, sliced beets, chopped red onion, and artichoke hearts. Add ¼ cup starchy beans and 5 sliced olives. Toss with 2 teaspoons olive oil and unlimited vinegar or fresh lemon juice (or 2 to 4 tablespoons reduced-calorie dressing).

### Turkey Burger with Creamy Coleslaw

Top a 5-ounce lean turkey burger (or veggie burger) with lettuce, tomato, onion, and optional mustard or 2 tablespoons ketchup. Serve on ½ whole grain bun (or in a 70-calorie whole wheat pita pocket). Enjoy with 1 serving Creamy Coleslaw (page 458) or unlimited steamed vegetables (broccoli, cauliflower, carrots, kale, spinach, etc.).

### Chilled Gazpacho with Curry Chicken Salad

Enjoy 1 serving Judy's Gazpacho (page 463) or 1 cup any prepared variety with 5 ounces canned chicken breast, well drained, mashed, and mixed with 1 tablespoon reduced-fat mayonnaise, minced onion to taste, 1 teaspoon curry powder, and ½ cup green peas. (Use frozen peas and simply rinse under running cold water to thaw.) Serve chicken salad on a bed of dark leafy greens.

### Hearty Vegetable Bean Soup with Pita

Enjoy 1 serving Hearty Vegetable Bean Soup (page 459) with 1 whole wheat pita cut into 4 triangles, lightly toasted, and topped with optional hummus or 2 teaspoons soft tub, trans-fat-free spread.

## DINNER OPTIONS

(500 TO 600 CALORIES)

### Baked Fish with Lemony Brussels Sprouts and Sweet Potato

Season 6 ounces fish fillet (wild salmon, flounder, cod, sole, tilapia, or trout) with 1 teaspoon olive oil, lemon juice, and preferred seasonings and bake in the oven. Enjoy with 1 serving Lemony Brussels Sprouts (page 460) or unlimited Brussels sprouts, asparagus, cauliflower, sugar snap peas, or broccoli (steamed or sautéed in 1 teaspoon olive oil), and 1 medium baked white or sweet potato topped with optional salsa.

### Healthy Chinese Takeout

Order 1 steamed seafood, tofu, or chicken and vegetable entrée (such as steamed chicken and broccoli) and request garlic, black bean, or ginger sauce on the side. Flavor with 1 to 2 tablespoons side sauce and toss thoroughly. Enjoy with 1 cup steamed brown rice.

### Chicken Curry and Vegetables with Brown Rice

Enjoy 1 serving Chicken Curry and Vegetables (page 178) with ½ cup cooked brown or brown basmati rice or ½ cup cooked whole wheat pasta.

### Tofu Salad with Snow Peas, Almonds, and Mandarin Oranges

Toss 8 ounces extra-firm tofu, cubed and chilled, with 3 cups baby spinach leaves, 1 cup steamed and chilled snow peas, ½ chopped tomato, and ½ cup mandarin oranges (canned in light syrup or juice). Drizzle with 1 teaspoon sesame oil and 1 tablespoon reduced-sodium soy sauce and top with 2 tablespoons slivered almonds. You may substitute chicken or shrimp for the tofu.

### Sautéed Shrimp with Tandoori Cauliflower

Sauté 6 to 8 ounces shrimp in 1 teaspoon olive oil and sprinkle with fresh lemon or lime juice. Enjoy with 2 servings Tandoori Cauliflower with yogurt topping (page 462).

### Poached Salmon with Rosemary-Roasted Vegetables

Enjoy 1 serving Easy! 3-Step Microwave Salmon (page 345) or 5 ounces wild salmon fillet, poached and topped with 1 tablespoon Dijon mustard and ½ teaspoon dried dill and drizzled with juice from ½ lemon. Enjoy with 2 servings Rosemary-Roasted Vegetables (page 461).

### Bean and Cheese Burrito

Sauté 1 cup sliced onions and bell peppers in oil spray until tender. Add ¾ cup black beans to the pan and cook until warmed through. Place the mixture in the center of a whole grain tortilla (150 calories or less) and top with ¼ cup (1 ounce) shredded reduced-fat cheese, 2 slices avocado, and optional salsa or hot sauce. Wrap up the tortilla and serve.

## SNACK OPTIONS

### 100 CALORIES OR LESS

◆ *Best Vegetable Snacks:* up to 2 cups raw or cooked bell peppers, broccoli, cauliflower, Brussels sprouts, cherry tomatoes, green beans, sugar snap peas, snow peas, carrots, or asparagus

◆ *Best Fruit Snacks:* 1 apple (with skin), guava, orange, blood orange, persimmon or peach; 2 plums, kiwifruit, clementines, or tangerines; ½ papaya, grape-fruit, cantaloupe, pomegranate, or mango; 1 cup berries (sliced strawberries, blueberries, boysenberries, blackberries, raspberries), cherries, or grapes (red, purple, or black); 1 cup cubed watermelon or pineapple; ½ cup lychees; 4 apricots; 20 whole strawberries

◆ 1 level tablespoon peanut or almond butter with celery sticks

◆ 10 almonds

◆ ½ cup fat-free cottage cheese with red, green, or yellow bell pepper strips

◆ 1 serving (1 cup) Judy's Gazpacho (page 463)

◆ 1 serving Creamy Coleslaw (page 458)

### 100 TO 200 CALORIES

◆ 10 almonds with 1 serving fruit (see Best Fruit Snacks)

◆ 1 cup boiled edamame (green soybeans in the pod)

◆ Whole nuts: 1 ounce (about ¼ cup) almonds, pecans, walnuts, peanuts, or other nuts of choice

◆ ½ cup sunflower seeds or pistachios in the shell

◆ ½ cup fat-free or 1% cottage cheese (or fat-free yogurt) mixed with ½ cup berries (or 2 tablespoons ground flaxseed or wheat germ)

◆ 70-calorie whole wheat pita with 1 level tablespoon peanut butter (or 2 tablespoons hummus)

◆ 1 serving Rosemary-Roasted Vegetables (page 461)

◆ 2 servings (2 cups) Judy's Gazpacho (page 463)

◆ 1 cup baby carrots and/or bell pepper strips with ¼ cup guacamole or hummus

◆ Sliced apple with 1 level tablespoon peanut or almond butter

◆ ½ cantaloupe filled with ½ cup fat-free or 1% cottage cheese (or fat-free yogurt)

◆ ½ small avocado drizzled with lime juice and lightly sprinkled with kosher salt

◆ 1 cup lentil or black bean soup

◆ 1 slice Green Tea Pound Cake (page 464)

◆ 1 Ginger-Spiced Pumpkin Muffin (page 180)

◆ 2 cups Strawberry-Kiwi Smoothie (page 114)

◆ 2 cups Tropical Mango-Citrus Smoothie (page 114)

◆ Berry smoothie: In a blender, mix ½ cup fat-free milk (or soy milk), ½ cup fat-free yogurt, ¾ cup fresh or frozen berries, and 3 to 5 ice cubes.

◆ Vanilla Pumpkin Yogurt Pudding: Mix 1 cup fat-free vanilla yogurt with ½ cup canned 100% pure pumpkin puree and optional ground cinnamon.

◆ Baked apple with 1 to 2 teaspoons sugar and cinnamon

# CREAMY COLESLAW

*Coleslaw, starring cabbage—one of the cruciferous vegetable superheroes—is the perfect addition to any meal. My low-calorie version calls for reduced-fat mayo and adds scallions and dried cranberries for terrific color, flavor, and—of course—additional cancer-fighting nutrients. For this recipe, you can either shred whole cabbage and carrots in the food processor or simply buy preshredded bags at your local grocery store. I personally love adding this slaw to my wrap sandwiches. Try this: Layer a whole wheat wrap with a few slices of tomato and turkey breast, and top with a few generous tablespoons of the coleslaw. Roll up the wrap and dig in.*

**MAKES 6 SERVINGS**

4 cups shredded cabbage

2 cups shredded carrots

½ cup chopped scallions

¼ cup dried cranberries

¼ cup reduced-fat mayonnaise

1 tablespoon sugar

1 tablespoon apple cider vinegar or orange juice

1 teaspoon Dijon mustard

½ teaspoon kosher salt

Ground black pepper to taste

Combine the cabbage, carrots, scallions, cranberries, mayonnaise, sugar, vinegar or juice, mustard, salt, and pepper in a large bowl and toss to mix.

**Per serving:** 62 calories, 1 g protein, 12 g carbohydrate, 1 g fat (0 g saturated), 0 mg cholesterol, 200 mg sodium, 2 g fiber; plus 21 mg vitamin C (35% DV), 3,100 mcg beta-carotene

# Hearty Vegetable Bean Soup

*With veggies rich in vitamin C, beta-carotene, quercetin, and lycopene, this soup packs a lot of nutrition in just one serving—and I promise you will not be disappointed with the taste.*

**MAKES 8 SERVINGS**

1 teaspoon olive oil

1 onion, sliced

2 leeks, chopped

2 cloves garlic, minced

3 small zucchini, chopped

2 large carrots, chopped

1 cup mushrooms, sliced

1 cup green beans, cut into 1" pieces

1 large potato (about 8 ounces), peeled and halved

3 tablespoons chopped fresh cilantro

4 cups low-sodium chicken or vegetable broth

2 cups crushed tomatoes (preferably no-salt-added)

1 can (15 ounces) stewed tomatoes (preferably no-salt-added)

1 can (15 ounces) navy or kidney beans, well rinsed and drained

2 teaspoons dried basil

2 teaspoons dried oregano

1 teaspoon kosher salt

1 package (7 ounces) frozen chopped spinach or kale

⅓ cup fresh parsley, chopped

Ground black pepper to taste

Heat the oil in a large nonstick pan over medium-high heat. Add the onion, leeks, and garlic and cook, stirring frequently, until soft. Add the zucchini, carrots, mushrooms, green beans, potato, cilantro, broth, crushed tomatoes, stewed tomatoes (with juice), navy or kidney beans, basil, oregano, and salt. Bring to a boil. Simmer for 25 minutes, or until the potato is cooked.

Transfer the potato to a food processor or blender with some of the cooking liquid and puree it. Return it to the pan and add the spinach or kale and parsley. Season to taste with black pepper and additional salt, if desired.

**Per serving:** 243 calories, 13 g protein, 46 g carbohydrate, 2 g fat (0 g saturated), 0 mg cholesterol, 196 mg sodium, 13 g fiber; plus 38 mg vitamin C (63% DV), 4,045 mcg beta-carotene, 15,770 mcg lycopene

# LEMONY BRUSSELS SPROUTS

*Brussels sprouts are nutritional winners no matter how they're prepared. This cruciferous vegetable is naturally loaded with cancer-fighting compounds, and my lemony version adds extra vitamin C and fantastic flavor.*

**MAKES 4 SERVINGS**

1 large lemon

1 tablespoon reduced-fat, soft tub, trans-fat-free spread

1 pound Brussels sprouts, trimmed and each cut in half lengthwise

¼ teaspoon kosher salt

1 tablespoon apple cider vinegar

Preheat the oven to 400°F. Zest and juice the lemon and set aside.

Coat a large ovenproof skillet with oil spray. Place over high heat and add the spread. When the spread foams, add the Brussels sprouts, cut sides down, and sprinkle with the salt. Reduce the heat to medium and cook for 5 to 6 minutes, or until the Brussels sprouts begin to brown. Add the lemon zest and juice and vinegar. Transfer the skillet to the oven and bake for 4 to 5 minutes, or until the sprouts are tender when pierced with a knife. Serve immediately.

**Per serving:** 68 calories, 4 g protein, 13 g carbohydrate, 1 g fat (0 g saturated), 0 mg cholesterol, 120 mg sodium, 6 g fiber; plus 102 mg vitamin C (170% DV), 510 mcg beta-carotene

# ROSEMARY-ROASTED VEGETABLES

*This dish is a cancer-fighting powerhouse! Thanks to selected vegetables seasoned with rosemary, it's downright delicious and great for your body at the same time.*

**MAKES 4 SERVINGS**

2 large tomatoes, chopped

2 carrots, thinly sliced

1 zucchini, thinly sliced

1 red bell pepper, chopped

1 cup small broccoli florets

1 red onion, thinly sliced

½ cup thawed frozen corn or fresh corn kernels

2 tablespoons reduced-fat, soft tub, trans-fat-free spread

¼ cup minced fresh rosemary

¼ cup balsamic vinegar

2 cloves garlic, minced

¼ teaspoon red-pepper flakes

¼ teaspoon kosher salt

Preheat the oven to 400°F. Line a baking sheet with aluminum foil or parchment paper.

In a large bowl, combine the tomatoes, carrots, zucchini, bell pepper, broccoli, onion, and corn. Add the spread and rub it over all the vegetables until well coated. Add the rosemary, vinegar, garlic, red-pepper flakes, and salt. Mix well. Spread out evenly on the prepared baking sheet. Sprinkle with 2 tablespoons of water.

Roast for 20 to 25 minutes, turning occasionally, until the vegetables are tender and the tomatoes begin to fall apart. Serve immediately.

**Per serving:** 106 calories, 3 g protein, 19 g carbohydrate, 3 g fat (0 g saturated), 0 mg cholesterol, 150 mg sodium, 4 g fiber; plus 85 mg vitamin C (140% DV), 3,565 mcg beta-carotene, 2,375 mcg lycopene

# TANDOORI CAULIFLOWER

*My twist on tandoori incorporates the medicinal benefits of curcumin (turmeric) and cauliflower. You may choose to enjoy seasoned cauliflower plain for a mere 65 calories or prepare the more decadent version with the yogurt-and-raisin topping. Either way, your body will reap the benefits and your kitchen will smell fantastic!*

**MAKES 4 SERVINGS**

1 lemon, juiced

1 teaspoon turmeric

1 head cauliflower (about 2 pounds), cut into florets

¼ teaspoon kosher salt

2 scallions, thinly sliced

**Yogurt Topping (Optional)**

1 cup low-fat or nonfat plain yogurt

1 tablespoon curry powder

¼ cup golden raisins or dried cherries (optional)

Kosher salt

Preheat the oven to 400°F. Line a baking sheet with aluminum foil or parchment paper.

Half-fill a large stockpot with water. Add the lemon juice and turmeric and bring to a boil. Add the cauliflower and cook for 5 to 6 minutes, or until the florets just begin to soften but are still crisp.

Drain the cauliflower well and spread on the prepared baking sheet. Coat with oil spray and sprinkle with the salt. Bake for 7 to 8 minutes, or until the cauliflower is lightly browned and fork-tender. Garnish with the scallions and serve immediately.

**To make the optional yogurt topping:** In a small bowl, mix the yogurt, curry powder, and raisins or cherries. Season with salt to taste. Before transferring the cauliflower to the oven, pour the yogurt topping over the florets to cover evenly. (Omit the oil spray.)

**Per serving, without topping:** 65 calories, 5 g protein, 14 g carbohydrate, 0 g fat, 0 mg cholesterol, 139 mg sodium, 6 g fiber; plus 76 mg vitamin C (127% DV)

**Per serving, with topping:** 135 calories, 8 g protein, 26 g carbohydrate, 1 g fat (0 g saturated), 0 mg cholesterol, 184 mg sodium, 7 g fiber; plus 77 mg vitamin C (129% DV)

## JUDY'S GAZPACHO

*Judy and Marvin Lieberman opened Great Barrington Bagels in Great Barrington, Massachusetts, in the middle of a snowstorm. The horrendous weather must have been a sign of good luck because their business is thriving. Part of the reason has to be Judy's gazpacho—hands down, it's the best I've ever tasted. I'm not alone in my enthusiasm. People come from all around the Berkshire community to buy her gazpacho by the gallon. This is the first time Judy has ever shared her secret recipe, and I am honored and excited to be able to share it with you, too. Although Judy will use only Sacramento brand tomato juice, I encourage you to make this with any low-sodium brand you can find to keep the salt in check. If you like, garnish each serving with a swirl of fat-free or reduced-fat sour cream and additional chopped onion, cucumber, and pepper.*

**MAKES 8 SERVINGS (ABOUT 1 CUP EACH)**

1 onion, sliced

1 cucumber, sliced

1 green bell pepper, sliced

1 clove garlic

4 cups tomato juice (preferably low-sodium)

¼ cup red wine vinegar

¼ cup olive oil

¼ teaspoon kosher salt

⅛ teaspoon ground red pepper

In a food processor or blender, puree the onion, cucumber, bell pepper, garlic, and 1 cup of the tomato juice. Transfer to a large bowl and add the vinegar, oil, salt, red pepper, and the remaining 3 cups tomato juice. Prepare the gazpacho a day in advance and refrigerate. Serve chilled.

**Per serving:** 100 calories, 1 g protein, 9 g carbohydrate, 7 g fat (1 g saturated), 0 mg cholesterol, 120 mg sodium, 1 g fiber; plus 48 mg vitamin C (79% DV), 1,058 mcg beta-carotene, 11,690 mcg lycopene

# GREEN TEA POUND CAKE

*Hooray—a reason to eat cake! With only 183 calories and 4 grams of fat per slice, this special pound cake offers great flavor plus a hit of medicinal green tea. Enjoy it as an afternoon snack with a cup of hot tea, or, better yet, serve it at a get-together with friends and spread the health.*

**MAKES 6 SERVINGS**

¾ cup whole wheat pastry flour

¾ cup cake flour

1½ teaspoons baking powder

1 teaspoon baking soda

¼ teaspoon kosher salt

¼ cup reduced-fat, soft tub, trans-fat-free spread

¼ cup brown sugar

2 egg whites

1 cup buttermilk

2 teaspoons matcha (powdered green tea), dissolved in 1 tablespoon hot water*

2 teaspoons vanilla extract

Preheat the oven to 350°F. Coat a 1-pound loaf pan with oil spray.

In a medium bowl, combine the pastry flour, cake flour, baking powder, baking soda, and salt. In a large bowl, beat the spread and brown sugar with an electric mixer on medium speed until fluffy. Add the egg whites and mix well. Mix in the buttermilk, green tea, and vanilla. On low speed, mix in the flour mixture until just combined. Do not overmix.

Bake for 30 to 35 minutes, or until the top begins to brown and a wooden pick comes out clean when inserted in the middle of the cake. Transfer to a wire rack and let cool for 5 minutes. Remove the cake from the pan and cool completely.

*Matcha can be found in the natural foods aisle of major supermarkets; it should not confused with regular green tea bags or loose green tea.*

**Per serving:** 183 calories, 6 g protein, 30 g carbohydrate, 4 g fat (1 g saturated), 0 mg cholesterol, 480 mg sodium, 2 g fiber

# PART 6

# RESOURCES

# DECODING A NUTRITION LABEL

Once you become comfortable reading food labels and interpreting the wealth of information they offer, making healthy food choices at the supermarket will be a breeze. Here's how to decode a nutrition label (see sample label on page 469).

1. **Serving size and servings per container.** Look here first. All the other information on the label is based on a single serving, so you need to know the size of a single serving and how many servings are contained in the package. You may be surprised. Some packages look small, but they could contain two or more servings. Serving sizes are standardized, so you can compare similar foods and choose the one with the best nutrient profile.

2. **Calories.** If you are watching your weight (as most of us are), calories are key. This number is the total number of calories in a single serving. If you eat two servings, multiply the number of calories by two; if you eat three servings, multiply the number of calories by three, and so on.

3. **Calories from fat.** This tells you the number of calories in a single serving that come from fat. Some foods—such as margarine, butter, and oil—are all fat, so this number will be the same as the total number of calories.

4. **Total fat.** This section specifies the amount of total fat, plus the amounts of the two most dangerous types of fats: saturated fats and trans fats. (These are displayed in grams. To convert to calories from fat, multiply by 9.) You'll notice that there is a second number for both total fat and saturated fat—% Daily Value. This shows what percent of your total daily calories (based on a 2,000-calorie diet) is contained in one serving. As long as you keep your calories in check, there's really no need to be overly concerned with total fat. However, you do want to focus on keeping the two problematic fats, saturated and trans fats, to a minimum. I advise limiting saturated fat intake to less than 10 percent of calories (that works out to *less* than 22 grams of saturated fat per day based on a 2,000-calorie diet). There is no safe amount of trans fats, so aim to eat as few grams per day as possible.

5. **Cholesterol.** Only animal products contain cholesterol, so don't get too excited if your breakfast cereal or favorite candy doesn't have any. The American Heart Association recommends that healthy adults limit their daily cholesterol intake to 300 milligrams or less. For people with heart disease, they advise less than 200 milligrams per day. (The % Daily Value is based on a 300-milligram daily allotment.)

6. **Sodium.** This tells you the amount of salt in a single serving. In general, people should aim to keep their daily sodium intake below 2,300 milligrams. However,

certain populations are advised to further reduce their intake to 1,500 milli-grams or less. These populations include people 51 years old and older, all African Americans (this ethnic group is at high risk of high blood pressure), and people who have high blood pressure, diabetes, or chronic kidney disease.

7. **Carbohydrates.** I divide carbohydrates into two broad categories—high-quality and low-quality. Your goal should be to eat more of the former and less of the latter. Food labels tell you the amount of total carbohydrates in one serving. The label also gives you a few clues to the general quality of the carbohydrate via two categories: dietary fiber and sugars.

    Dietary fiber typically accompanies high-quality carbohydrates like whole grains, beans, lentils, vegetables, and fruits. Experts recommend that you consume 25 to 35 grams of total fiber daily.

    The sugars category can be tricky, since it includes naturally occurring sugars from unsweetened dairy and fruit, as well as added sugar from syrups, honey, high-fructose corn syrup, evaporated cane juice, and other sweeteners. When a product is high in sugar, it's typically easy to figure out where the sugar is coming from by examining the ingredients list. I advise choosing breakfast cereals with less than 8 grams of sugar per serving and 6-ounce flavored yogurt containers with less than 20 grams of sugar.

8. **Protein.** Take your weight in pounds and divide it in half. That's approximately how many grams of protein you should eat per day. This listing will help you figure out how much protein is contained in packaged foods.

9. **Vitamins and minerals.** Below the thick dividing line under Protein is the space for listing select vitamins and minerals and the percentage of the Recommended Daily Value contained in one serving. This can be helpful if you want to boost your intake of particular nutrients.

10. **Goals for certain calorie diets.** Some of the larger food labels also contain a small chart that lists recommended goals for various nutrients based on both a 2,000-calorie diet and a 2,500-calorie diet. These are simply reminders, and they do not provide additional information specific to that food.

11. **Calorie guide.** Some larger food labels also contain an informational section that lists the calories per gram for fat (9 calories per gram), carbohydrate (4 calories per gram), protein (4 calories per gram), and alcohol (7 calories per gram). This is strictly informational and not specific to any one food.

12. **Ingredients.** Somewhere outside the Nutrition Facts box is a list of ingredients, in descending order of predominance according to weight. That means that the first food listed is the most abundant (by weight).

13. **Special notations.** Look for special notations that might tell you more about the product, such as "enriched" or "fortified" (which tells you that extra vitamins or minerals have been added or replaced after processing), "contains

wheat ingredients" (which means it isn't safe for people with celiac disease or wheat sensitivities), or "may contain peanuts" (as a warning to people with peanut allergies).

14. **Contact information.** All labels must include a way for you to contact the company, such as the company name, address, telephone number, and/or Web site address. Don't hesitate to contact the company if you have questions about its products.

**① Nutrition Facts**
Serving Size
Servings Per Container

**Amount Per Serving**

| | |
|---|---|
| **② Calories** 0 | Calories from Fat 0 **③** |

% Daily Value*

| | |
|---|---|
| **④ Total Fat** 0g | 0% |
| Saturated Fat 0g | 0% |
| Trans Fat 0g | |
| **⑤ Cholesterol** 0mg | 0% |
| **⑥ Sodium** 0mg | 0% |
| **⑦ Total Carbohydrate** 0g | 0% |
| Dietary Fiber 0g | 0% |
| Soluble Fiber 0g | 0% |
| Insoluble Fiber 0g | 0% |
| Sugars 0g | |
| **⑧ Protein** 0g | |

| | | | |
|---|---|---|---|
| Vitamin A 0% | • | Vitamin C 0% | |
| Calcium 0% | • | Iron 0% | |
| **⑨** Phosphorus 0% | • | Magnesium 0% | |

* Percent Daily Values are based on a 2,000 calorie diet. Your daily values may be higher or lower depending on your calorie needs:

| | Calories: | 2,000 | 2,500 |
|---|---|---|---|
| **⑩** Total Fat | Less than | 0g | 0g |
| Sat Fat | Less than | 0g | 0g |
| Cholesterol | Less than | 0mg | 0mg |
| Sodium | Less than | 0mg | 0mg |
| Potassium | | 0mg | 0mg |
| Total Carbohydrate | | 0g | 0g |
| Dietary Fiber | | 0g | 0g |

**⑪** Calories per gram:
Fat 0 • Carbohydrate 0 • Protein 0

**⑫ INGREDIENTS:** Whole Wheat Flour, (Stone Ground Whole Oats, Hard Red Winter Wheat, Rye, Long Grain Brown Rice, Triticale, Buckwheat, Barley, Sesame Seeds), Malted Barley, Salt, Yeast, Mixed Tocopherols (Natural Vitamin E) for Freshness.

**⑬ CONTAINS WHEAT INGREDIENTS**

**⑭** DISTRIBUTED BY
COMPANY NAME
ADDRESS
CITY, STATE, ZIP
WEB ADDRESS

# REFERENCES

## WEIGHT LOSS, Chapter 3

Andrade A, Minaker T, Melanson K. Eating rate and satiation. Presentation at the 2006 Annual Scientific Meeting of NAASO: The Obesity Society. Boston, MA: October 20–24, 2006.

Czernichow S, Bertrais S, Preziosi P, et al. Indicators of abdominal obesity in middle-aged participants of the SU.VI.MAX study: relationships with educational level, smoking status and physical inactivity. *Diabetes Metabolism* 2004; 30(2):153–59.

Davis JN, Hodges VA, Gillham MB. Normal-weight adults consume more fiber and fruit than their age- and height-matched overweight/obese counterparts. *Journal of the American Dietetic Association* 2006; 106(6):833–40.

Gillum RF, Sempos CT. Ethnic variation in validity of classification of overweight and obesity using self-reported weight and height in American women and men: the Third National Health and Nutrition Examination Survey. *Nutrition Journal* [serial online] 2005; 4:27.

Gray DS, Fujioka K. Use of relative weight and body mass index for the determination of adiposity. *Journal of Clinical Epidemiology* 1991; 44(6):545–50.

Harrison GG. Height-weight tables. *Annals of Internal Medicine* 1985; 103(6 part 2):989–94.

Howard BV, Manson JE, Stefanick, ML, et al. Low-fat dietary pattern and weight change over 7 years: the Women's Health Initiative dietary modification trial. *Journal of the American Medical Association* 2006; 295(1):39–49.

Howarth NC, Huang TT, Roberts SB, McCrory MA. Dietary fiber and fat are associated with excess weight in young and middle-aged US adults. *Journal of the American Dietetic Association* 2005; 105(9):1365–72.

Howarth NC, Saltzman E, Roberts SB. Dietary fiber and weight regulation. *Nutrition Reviews* 2001; 59(5): 129–39.

Littman AJ, Kristal AR, White E. Effects of physical activity intensity, frequency, and activity type on 10-y weight change in middle-aged men and women. *International Journal of Obesity* 2005; 29(5):524–33.

Monti V, Carlson JJ, Hunt SC, Adams TD. Relationship of ghrelin and leptin hormones with body mass index and waist circumference in a random sample of adults. *Journal of the American Dietetic Association* 2006; 106(6):822–28.

Nelson LH, Tucker LA. Diet composition related to body fat in a multivariate study of 203 men. *Journal of the American Dietetic Association* 1996; 96(8):771–77.

Schoeller DA, Buchholz AC. Energetics of obesity and weight control: does diet composition matter? *Journal of the American Dietetic Association* 2005; 105(5 Suppl 1):S24–S28.

St Jeor ST, Howard BV, Prewitt TE, et al. Dietary protein and weight reduction: a statement for health care professionals from the Nutrition Committee of the Council on Nutrition, Physical Activity, and Metabolism of the American Heart Association. *Circulation* 2001; 104(15):1869–74.

Weigley ES. Average? Ideal? Desirable? A brief overview of height-weight tables in the United States. *Journal of the American Dietetic Association* 1984; 84(4):417–23.

Willett WC. The Mediterranean diet: science and practice. *Public Health Nutrition* 2006; 9(1A):105–10.

Williams PT, Pate RR. Cross-sectional relationships of exercise and age to adiposity in 60,617 male runners. *Medicine and Science in Sports and Exercise* 2005; 37(8):1329–37.

Williams PT, Satariano WA. Relationships of age and weekly running distance to BMI and circumferences in 41,582 physically active women. *Obesity Research* 2005; 13(8):1370–80.

Williams PT, Wood PD. The effects of changing exercise levels on weight and age-related weight gain. *International Journal of Obesity* 2006; 30(3):543–51.

Yao M, Roberts SB. Dietary energy density and weight regulation. *Nutrition Reviews* 2001; 59(8 Pt 1):247–58.

Zemel MB. The role of dairy foods in weight management. *Journal of the American College of Nutrition* 2005; 24(6 Suppl):537S–546S.

## BEAUTIFUL SKIN, Chapter 4

Adebamowo CA, Spiegelman D, Berkey CS, et al. Milk consumption and acne in teenaged boys. *Journal of the American Academy of Dermatology* 2008; 58(5):794–95.

Adebamowo CA, Spiegelman D, Danby FW, et al. High school dietary dairy intake and teenage acne. *Journal of the American Academy of Dermatology* 2005; 52(2):207–14.

Camouse MM, Domingo DS, Swain FR, et al. Topical application of green and white tea extracts provides protection from solar-stimulated ultraviolet light in human skin. *Experimental Dermatology* 2009; 18(6):522–26.

Duffield-Lillico AJ, Slate EH, Reid ME, et al. Selenium supplementation and secondary prevention of non-melanoma skin cancer in a randomized trial. *Journal of the National Cancer Institute* 2003; 95(19):1477–81.

Elmets CA, Sing D, Tubesing K, et al. Cutaneous photoprotection from ultraviolet injury by green tea polyphenols. *Journal of the American Academy of Dermatology* 2001; 44(3):425–32.

Hakim IA, Harris RB, Ritenbaugh C. Fat intake and risk of squamous cell carcinoma of the skin. *Nutrition and Cancer* 2000; 36(2):155–62.

Schwartz JR, Marsh RG, Draelos ZD. Zinc and skin health: overview of physiology and pharmacology. *Dermatologic Surgery* 2005; 31(7 Pt 2):837–47.

Sies HO, Stahl W. Nutritional protection against skin damage from sunlight. *Annual Review of Nutrition* 2004; 24:173–200.

Skolnik P, Eaglstein WH, Ziboh VA. Human essential fatty acid deficiency: treatment by topical application of linoleic acid. *Archives of Dermatology* 1977; 113(7):939–41.

Steele VE, Kelloff GJ, Balentine D, et al. Comparative chemopreventive mechanisms of green tea, black tea and selected polyphenol extracts measured by in vitro bioassays. *Carcinogenesis* 2000; 21(1):63–67.

Wilson D, Varigos G, Ackland ML. Apoptosis may underlie the pathology of zinc-deficient skin. *Immunology and Cell Biology* 2006; 84(1):28–37.

## HEALTHY HAIR, Chapter 5

Birch MP, Lalla SC, Messenger AG. Female pattern hair loss. *Clinical and Experimental Dermatology* 2002; 27(5):383–88.

Corazza GR, Andreani ML, Venturo N, et al. Celiac disease and alopecia areata: report of a new association. *Gastroenterology* 1995; 109(4):1333–37.

Harkey MR. Anatomy and physiology of hair. *Forensic Science International* 1993; 63(1-3):9–18.

Rushton DH. Nutritional factors and hair loss. *Clinical and Experimental Dermatology* 2002; 27(5):396–404.

Springer K, Brown M, Stulberg DL. Common hair loss disorders. *American Family Physician* 2003; 68(1):93–102.

Trost LB, Bergfeld WF, Calogeras E. The diagnosis and treatment of iron deficiency and its potential relationship to hair loss. *Journal of the American Academy of Dermatology* 2006; 54(5):824–44.

Wiedemeyeer K, Schill WB, Loser C. Diseases on hair follicles leading to hair loss part: nonscarring alopecias. *Skinmed* 2004; 3(4):209–14.

## FEEDING A BEAUTIFUL SMILE, Chapter 6

Adegboye AR, Fiehn NE, Twetman S, et al. Low calcium intake is related to increased risk of tooth loss in men. *Journal of Nutrition* 2010; 140(10):1864–68.

Bergstrom J. Cigarette smoking as a risk factor in chronic periodontal disease. *Community Dentistry and Oral Epidemiology* 1989; 17(5):245–47.

Briggs JE, McKeown PP, Crawford VL, et al. Angiographically confirmed coronary heart disease and periodontal disease in middle-aged males. *Journal of Periodontology* 2006; 77(1):95–102.

Bsoul SA, Terezhalmy GT. Vitamin C in health and disease. *Journal of Contemporary Dental Practice* 2004; 5(2):1–13.

Hamilton-Miller JMT. Anti-cariogenic properties of tea (*Camellia sinensis*). *Journal of Medical Microbiology* 2001; 50(4):299–302.

Kushiyama M, Shimazaki Y, Murakami M, et al. Relationship between intake of green tea and periodontal disease. *Journal of Periodontology* 2009; 80(3):372–77.

Nishida M, Grossi SG, Dunford RG, et al. Calcium and the risk for periodontal disease. *Journal of Periodontology* 2000; 71(7):1057–66.

Nishida M, Grossi SG, Dunford RG, et al. Dietary vitamin C and the risk for periodontal disease. *Journal of Periodontology* 2000; 71(8):1215–23.

Parry J, Shaw L, Arnaud MJ, et al. Investigation of mineral waters and soft drinks in relation to dental erosion. *Journal of Oral Rehabilitation* 2001; 28(8):766–72.

Wang PL, Shirasu S, Shinohara M, et al. Salivary amylase activity of rats fed a low calcium diet. *Japanese Journal of Pharmacology* 1998; 78(3):279–83.

## CARDIOVASCULAR DISEASE, Chapter 7

Andersen LF, Jacobs Jr DR, Carlsen MH, Blomhoff R. Consumption of coffee is associated with reduced risk of death attributed to inflammatory and cardiovascular diseases in the Iowa Women's Health Study. *American Journal of Clinical Nutrition* 2006; 82(5):1039-46.

Austin MA, Hokanson JE, Edwards KL. Hypertriglyceridemia as a cardiovascular risk factor. *American Journal of Cardiology* 1998; 81(4A):7B-12B.

Blache D, Devaux S, Joubert O, et al. Long-term moderate magnesium-deficient diet shows relationships between blood pressure, inflammation and oxidant stress defense in aging rats. *Free Radical Biology & Medicine* 2006; 41(2):277-84.

Borek C. Garlic reduces dementia and heart-disease risk. *Journal of Nutrition* 2006; 136(3 Suppl):S810-S812.

Brown CD, Higgins M, Donato KA, et al. Body mass index and the prevalence of hypertension and dyslipidemia. *Obesity Research* 2000; 8(9):605-19.

Brown L, Rosner B, Willett WW, Sacks FM. Cholesterol-lowering effects of dietary fiber: a meta-analysis. *American Journal of Clinical Nutrition* 1999; 69(1):30-42.

Chrysohoou C, Panagiotakos DB, Pitsavos C, et al. The association between pre-hypertension status and oxidative stress markers related to atherosclerotic disease: The ATTICA study. *Atherosclerosis* 2007; 192(1):169-76.

Davidson MH, Maki KC, Umporowicz DM, et al. Safety and tolerability of esterified phytosterols administered in reduced-fat spread and salad dressing to healthy adult men and women. *Journal of the American College of Nutrition* 2001; 20(4):307-19.

Ding EL, Hutfless SM, Ding X, Girotra S. Chocolate and prevention of cardiovascular disease: a systematic review. *Nutrition and Metabolism* (London) [online] 2006; 3:2.

Flint AJ, Hu FB, Glynn RJ, et al. Whole grains and incident hypertension in men. *American Journal of Clinical Nutrition* 2009; 90(3):493-98.

Gardner CD, Lawson LD, Block E, et al. Effect of raw garlic vs commercial garlic supplements on plasma lipid concentrations in adults with moderate hypercholesterolemia: a randomized clinical trial. *Archives of Internal Medicine* 2007; 167(4):346-53.

Gill JM, Mees GP, Frayn KN, Hardman AE. Moderate exercise, postprandial lipaemia and triacylglycerol clearance. *European Journal of Clinical Investigation* 2001; 31(3):201-07.

Gonen A, Harats D, Rabinkov A, et al. The antiatherogenic effect of allicin: possible mode of action. *Pathobiology* 2005; 72(6):325-34.

Gordon RY, Cooperman T, Obermeyer W, et al. Marked variability of monacolin levels in commercial red yeast rice products: buyer beware! *Archives of Internal Medicine* 2010; 170(19):1722-27.

Grubben MJ, Boers GH, Blom HJ, et al. Unfiltered coffee increases plasma homocysteine concentrations in healthy volunteers: a randomized trial. *American Journal of Clinical Nutrition* 2000; 71(2):480-84.

Guyton JR. Extended-release niacin for modifying the lipoprotein profile. *Expert Opinion on Pharmacotherapy* 2004; 5(6):1385-98.

Halperin RO, Sesso HD, Ma J, et al. Dyslipidemia and the risk of incident hypertension in men. *Hypertension* 2006; 47(1):45-50.

He K, Liu K, Daviglus ML, et al. Magnesium intake and incidence of metabolic syndrome among young adults. *Circulation* 2006; 113(13):1675–82.

Hendriks HF, Brink EJ, Meijer GW, et al. Safety of long-term consumption of plant sterol esters-enriched spread. *European Journal of Clinical Nutrition* 2003; 57(5):681–92.

Hokanson JE, Austin MA. Plasma triglyceride level is a risk factor for cardiovascular disease independent of high-density lipoprotein cholesterol level: a meta-analysis of population-based prospective studies. *Journal of Cardiovascular Risk* 1996; 3(2):213–19.

Hu FB, Manson JE, Willett WC. Types of dietary fat and risk of coronary heart disease: a critical review. *Journal of the American College of Nutrition* 2001; 20(1):5–19.

Hu FB, Rimm EB, Stampfer MJ, et al. Prospective Study of major dietary patterns and risk of coronary heart disease in men. *American Journal of Clinical Nutrition* 2000; 72(4):912–21.

Jakobsen MU, Dethlefsen C, Joensen AM, et al. Intake of carbohydrates compared with intake of saturated fatty acids and risk of myocardial infarction: importance of the glycemic index. *American Journal of Clinical Nutrition* 2010; 91(6):1764–68.

Jakobsen MU, O'Reilly EJ, Heitmann BL. Major types of dietary fat and risk of coronary heart disease: a pooled analysis of 11 cohort studies. *American Journal of Clinical Nutrition* 2009; 89(5):1425–32.

Jorde R, Bonaa KH. Calcium from dairy products, vitamin D intake, and blood pressure: the Tromso Study. *American Journal of Clinical Nutrition* 2000; 71(6):1530–35.

Katsanos CS. Prescribing aerobic exercise for the regulation of postprandial lipid metabolism: current research and recommendations. *Sports Medicine* 2006; 36(7):547–60.

Klag MJ, Wang NY, Meoni LA, et al. Coffee intake and risk of hypertension: the Johns Hopkins precursors study. *Archives of Internal Medicine* 2002; 162(6):657–62.

Kolovou GD, Salpea KD, Anagnostopoulou KK, Mikhailidis DP. Alcohol use, vascular disease, and lipid-lowering drugs. *Journal of Pharmacology and Experimental Therapeutics* 2006; 318(1):1–7.

Lavie CJ, Milani RV, Ventura HO. Obesity and cardiovascular disease: risk factor, paradox, and impact of weight loss. *Journal of the American College of Cardiology* 2009; 53(21):1925–32.

Lee KW, Lip GYH. The role of omega-3 fatty acids in the secondary prevention of cardiovascular disease. *Quarterly Journal of Medicine* 2003; 96;465–80.

Lichtenstein A, Appel LJ, Brands M, et al. Diet and lifestyle recommendations revision 2006: a scientific statement from the American Heart Association Nutrition Committee. *Circulation* 2006; 114(1):82–96.

Lopez-Garcia E, van Dam RM, Willett WC, et al. Coffee consumption and coronary heart disease in men and women: a prospective cohort study. *Circulation* 2006; 113(17):2045–53.

Lovallo WR, Wilson MF, Vincent AS, et al. Blood pressure response to caffeine shows incomplete tolerance after short-term regular consumption. *Hypertension* 2004; 43(4):760–65.

Lu Z, Chen TC, Zhang A, et al. An evaluation of the vitamin $D_3$ content in fish: is the vitamin D content adequate to satisfy the dietary requirement for vitamin D? *Journal of Steroid Biochemistry and Molecular Biology* 2007; 103(3-5):642–44.

Makela P, Valkonen T, Martelin T. Contribution of deaths related to alcohol use of socioeconomic variation in mortality: register based follow up study. *British Medical Journal* 1997; 315(7102):211–16.

Maki KC, Davidson MH, Umporowicz DM, et al. Lipid responses to plant-sterol-enriched reduced-fat spreads incorporated into a National Cholesterol Education Program Step I diet. *American Journal of Clinical Nutrition* 2001; 74(1):33–43.

McTigue K, Larson JC, Valoski A, et al. Mortality and cardiac and vascular outcomes in extremely obese women. *Journal of the American Medical Association* 2006; 296(1):79–86.

Mellen PB, Walsh TF, Herrington DM. Whole grain intake and cardiovascular disease: a meta-analysis. *Nutrition, Metabolism, and Cardiovascular Diseases* 2008; 18(4):283–90.

Mozaffarian D, Micha R, Wallace S. Effects on coronary heart disease of increasing polyunsaturated fat in place of saturated fat: a systematic review and meta-analysis of randomized controlled trials. *Public Library of Science Medicine* 2010; 7(3):e1000252.

Mozaffarian D, Rimm EB. Fish intake, contaminants, and human health: evaluating the risks and the benefits. *Journal of the American Medical Association* 2006; 296(15):1885–99.

Myers MG. Effect of caffeine on blood pressure beyond the laboratory. *Hypertension* 2004; 43(4):724–25.

Nam BH, Kannel WB, D'Agostino RB. Search for an optimal atherogenic lipid risk profile: from the Framingham Study. *American Journal of Cardiology* 2006; 97(3):372–75.

Oh K, Hu FB, Manson JE, et al. Dietary fat intake and risk of coronary heart disease in women: 20 years of follow-up of the nurses' health study. *American Journal of Epidemiology* 2005; 161(7):672–79.

Reilly MP, Wolfe ML, Localoi AR, Rader, DJ. C-reactive protein and coronary artery calcification: the study of inherited risk of coronary atherosclerosis (SIRCA). *Arteriosclerosis, Thrombosis, and Vascular Biology* 2003; 23:1851–56.

Ridker PM, Stampfer MJ, Rifai N. Novel risk factors for systemic atherosclerosis: a comparison of C-reactive protein, fibrinogen, homocysteine, lipoprotein(a), and standard cholesterol screening as predictors of peripheral arterial disease. *Journal of the American Medical Association* 2001; 285(19):2481–85.

Ried K, Frank OR, Stocks NP, et al. Effect of garlic on blood pressure: a systematic review and meta-analysis. *BMC Cardiovascular Disorders* 2008; 8:13.

Rimm EB, Williams P, Fosher K, et al. Moderate alcohol intake and lower risk of coronary heart disease: meta-analysis of effects on lipids and haemostatic factors. *British Medical Journal* 1999; 319(7224):1523–28.

Sacks FM, Lichtenstein A, Van Horn L, et al. Soy protein, isoflavones, and cardiovascular health: an American Heart Association Science Advisory for Professionals from the Nutrition Committee. *Circulation* 2006; 113(7):1034–44.

Salonen JT, Lakka TA, Lakka HM, et al. Hyperinsulinemia is associated with the incidence of hypertension and dyslipidemia in middle-aged men. *Diabetes* 1998; 47(2):270–75.

Sesso HD, Buring JE, Chown MJ, et al. A prospective study of plasma lipid levels and hypertension in women. *Archives of Internal Medicine* 2005; 165(20):2420–27.

Sesso HD, Buring JE, Rifai N, et al. C-reactive protein and the risk of developing hypertension. *Journal of the American Medical Association* 2003; 290(22):2945–51.

Shai I, Rimm EB, Hankinson SE, et al. Multivariate assessment of lipid parameters as predictors of coronary heart disease among postmenopausal women: potential implications for clinical guidelines. *Circulation* 2004; 110(18):2824–30.

Siri-Tarino PW, Sun Q, Hu FB, et al. Meta-analysis of prospective cohort studies evaluating the association of saturated fat with cardiovascular disease. *American Journal of Clinical Nutrition* 2010; 91(3):535–46.

Strazzullo P, D'Elia L, Kandala NB, et al. Salt intake, stroke, and cardiovascular disease: meta-analysis of prospective studies. *British Medical Journal* 2009; 339:b4567. [Epub]

Tanne D, Koren-Morag N, Graff E, Goldbourt U. Blood lipids and first-ever ischemic stroke/transient ischemic attack in the bezafibrate infarction prevention (BIP) registry: high triglycerides constitute an independent risk factor. *Circulation* 2001; 104:2892–97.

Thomson M, Al-Qattan KK, Bordia T, Ali M. Including garlic in the diet may help lower blood glucose, cholesterol, and triglycerides. *Journal of Nutrition* 2006: 136(3 Suppl):S800–S802.

Tighe P, Duthie G, Vaughan N, et al. Effect of increased consumption of whole-grain foods on blood pressure and other cardiovascular risk markers in healthy middle-aged persons: a randomized controlled trial. *American Journal of Clinical Nutrition* 2010; 92(4):733–40.

Tobias K, Moore SC, Gaziano M, et al. Healthy lifestyle and the risk of stroke in women. *Archives of Internal Medicine* 2006; 166(13):1403–09.

Wang L, Gaziano JM, Liu S, et al. Whole- and refined-grain intakes and the risk of hypertension in women. *American Journal of Clinical Nutrition* 2007; 86(2):472–79.

Welsh JA, Sharma A, Abramson JL, et al. Caloric sweetener consumption and dyslipidemia among US adults. *Journal of the American Medical Association* 2010; 303(15):1490–97.

Weststrate JA, Meijer GW. Plant sterol-enriched margarines and reduction of plasma total- and LDL-cholesterol concentrations in normocholesterolaemic and mildly hypercholesterolaemic subjects. *European Journal of Clinical Nutrition* 1998; 52(5):334–43.

Wexler R, Aukerman G. Nonpharmacologic strategies for managing hypertension. *American Family Physician* 2006; 73(11):1953–56.

Wilburn AJ, King DS, Glisson J, et al. The natural treatment of hypertension. *Journal of Clinical Hypertension* (Greenwich) 2004; 6(5):219–21.

Wildman RP, Sutton-Tyrrell K, Newman AB, et al. Lipoprotein levels are associated with incident hypertension in older adults. *Journal of the American Geriatric Society* 2004; 52(6):916–21.

## ARTHRITIS, Chapter 8

Ahmed S, Wang N, Lalonde M, et al. Green tea polyphenol epigallocatechin-3-gallate (EGCG) differentially inhibits interleukin-1 beta-induced expression of matrix metalloproteinase-1 and -13 in human chondrocytes. *Journal of Pharmacology and Experimental Therapeutics* 2004; 308(2):767–73.

Altman RD, Marcussen KC. Effects of a ginger extract on knee pain in patients with osteoarthritis. *Arthritis and Rheumatism* 2001; 44(11):2531–38.

Belch J, Hill A. Evening primrose oil and borage oil in rheumatologic conditions. *American Journal of Clinical Nutrition* 2000; 71(Suppl):S352–S356.

Cameron M, Gagnier JJ, Little CV, et al. Evidence of effectiveness of herbal medicinal products in the treatment of arthritis. Part 2: Rheumatoid arthritis. *Phytotherapy Research* 2009; 23(12):1647–62.

Chaganti RK, Parimi N, Cawthon P, et al. Association of 25-hydroxyvitamin D with prevalent osteoarthritis of the hip in elderly men: the osteoporotic fractures in men study. *Arthritis and Rheumatism* 2010; 62(2):511–14.

Chainani-Wu N. Safety and anti-inflammatory activity of curcumin: a component of turmeric (Curcumalonga). *Journal of Alternative and Complementary Medicine* 2003; 9(1):161–68.

Choi HK. A prescription for lifestyle change in patients with hyperuricemia and gout. *Current Opinion in Rheumatology* 2010; 22(2):165–72.

Choi HK. Dietary risk factors for rheumatic diseases. *Current Opinion in Rheumatology* 2005; 17(2):141–46.

Choi HK, Atkinson K, Karlson EW, et al. Alcohol intake and risk of incident gout in men: a prospective study. *Lancet* 2004; 363:1277–81.

Choi HK, Atkinson K, Karlson EW, et al. Purine-rich foods, dairy and protein intake, and the risk of gout in men. *New England Journal of Medicine* 2004; 350(11):1093–03.

Choi HK, Atkinson K, Karlson EW. Alcohol intake and risk of incident gout in men: a prospective study. *Lancet* 2004; 363(9417):1251–52.

Choi HK, Curhan G. Coffee consumption and risk of incident gout in women: the Nurses' Health Study. *American Journal of Clinical Nutrition* 2010; 92(4):922–27.

Choi HK, Curhan G. Gout: epidemiology and lifestyle choices. *Current Opinion in Rheumatology* 2005; 17(3):341–45.

Choi HK, Curhan G. Soft drinks, fructose consumption, and the risk of gout in men: prospective cohort study. *British Medical Journal* 2008; 336(7639):309–12.

Choi HK, Willett W, Curhan G. Coffee consumption and risk of incident gout in men: a prospective study. *Arthritis and Rheumatism* 2007; 56(6):2.

Cleland LG, James MJ, Proudman SM. Fish oil: what the prescriber needs to know. *Arthritis Research & Therapy* 2005; 8(1):202.

Cleland LG, James MJ, Proudman SM. The role of fish oils in the treatment of rheumatoid arthritis. *Drugs* 2003; 63(9):845–53.

De Silva V, El-Metwally A, Ernst E, et al. Evidence for the efficacy of complementary and alternative medicines in the management of osteoarthritis: a systematic review. *Rheumatology* 2011; 50(5):911–20.

Ding C, Cicuttini F, Scott F, et al. Natural history of knee cartilage defects and factors affecting change. *Archives of Internal Medicine* 2006; 166(6):651–58.

Funk JL, Oyarzo JN, Frye JB, et al. Turmeric extracts containing curcuminoids prevent experimental rheumatoid arthritis. *Journal of Natural Products* 2006; 69(3):351–55.

Grant WB. Epidemiology of disease risks in relation to vitamin D insufficiency. *Progress in Biophysics and Molecular Biology* 2006; 92(1):65–79.

Hochberg M, Lixing L, Barker B, et al. Traditional Chinese acupuncture is effective as adjunctive therapy in patients with osteoarthritis of the knee. *Arthritis and Rheumatism* 2001; 44:819–25.

Hooper MM, Stellato TA, Hallowell PT, et al. Musculoskeletal findings in obese subjects before and after weight loss following bariatric surgery. *International Journal of Obesity* (Lond) [serial online] 2006; Apr 25.

Ishikawa Y, Kitamura M. Bioflavonoid quercetin inhibits mitosis and apoptosis of glomerular cells in vitro and in vivo. *Biochemical and Biophysical Research Communications* 2000; 279(2):629–34.

Kopp W. The atherogenic potential of dietary carbohydrate. *Preventive Medicine* 2006; 42(5):336–42.

Kraus VB, Huebner JL, Stabler T, et al. Ascorbic acid increases severity of spontaneous knee osteoarthritis in a guinea pig model. *Arthritis and Rheumatism* 2004; 50(6):1822–31.

Lee SJ, Terkeltaub RA, Kavanaugh A. Recent developments in diet and gout. *Current Opinion in Rheumatology* 2006; 18(2):193–98.

Luk AJ, Simkin PA. Epidemiology of hyperuricemia and gout. *American Journal of Managed Care* 2005; 11(15 Suppl):S435–S442.

Martinez-Dominguez E, de la Puerta R, Ruiz-Gutierrez V. Protective effects upon experimental inflammation models of a polyphenol-supplemented virgin olive oil diet. *Inflammation Research* 2001; 50(2):102–6.

Messier SP, Gutekunst DJ, Davis C, DeVita P. Weight loss reduces knee-joint loads in overweight and obese older adults with knee osteoarthritis. *Arthritis and Rheumatism* 2005; 52(7):2026–32.

Messier SP, Loeser RF, Miller GD, et al. Exercise and dietary weight loss in overweight and obese older adults with knee osteoarthritis: the arthritis, diet, and activity promotion trial. *Arthritis and Rheumatism* 2004; 50(5):1501–10.

Morelli V, Naquin C, Weaver, V. Alternative therapies for traditional disease states: osteoarthritis. *American Family Physician* 2003; 67(2):339–44.

Najm WI, Reinsch S, Hoehler F, et al. S-Adenosyl methionine (SAMe) versus celecoxib for the treatment of osteoarthritis symptoms: a double-blind cross-over trial. *BMC Musculoskeletal Disorders* [serial online] 2004; 5:6.[Epub]

Padyukov L, Silva C, Stolt P, et al. A gene-environment interaction between smoking and shared epitope genes in HLA-DR provides a high risk of seropositive rheumatoid arthritis. *Arthritis and Rheumatism* 2004; 50(10):3085–92.

Pattison DJ, Silman AJ, Goodson NJ, et al. Vitamin C and the risk of developing inflammatory polyarthritis: prospective nested case-control study. *Annals of the Rheumatic Diseases* 2004; 63(7):843–47.

Pattison DJ, Symmons DP, Lunt M, et al. Dietary beta-cryptoxanthin and inflammatory polyarthritis: results from a population-based prospective study. *American Journal of Clinical Nutrition* 2005; 82(2):451–55.

Pattison DJ, Symmons DPM, Lunt M, et al. Dietary risk factors for the development of inflammatory polyarthritis: evidence for a role of high level of red meat consumption. *Arthritis and Rheumatism* 2004; 50(12):3804–12.

Piscoya J, Rodriguez Z, Bustamante SA, et al. Efficacy and safety of freeze-dried cat's claw in osteoarthritis of the knee: mechanisms of action of the species *Uncaria guianensis*. *Inflammation Research* 2001; 50(9):442–48.

Sato M, Miyazaki T, Kambe F. Quercetin, a bioflavonoid, inhibits the induction of interleukin 8 and monocyte chemoattractant protein-1 expression by tumor necrosis factor-alpha in cultured human synovial cells. *Journal of Rheumatology* 1997; 24(9):1680–84.

Sawitzke AD, Shi H, Finco MF, et al. Clinical efficacy and safety of glucosamine, chondroitin sulphate, their combination, celecoxib or placebo taken to treat osteoarthritis of the knee: 2-year results from GAIT. *Annals of the Rheumatic Diseases* 2010; 69(8):1459–64.

Sawitzke AD, Shi H, Finco MF, et al. The effect of glucosamine and/or chondroitin sulfate on the progression of knee osteoarthritis: a report from the glucosamine/chondroitin arthritis intervention trial. *Arthritis and Rheumatism* 2008; 58(10):3183–91.

Schlesinger N. Dietary factors and hyperuricaemia. *Current Pharmaceutical Design* 2005; 11(32):4133–38.

Shishodia S, Sethi G, Aggarwal BB. Curcumin: getting back to the roots. *Annals of the New York Academy of Sciences* 2005; 1056:206–17.

Teixeira S. Bioflavonoids: proanthocyanidins and quercetin and their potential roles in treating musculoskeletal conditions. *Journal of Orthopaedic and Sports Physical Therapy* 2002; 32(7):357–63.

Yoon JH, Baek SJ. Molecular targets of dietary polyphenols with anti-inflammatory properties. *Yonsei Medical Journal* 2005; 46(5):585–96.

## TYPE 2 DIABETES, Chapter 9

Agardh EE, Carlsson S, Ahlbom A, et al. Coffee consumption, type 2 diabetes and impaired glucose tolerance in Swedish men and women. *Journal of Internal Medicine* 2004; 255(6):645–52.

Althuis MD, Jordan NE, Ludington EA, Wittes JT. Glucose and insulin responses to dietary chromium supplements: a meta-analysis. *American Journal of Clinical Nutrition* 2002; 76(1):148–55.

American Diabetes Association. Standards of medical care in diabetes—2010. *Diabetes Care* 2010; 33(Suppl 1):S11–S61.

Carlsson S, Hammar N, Grill V, Kaprio J. Alcohol consumption and the incidence of type 2 diabetes: a 20-year follow-up of the Finnish Twin Cohort Study. *Diabetes Care* 2003; 26(10):2785–90.

Colberg SR, Sigal RJ, Fernhall B, et al. Exercise and type 2 diabetes: the American College of Sports Medicine and the American Diabetes Association: joint position statement. *Diabetes Care* 2010; 33(12):e147–67.

Davies M, Brophy S, Williams R, Taylor A. The prevalence, severity, and impact of painful diabetic peripheral neuropathy in type 2 diabetes. *Diabetes Care* 2006; 29(7):1518–22.

Fung TT, Hu FB, Pereira MA, et al. Whole-grain intake and the risk of type 2 diabetes: a prospective study in men. *American Journal of Clinical Nutrition* 2002; 76(3):535–40.

Gerhard GT, Ahmann A, Meeuws K, et al. Effects of a low-fat diet compared with those of a high-monoun-saturated fat diet on body weight, plasma lipids and lipoproteins, and glycemic control in type 2 diabetes. *American Journal of Clinical Nutrition* 2004; 80(3):668–73.

Gillen LJ, Tapsell LC, Patch CS, et al. Structured dietary advice incorporating walnuts achieves optimal fat and energy balance in patients with type 2 diabetes mellitus. *Journal of the American Dietetic Association* 2005; 105(7):1087–96.

Gumbiner B, Low CC, Reaven PD. Effects of a monounsaturated fatty acid–enriched hypocaloric diet on cardiovascular risk factors in obese patients with type 2 diabetes. *Diabetes Care* 1998; 21(1):9–15.

Haag M, Dippenaar NG. Dietary fats, fatty acids and insulin resistance: short review of a multifaceted connection. *Medical Science Monitor* 2005; 11(12):RA359–67.

Harsch IA, Schahin SP, Bruckner K, et al. The effect of continuous positive airway pressure treatment on insulin sensitivity in patients with obstructive sleep apnoea syndrome and type 2 diabetes. *Respiration* 2004; 71(3):252–59.

Hasanain B, Mooradian AD. Antioxidant vitamins and their influence in diabetes mellitus. *Current Diabetes Reports* 2002; 2(5):448–56.

Howard AA, Arnsten JH, Gourevitch MN. Effect of alcohol consumption on diabetes mellitus: a systematic review. *Annals of Internal Medicine* 2004; 140(3):211–19.

Hu FB, Manson JE, Stampfer MJ, et al. Diet, lifestyle, and the risk of type 2 diabetes mellitus in women. *New England Journal of Medicine* 2001; 345(11):790–97.

Huxley R, Lee CM, Barzi F, et al. Coffee, decaffeinated coffee, and tea consumption in relation to incident type 2 diabetes mellitus: a systematic review with meta-analysis. *Archives of Internal Medicine* 2009; 169(22):2053–63.

Ip MSM, Lam B, Ng MMT, et al. Obstructive sleep apnea is independently associated with insulin resistance. *American Journal of Respiratory and Critical Care Medicine* 2002; 165(5):670–76.

Khader YS, Dauod AS, El-Qaderi SS, et al. Periodontal status of diabetics compared with nondiabetics: a meta-analysis. *Journal of Diabetes Complications* 2006; 20(1):59–68.

Khan A, Safdar M, Ali Khan MM, et al. Cinnamon improves glucose and lipids of people with type 2 diabetes. *Diabetes Care* 2003; 26(12):3215–18.

Kim DJ, Xun P, Liu K, et al. Magnesium intake in relation to systemic inflammation, insulin resistance, and the incidence of diabetes. *Diabetes Care* 2010; 33(12):2604–10.

Kiran M, Arpak N, Unsal E, Erdogan MF. The effect of improved periodontal health on metabolic control in type 2 diabetes mellitus. *Journal of Clinical Periodontology* 2005; 32(3):266–72.

Kleefstra N, Houweling ST, Jansman FG, et al. Chromium treatment has no effect in patients with poorly controlled, insulin-treated type 2 diabetes in an obese Western population: a randomized, double-blind, placebo-controlled trial. *Diabetes Care* 2006; 29(3):521–25.

Knowler WC, Barrett-Connor E, Fowler SE, et al. Diabetes Prevention Program Research Group. Reduction in the incidence of type 2 diabetes with lifestyle intervention or metformin. *New England Journal of Medicine* 2002; 346(6):393–403.

Liese AD, Schulz M, Fang F, et al. Dietary glycemic index and glycemic load, carbohydrate and fiber intake, and measures of insulin sensitivity, secretion, and adiposity in the Insulin Resistance Atherosclerosis Study. *Diabetes Care* 2005; 28(12):2832–38.

Lopez-Garcia E, van Dam RM, Willett WC, et al. Coffee consumption and coronary heart disease in men and women: a prospective cohort study. *Circulation* 2006; 113(17):2045–53.

Lopez-Ridaura R, Willett WC, Rimm EB, et al. Magnesium intake and risk of type 2 diabetes in men and women. *Diabetes Care* 2004; 27(1):134–40.

Mang B, Wolters M, Schmitt B, et al. Effects of a cinnamon extract on plasma glucose, HbA, and serum lipids in diabetes mellitus type 2. *European Journal of Clinical Investigation* 2006; 36(5):340–44.

Meyer KA, Kushi LH, Jacobs Jr DR, Folsom AR. Dietary fat and incidence of type 2 diabetes in older Iowa women. *Diabetes Care* 2001; 24(9):1528–35.

Montonen J, Knekt P, Jarvinen R, et al. Whole-grain and fiber intake and the incidence of type 2 diabetes. *American Journal of Clinical Nutrition* 2003; 77(3):622–29.

Mooren FC, Kruger K, Volker K, et al. Oral magnesium supplementation reduces insulin resistance in non-diabetic subjects—a double-blind, placebo-controlled, randomized trial. *Diabetes, Obesity, and Metabolism* 2011; 13(3):281–84.

Ostman E, Granfeldt, Y, Persson L, Bjorck I. Vinegar supplementation lowers glucose and insulin responses and increases satiety after a bread meal in healthy subjects. *European Journal of Clinical Nutrition* 2005; 59(9):983–88.

Partanen J, Niskanen L, Lehtinen J, et al. Natural history of peripheral neuropathy in patients with non-insulin-dependent diabetes mellitus. *New England Journal of Medicine* 1995; 333(2):89–94.

Pereira MA, Parker ED, Folsom AR. Coffee consumption and risk of type 2 diabetes mellitus: an 11-year prospective study of 28,812 postmenopausal women. *Archives of Internal Medicine* 2006; 166(12):1311–16.

Pittas AG, Dawson-Hughes B, Li T, et al. Vitamin D and calcium intake in relation to type 2 diabetes in women. *Diabetes Care* 2006; 29(3):650–56.

Rasmussen OW, Thomsen C, Hansen KW, et al. Effects on blood pressure, glucose, and lipid levels of a high-monounsaturated fat diet compared with a high-carbohydrate diet in NIDDM subjects. *Diabetes Care* 1993; 16(12):1565–71.

Rodrigues DC, Taba MJ, Novaes AB, et al. Effect of non-surgical periodontal therapy on glycemic control in patients with type 2 diabetes mellitus. *Journal of Periodontology* 2003; 74(9):1361–67.

Salmeron J, Hu FB, Manson JE, et al. Dietary fat intake and risk of type 2 diabetes in women. *American Journal of Clinical Nutrition* 2001; 73(6):1019–26.

Thomas DE, Elliott EJ, Naughton GA. Exercise for type 2 diabetes mellitus (review). *Cochrane Review* [serial online] 2006; 3.

Tuomilehto J, Lindstrom J, Eriksson JG, et al. Prevention of type 2 diabetes mellitus by changes in lifestyle among subjects with impaired glucose tolerance. *New England Journal of Medicine* 2001; 334(18):1343–50.

van Dam RM, Pasman WJ, Verhoef P. Effects of coffee consumption on fasting blood glucose and insulin concentrations: randomized controlled trials in healthy volunteers. *Diabetes Care* 2004; 27(12):2990–92.

van Dam RM, Willett WC, Manson JE, Hu FB. Coffee, caffeine, and risk of type 2 diabetes. *Diabetes Care* 2006; 29(2):308–403.

Wannamethee SG, Camargo Jr CA, Manson JE, et al. Alcohol drinking patterns and risk of type 2 diabetes mellitus among younger women. *Archives of Internal Medicine* 2003; 163(11):1329–36.

Wiernsperger N, Nivoit P, Bouskela E. Obstructive sleep apnea and insulin resistance: a role for microcirculation? *Clinics* 2006; 61(3):253–66.

Wing RR, Venditti E, Jakicic JM, et al. Lifestyle intervention in overweight individuals with a family history of diabetes. *Diabetes Care* 1998; 21(3):350–59.

Yeh GY, Eisenberg DM, Kaptchuk TJ, Phillips RS. Systematic review of herbs and dietary supplements for glycemic control in diabetes. *Diabetes Care* 2003; 26(4):1277–94.

## OSTEOPOROSIS, Chapter 10

Bacon L, Stern JS, Keim, NL, Van Loan MD. Low bone mass in premenopausal chronic dieting women. *European Journal of Clinical Nutrition* 2004; 58(6):966–71.

Bonjour JP. Dietary protein: an essential nutrient for bone health. *Journal of the American College of Nutrition* 2005; 24(6 Suppl):S526–S536.

Booth SL, Tucker KL, Chen H, et al. Dietary vitamin K intakes are associated with hip fracture but not with bone mineral density in elderly men and women. *American Journal of Clinical Nutrition* 2000; 71(5):1201–08.

Cao JJ, Nielsen FH. Acid diet (high-meat protein) effects on calcium metabolism and bone health. *Current Opinion in Clinical Nutrition and Metabolic Care* 2010; 13(6):698–702.

Dawson-Hughes B, Harris SS, Palermo NJ, et al. Treatment with potassium bicarbonate lowers calcium excretion and bone resorption in older men and women. *Journal of Clinical Endocrinology and Metabolism* 2009; 94(1):96–102.

Feskanich D, Weber P, Willett WC, et al. Vitamin K intake and hip fractures in women: A prospective study. *American Journal of Clinical Nutrition* 1999; 69(1):74–79.

Guadalupe-Grau A, Fuentes T, Guerra B, et al. Exercise and bone mass in adults. *Sports Medicine* 2009; 39(6):439–68.

Ikeda Y, Iki M, Morita A, et al. Intake of fermented soybeans, natto, is associated with reduced bone loss in postmenopausal women: Japanese Population-Based Osteoporosis Study (JPOS). *Journal of Nutrition* 2006; 136(5):1323–28.

Ilich JZ, Brownbill RA, Tamorini L, Crncevic-Orlic Z. To drink or not to drink: how are alcohol, caffeine and past smoking related to bone mineral density in elderly women? *Journal of the American College of Nutrition* 2002; 21(6):526–44.

Ilich JZ, Kerstetter JE. Nutrition in bone health revisited: A story beyond calcium. *Journal of the American College of Nutrition* 2000; 19(6):715–37.

Jacka FN, Pasco JA, Henry MJ, et al. Depression and bone mineral density in a community sample of peri-menopausal women: Geelong Osteoporosis Study. *Menopause* 2005; 12(1):88–91.

Judge JO, Kleppinger A, Kenny A, et al. Home-based resistance training improves femoral bone mineral density in women on hormone therapy. *Osteoporosis International* 2005; 16(9):1096–08.

Kamer AR, El-Ghorab N, Marzec N, et al. Nicotine induced proliferation and cytokine release in osteoblastic cells. *International Journal of Molecular Medicine* 2006; 17(1):121–27.

Kerstetter JE, O'Brien KO, Caseria DM, et al. The impact of dietary protein on calcium absorption and kinetic measures of bone turnover in women. *Journal of Clinical Endocrinology and Metabolism* 2005; 90(1):26–31.

Kerstetter JE, O'Brien KO, Insogna KL. Dietary protein, calcium metabolism, and skeletal homeostasis revisited. *American Journal of Clinical Nutrition* 2003; 78(3 suppl):S584–S592.

Kerstetter JE, O'Brien KO, Insogna KL. Low protein intake: the impact on calcium and bone homeostasis in humans. *Journal of Nutrition* 2003; 133(3):S855–S861.

Lanham-New SA. The balance of bone health: tipping the scales in favor of potassium-rich, bicarbonate-rich foods. *Journal of Nutrition* 2008; 138(1):S172–S177.

Macdonald HM, New SA, Fraser, et al. Low dietary potassium intakes and high dietary estimates of net endogenous acid production are associated with low bone mineral density in premenopausal women and increased markers of bone resorption in postmenopausal women. *American Journal of Clinical Nutrition* 2005; 81(4):923–33.

Macdonald HM, New SA, Golden MHN, et al. Nutritional associations with bone loss during the menopausal transition: evidence of a beneficial effect of calcium, alcohol, and fruit and vegetable nutrients and of a detrimental effect of fatty acids. *American Journal of Clinical Nutrition* 2004; 79(1):155–65.

Mussolino ME. Depression and hip fracture risk: the NHANES I epidemiologic follow-up study. *Public Health Reports* 2005; 120(1):71–75.

National Institutes of Health. Osteoporosis Prevention, Diagnosis, and Therapy. *NIH Consensus Statement* [Online] 2000; March 27–29; 17(1):1–36.

New SA, Robins SP, Campbell MK, et al. Dietary influences on bone mass and bone metabolism: Further evidence of a positive link between fruit and vegetable consumption and bone health? *American Journal of Clinical Nutrition* 2000; 71(1):142–51.

Nieves JW. Osteoporosis: the role of micronutrients. *American Journal of Clinical Nutrition* 2005; 81(5):S1232–S1239.

Rapuri PB, Gallagher JC, Balhorn KE, Ryschon KL. Alcohol intake and bone metabolism in elderly women. *American Journal of Clinical Nutrition* 2000; 72(5):1206–13.

Reinwald S, Weaver CM. Soy isoflavones and bone health: a double-edged sword? *Journal of Natural Products* 2006; 69(3):450–59.

Ryder KM, Shorr RI, Bush AJ, et al. Magnesium intake from food and supplements is associated with bone mineral density in healthy older white subjects. *Journal of the American Geriatric Society* 2005; 53(11):1875–80.

Sahni S, Hannan MT, Gagnon D, et al. High vitamin C intake is associated with lower 4-year bone loss in elderly men. *Journal of Nutrition* 2008; 138(10):1931–38.

Suominen H. Muscle training for bone strength. *Aging Clinical and Experimental Research* 2006; 18(2):85–93.

Tucker KL, Hannan MT, Chen H, et al. Potassium, magnesium, and fruit and vegetable intakes are associated with greater bone mineral density in elderly men and women. *American Journal of Clinical Nutrition* 1999; 69(4):727–36.

Weber P. Vitamin K and bone health. *Nutrition* 2001; 17(10):880–87.

Yaegashi Y, Onoda T, Tanno K, et al. Association of hip fracture incidence and intake of calcium, magnesium, vitamin D, and vitamin K. *European Journal of Epidemiology* 2008; 23(3):219–25.

Zehnacker CH, Bemis-Dougherty A. Effect of weighted exercises on bone mineral density in post menopausal women. A systematic review. *Journal of Geriatric Physical Therapy* 2007; 30(2):79–88.

## VISION, Chapter 11

Chiu CJ, Milton RC, Klein R, et al. Dietary carbohydrate and the progression of age-related macular degeneration: a prospective study from the Age-Related Eye Disease Study. *American Journal of Clinical Nutrition* 2007; 86(4):1210–18.

Chiu CJ, Milton RC, Klein R, et al. Dietary compound score and risk of age-related macular degeneration in the age-related eye disease study. *Ophthalmology* 2009; 116(5):939–46.

Chiu CJ, Taylor A. Nutritional antioxidants and age-related cataract and maculopathy. *Experimental Eye Research* 2007; 84(2):229–45.

Christen WG, Glynn RJ, Chew EY, et al. Folic acid, pyridoxine, and cyanocobalamin combination treatment and age-related macular degeneration in women: the Women's Antioxidant and Folic Acid Cardiovascular Study. *Archives of Internal Medicine* 2009; 169(4):335–41.

Christen WG, Glynn RJ, Chew EY, et al. Vitamin E and age-related cataract in a randomized trial of women. *Ophthalmology* 2008; 115(5):822–29.

Christen WG, Liu S, Glynn RJ, et al. Dietary carotenoids, vitamins C and E, and risk of cataract in women: a prospective study. *Archives of Ophthalmology* 2008; 126(1):102–09.

Ferrigno L, Aldigeri R, Rosmini F, et al. Associations between plasma levels of vitamins and cataract in the Italian-American Clinical Trial of Nutritional Supplements and Age-Related Cataract (CTNS): CTNS Report #2. *Ophthalmic Epidemiology* 2005; 12(2):71–80.

Gale CR, Hall NF, Phillips DIW, Martyn CN. Lutein and zeaxanthin status and risk of age-related macular degeneration. *Investigative Ophthalmology & Visual Science* 2003; 44(6):2461–65.

Jacques PF, Taylor A, Moeller S, et al. Long-term nutrient intake and 5-year change in nuclear lens opacities. *Archives of Ophthalmology* 2005; 123(4):517–26.

Kuzniarz M, Mitchell P, Cumming RG, Flood VM. Use of vitamin supplements and cataract: the Blue Mountains Eye Study. *American Journal of Ophthalmology* 2001; 132(1):19–26.

Leske MC, Chylack LT Jr, Wu SY. The Lens Opacities Case-Control Study. Risk factors for cataract. *Archives of Ophthalmology* 1991; 109(2):244–51.

McNeil JJ, Robman L, Tikellis G, et al. Vitamin E supplementation and cataract: randomized controlled trial. *Ophthalmology* 2004; 111(1):75–84.

Moeller SM, Taylor A, Tucker KL, et al. Overall adherence to the Dietary Guidelines for Americans is associated with reduced prevalence of early age-related nuclear lens opacities in women. *Journal of Nutrition* 2004; 134(7):1812–19.

Newsome DA, Rothman RJ. Zinc uptake in vitro by human retinal pigment epithelium. *Investigative Ophthalmology and Visual Science* 1987; 28(11):1795–99.

Richer S, Stiles W, Statkute L, et al. Double-masked, placebo-controlled, randomized trial of lutein and antioxidant supplementation in the intervention of atrophic age-related macular degeneration: the Veterans LAST study (Lutein Antioxidant Supplementation Trial). *Optometry* 2004; 76(4):216–30.

Robertson JM, Donner AP, Trevithick JR. A possible role for vitamins C and E in cataract prevention. *American Journal of Clinical Nutrition* 1991; 53(1 Suppl):S346–S351.

Sangiovanni JP, Agron E, Meleth AD, et al. {omega}-3 Long-chain polyunsaturated fatty acid intake and 12-y incidence of neovascular age-related macular degeneration and central geographic atrophy: AREDS report 30, a prospective cohort study from the Age-Related Eye Disease Study. *American Journal of Clinical Nutrition* 2009; 90(6):1601–07.

Santosa S, Jones PJH. Oxidative stress in ocular disease: does lutein play a protective role? *Canadian Medical Association Journal* 2005; 173(8):861–62.

Schaumberg DA, Liu S, Seddon JM, et al. Dietary glycemic load and risk of age-related cataract. *American Journal of Clinical Nutrition* 2004; 80(2):489–95.

Sperduto RD, Hu TS, Milton RC, et al. The Linxian cataract studies. Two nutrition intervention trials. *Archives of Ophthalmology* 1993; 111(9):1246–53.

Tan AG, Mitchell P, Flood VM, et al. Antioxidant nutrient intake and the long-term incidence of age-related cataract: the Blue Mountains Eye Study. *American Journal of Clinical Nutrition* 2008; 87(6):1899–05.

Tan J, Wang JJ, Flood V, et al. Carbohydrate nutrition, glycemic index, and the 10-y incidence of cataract. *American Journal of Clinical Nutrition* 2007; 86(5):1502–08.

Tan JS, Wang JJ, Flood V, et al. Dietary fatty acids and the 10-year incidence of age-related macular degeneration: the Blue Mountains Eye Study. *Archives of Ophthalmology* 2009; 127(5):656–65.

Tavani A, Negri E, La Vecchia C. Food and nutrient intake and risk of cataract. *Annals of Epidemiology* 1996; 6(1):11–16.

Thiagarajan G, Chandani S, Sundari CS, et al. Antioxidant properties of green and black tea, and their potential ability to retard the progression of eye lens cataract. *Experimental Eye Research* 2001; 73(3):393–401.

van Leeuwen R, Boekhoorn S, Vingerling JR, et al. Dietary intake of antioxidants and risk of age-related macular degeneration. *Journal of the American Medical Association* 2005; 294(24):3101–07.

Vinson JA, Zhang J. Black and green teas equally inhibit diabetic cataracts in a streptozotocin-induced rat model of diabetes. *Journal of Agricultural and Food Chemistry* 2005; 53(9):3710–13.

Yang CS, Landau JM. Effects of tea consumption on nutrition and health. *Journal of Nutrition* 2000; 130(10):2409–12.

## MEMORY, Chapter 12

Albanese E, Dangour AD, Uauy R, et al. Dietary fish and meat intake and dementia in Latin America, China, and India: a 10/66 Dementia Research Group population-based study. *American Journal of Clinical Nutrition* 2009; 90(2):392–400.

Andres-Lacueva C, Shukitt-Hale B, Galli RL, et al. Anthocyanins in aged blueberry-fed rats are found centrally and may enhance memory. *Nutritional Neuroscience* 2005; 8(2):111–20.

Bassuk SS, Glass TA, Berkman LF. Social disengagement and incident cognitive decline in community-dwelling elderly persons. *Annals of Internal Medicine* 1999; 131(3):165–73.

Beydoun MA, Kaufma JS, Satia JA, et al. Plasma n-3 fatty acids and the risk of cognitive decline in older adults: the Atherosclerosis Risk in Communities Study. *American Journal of Clinical Nutrition* 2007; 85(4):1103–11.

Casadesus G, Shukitt-Hale B, Stellwagen HM, et al. Modulation of hippocampal plasticity and cognitive behavior by short-term blueberry supplementation in aged rats. *Nutritional Neuroscience* 2004; 7(5-6):309–16.

Collins MA, Neafsey EJ, Mukamal KJ, et al. Alcohol in moderation, cardioprotection, and neuroprotection: epidemiological considerations and mechanistic studies. *Alcoholism, Clinical and Experimental Research* 2009; 33(2):206–19.

Dang-Vu TT, Desseilles M, Peigneux P, Maquet P. A role for sleep in brain plasticity. *Pediatric Rehabilitation* 2006; 9(2):98–118.

Devore EE, Grodstein F, van Rooij FJ, et al. Dietary intake of fish and omega-3 fatty acids in relation to long-term dementia risk. *American Journal of Clinical Nutrition* 2009; 90(1):170–76.

Devore EE, Stampfer MJ, Breteler MM, et al. Dietary fat intake and cognitive decline in women with type 2 diabetes. *Diabetes Care* 2009; 32(4):635–40.

Erickson KI, Voss MW, Prakash RS, et al. Exercise training increases size of hippocampus and improves memory. *Proceedings of the National Academy of Sciences USA* 2011; 108(7):3017–22.

Eskelinen MH, Ngandu T, Tuomilehto J, et al. Midlife coffee and tea drinking and the risk of late-life dementia: a population-based CAIDE study. *Journal of Alzheimer's Disease* 2009; 16(1):85–91.

Geng J, Dong J, Ni H, et al. Ginseng for cognition. *Cochrane Database of Systematic Reviews* 2010; 12:CD007769.

Gu Y, Nieves JW, Stern Y, et al. Food combination and Alzheimer disease risk: a protective diet. *Archives of Neurology* 2010; 67(6):699–706.

Jennings JR, Muldoon MF, Ryan C, et al. Reduced cerebral blood flow response and compensation among patients with untreated hypertension. *Neurology* 2005; 64(8):1358–65.

Jones N, Rogers PJ. Preoccupation, food, and failure: an investigation of cognitive performance deficits in dieters. *International Journal of Eating Disorders* 2003; 33(2):185–92.

Kang JH, Ascherio A, Grodstein F. Fruit and vegetable consumption and cognitive decline in aging women. *Annals of Neurology* 2005; 57(5):713–20.

Krikorian R, Shidler MD, Nash TA, et al. Blueberry supplementation improves memory in older adults. *Journal of Agricultural and Food Chemistry* 2010; 58(7):3996–4000.

Kuller LH, Margolis KL, Gaussoin SA, et al. Relationship of hypertension, blood pressure, and blood pressure control with white matter abnormalities in the Women's Health Initiative Memory Study (WHIMS)-MRI trial. *Journal of Clinical Hypertension* 2010; 12(3):203–12.

Luchsinger JA, Tang MX, Siddiqui M, et al. Alcohol intake and risk of dementia. *Journal of the American Geriatrics Society* 2004; 52(4):540–46.

Mahoney CR, Taylor HA, Kanarek RB, Samuel P. Effect of breakfast composition on cognitive processes in elementary school children. *Physiology and Behavior* 2005; 85(5):635–45.

Maquet P. The role of sleep in learning and memory. *Science* 2001; 294(5544):1048–52.

Matsuzaki T, Sasaki K, Tanizaki Y, et al. Insulin resistance is associated with the pathology of Alzheimer disease: the Hisayama study. *Neurology* 2010; 75(9):764–70.

Morris MC, Evans DA, Tangney CC, et al. Fish consumption and cognitive decline with age in a large community study. *Archives of Neurology* 2005; 62(12):1849–53.

Mosavi Jazayeri SM, Amani R, Mugahi NK. Effects of breakfast on memory in healthy young adults. *Asia Pacific Journal of Clinical Nutrition* 2004; 13(Suppl):S130.

O'Brien LT, Hummert ML. Memory performance of late middle-aged adults: contrasting self-stereotyping and stereotype threat accounts of assimilation to age stereotypes. *Social Cognition* 2006; 24(3):338–58.

Ritchie K, Carriere I, de Mendonca A, et al. The neuroprotective effects of caffeine: a prospective population study (the Three City Study). *Neurology* 2007; 69(6):536–45.

Rovio S, Karebolt I, Helkala EL, et al. Leisure-time physical activity at midlife and the risk of dementia and Alzheimer's disease. *Lancet Neurology* 2005; 4(11):705–11.

Scarmeas N, Stern Y, Mayeux R, et al. Mediterranean diet and mild cognitive impairment. *Archives of Neurology* 2009; 66(2):216–25.

Singh A, Naidu PS, Kulkarni SK. Reversal of aging and chronic ethanol-induced cognitive dysfunction by quercetin a bioflavonoid. *Free Radical Research* 2003; 37(11):1245–52.

Singh M. Essential fatty acids, DHA and human brain. *Indian Journal of Pediatrics* 2005; 72(3):239–42.

Sing-Manoux A, Gimeno D, Kivimaki M, et al. Low HDL cholesterol is a risk factor for deficit and decline in memory in midlife: the Whitehall II study. *Arteriosclerosis, Thrombosis, and Vascular Biology* 2008; 28(8):1556–62.

Snitz BE, O'Meara ES, Carlson MC, et al. Ginkgo biloba for preventing cognitive decline in older adults. *Journal of the American Medical Association* 2009; 302(24):2663–70.

Solfrizzi V, Panza F, Capurso A. The role of diet in cognitive decline. *Journal of Neural Transmission* 2003; 110(1):95–110.

Solomon A, Kivipelto M, Wolozin B, et al. Midlife serum cholesterol and increased risk of Alzheimer's and vascular dementia three decades later. *Dementia and Geriatric Cognitive Disorders* 2009; 28(1):75–80.

Vakhapova V, Cohen T, Richter Y, et al. Phosphatidylserine containing omega-3 fatty acids may improve memory abilities in non-demented elderly with memory complaints: a double-blind placebo-controlled trial. *Dementia and Geriatric Cognitive Disorders* 2010; 29(5):467–74.

van de Rest O, Geleijnse JM, Kok FJ, et al. Effect of fish oil on cognitive performance in older subjects: a randomized, controlled trial. *Neurology* 2008; 71(6):430–38.

van de Rest O, Spiro A 3rd, Krall-Kaye E, et al. Intakes of (n-3) fatty acids and fatty fish are not associated with cognitive performance and 6-year cognitive change in men participating in the Veterans Affairs Normative Aging Study. *Journal of Nutrition* 2009; 139(12):2329–36.

van Gelder BM, Buijsse B, Tijhuis M, et al. Coffee consumption is inversely associated with cognitive decline in elderly European men: the FINE Study. *European Journal of Clinical Nutrition* 2007; 61(2):226–32.

van Gelder BM, Tijhuis M, Kalmijn S, et al. Fish consumption, n-3 fatty acids, and subsequent 5-y cognitive decline in elderly men: the Zutphen Elderly Study. *American Journal of Clinical Nutrition* 2007; 85(4):1142–47.

Wang BS, Wang H, Wei ZH, et al. Efficacy and safety of natural acetylcholinesterase inhibitor huperzine A in the treatment of Alzheimer's disease: an updated meta-analysis. *Journal of Neural Transmission* 2009; 116(4):457–65.

Wesnes KA, Pincock C, Richardson D, et al. Breakfast reduces declines in attention and memory over the morning in schoolchildren. *Appetite* 2003; 41(3):329–31.

Whitmer RA, Gustafson DR, Barrett-Connor E, et al. Central obesity and increased risk of dementia more than three decades later. *Neurology* 2008; 71(14):1057–64.

Winocur G, Greenwood CF. The effects of high fat diets and environmental influences on cognitive performance in rats. *Behavioural Brain Research* 1999; 101(2):153–61.

Wu W, Brickman AM, Luchsinger J, et al. The brain in the age of old: the hippocampal formation is targeted differentially by diseases of late life. *Annals of Neurology* 2008; 64(6):698–706.

Xu W, Qiu C, Gatz M, et al. Mid- and Late-Life Diabetes in Relation to the Risk of Dementia. *Diabetes* 2009; 58(1):71–77.

Yeung SE, Fischer AL, Dixon RA. Exploring effects of type 2 diabetes on cognitive functioning in older adults. *Neuropsychology* 2009; 23(1):1–9.

Zimmerman FJ, Christakis DA. Children's television viewing and cognitive outcomes: a longitudinal analysis of national data. *Archives of Pediatric and Adolescent Medicine* 2005; 159(7):619–25.

## MOOD, Chapter 13

Beydoun MA, Shroff MR, Beydoun HA, et al. Serum folate, vitamin B-12, and homocysteine and their association with depressive symptoms among US adults. *Psychosomatic Medicine* 2010; 72(9):862–73.

Bottiglieri T. Homocysteine and folate metabolism in depression. *Progress in Neuropsychopharmacology & Biological Psychiatry* 2005; 29(7):1103–12.

Brinkworth GD, Buckley JD, Noakes M, et al. Long-term effects of a very low-carbohydrate diet and a low-fat diet on mood and cognitive function. *Archives of Internal Medicine* 2009; 169(20):1873–80.

Coppen A, Bolander-Gouaille C. Treatment of depression: time to consider folic acid and vitamin B12. *Journal of Psychopharmacology* 2005; 19(1):59–65.

Diehl DJ, Gershon S. The role of dopamine in mood disorders. *Comprehensive Psychiatry* 1992; 33(2):115–20.

Gariballa S, Forster S. Effects of dietary supplements on depressive symptoms in older patients: a randomised double-blind placebo-controlled trial. *Clinical Nutrition* 2007; 26(5):545–51.

Gloth FM 3rd, Alam W, Hollis B. Vitamin D vs broad spectrum phototherapy in the treatment of seasonal affective disorder. *Journal of Nutrition, Health and Aging* 1999; 3(1):5–7.

Hintikka J, Tolmunen T, Tanskanen A, et al. High vitamin B12 level and good treatment outcome may be associated in major depressive disorder. *BMC Psychiatry* 2003; 3:17.

Hypericum Depression Trial Study Group. Effect of *Hypericum perforatum* (St John's wort) in major depressive disorder: a randomized controlled trial. *Journal of the American Medical Association* 2002; 287(14):1807–14.

Jorde R, Sneve M, Figenschau Y, et al. Effects of vitamin D supplementation on symptoms of depression in overweight and obese subjects: randomized double blind trial. *Journal of Internal Medicine* 2008; 264(6):599–609.

Kim JM, Stewart R, Kim SW, et al. Predictive value of folate, vitamin B12 and homocysteine levels in late-life depression. *British Journal of Psychiatry* 2008; 192(4):268–74.

Lansdowne AT, Provost SC. Vitamin D3 enhances mood in healthy subjects during winter. *Psychopharmacology* (Berl) 1998; 135(4):319–23.

Lee S, Gura KM, Kim S, et al. Current clinical applications of omega-6 and omega-3 fatty acids. *Nutrition in Clinical Practice* 2006; 21(4):323–41.

Lin PY, Su KP. A meta-analytic review of double-blind, placebo-controlled trials of antidepressant efficacy of omega-3 fatty acids. *Journal of Clinical Psychiatry* 2007; 68(7):1056–61.

Linde K, Berner MM, Kriston L. St John's wort for major depression. *Cochrane Database of Systematic Reviews* 2008; 4:CD000448.

Papakostas GI, Mischoulon D, Shyu I, et al. S-adenosylmethionine (SAMe) augmentation of serotonin reuptake inhibitors for antidepressant nonresponders with major depressive disorder: a double-blind, randomized clinical trial. *American Journal of Psychiatry* 2018; 167(8):942–48.

Parker G, Gibson NA, Brotchie H, et al. Omega-3 fatty acids and mood disorders. *American Journal of Psychiatry* 2006; 163(6):969–78.

Shelton RC, Keller MB, Gelenberg A, et al. Effectiveness of St John's wort in major depression: a randomized controlled trial. *Journal of the American Medical Association* 2001; 285(15):1978–86.

Skarupski KA, Tangney C, Li H, et al. Longitudinal association of vitamin B-6, folate, and vitamin B-12 with depressive symptoms among older adults over time. *American Journal of Clinical Nutrition* 2010; 92(2):330–35.

Sontrop J, Campbell MK. Omega-3 polyunsaturated fatty acids and depression: a review of the evidence and a methodological critique. *Preventive Medicine* 2006; 42(1):4–13.

Szegedi A, Kohnen R, Dienel A, Kieser M. Acute treatment of moderate to severe depression with hypericum extract WS 5570 (St John's wort): randomized controlled double blind non-inferiority trial versus paroxetine. *British Medical Journal* [serial online] 2005; 330(7490):503.

Tolmunen T, Hintikka J, Ruusunen A, et al. Dietary folate and the risk of depression in Finnish middle-aged men. *Psychotherapy and Psychosomatics* 2004; 73(6):334–39.

Trivedi MH, Greer TL, Grannemann BD, et al. Exercise as an augmentation strategy for treatment of major depression. *Journal of Psychiatric Practice* 2006; 12(4):205–13.

Vieth R, Kimball S, Hu A, Walfish PG. Randomized comparison of the effects of the vitamin D3 adequate intake versus 100 mcg (4000 IU) per day on biochemical responses and the wellbeing of patients. *Nutrition Journal* [serial online] 2004; 3:8.

## MIGRAINE HEADACHES, Chapter 14

Allais G, Bussone G, De Lorenzo C, et al. Advanced strategies of short-term prophylaxis in menstrual migraine: state of the art and prospects. *Neurological Science* 2005: 26(Suppl2):S125–S129.

Bic Z, Blix GG, Hopp HP, et al. The influence of a low-fat diet on incidence and severity of migraine headaches. *Journal of Women's Health and Gender-Based Medicine* 1999; 8(5):623–30.

Bigal ME, Liberman JN, Lipton RB. Obesity and migraine: a population study. *Neurology* 2006; 66:545–50.

Biondi DM. Physical treatments for headache: a structured review. *Headache* 2005; 45(6):738–46.

Boardman HF, Thomas E, Millson DS, Croft PR. Psychological, sleep, lifestyle and comorbid associations with headache. *Headache* 2005; 45(6):657–69.

Crawford P, Simmons M. What dietary modifications are indicated for migraines? *Journal of Family Practice* 2006; 55(1):62–64.

Diener HC, Pfaffenrath V, Pageler L, et al. The fixed combination of acetylsalicylic acid, paracetamol and caffeine is more effective than single substances and dual combination for the treatment of headache: a multicentre, randomized, double-blind, singe-dose, placebo-controlled parallel group study. *Cephalalgia* 2005; 25(10):776–87.

Goldstein J, Silberstein SD, Saper JR, et al. Acetaminophen, aspirin, and caffeine versus sumatriptan succinate in the early treatment of migraine: results from the ASSET trial. *Headache* 2005; 45(8):973–82.

Harel Z, Gascon G, Riggs S, et al. Supplementation with omega-3 polyunsaturated fatty acids in the management of recurrent migraines in adolescents. *Journal of Adolescent Health* 2002; 31(2):154–61.

Hershey AD, Powers SW, Vockell AL, et al. Coenzyme Q10 deficiency and response to supplementation in pediatric and adolescent migraine. *Headache* 2007; 47(1):73–80.

Maizels M, Blumenfeld A, Burchette R. A combination of riboflavin, magnesium, and feverfew for migraine prophylaxis: a randomized trial. *Headache* 2006; 46(3):531.

Mather M. Migraines and tannins—any relationship? *Headache* 1997; 37(8):529.

Meskunas CA, Tepper SJ, Rapoport AM, et al. Medications associated with probable medication overuse headache reported in a tertiary care headache center over a 15-year period. *Headache* 2006; 46(5):766–72.

Millichap JG, Yee MM. The diet factor in pediatric and adolescent migraine. *Pediatric Neurology* 2003; 28(1):9–15.

Modi S, Lowder DM. Medications for migraine prophylaxis. *American Family Physician* 2006; 73(1):72–78.

Nadelson C. Sport and exercise-induced migraines. *Current Sports Medicine Reports* 2006; 5(1):29–33.

Rasura M, Spalloni A, Ferrari M, et al. A case series of young stroke in Rome. *European Journal of Neurology* 2006; 13(2):146–52.

Robberstad L, Dyb G, Hagen K, et al. An unfavorable lifestyle and recurrent headaches among adolescents: the HUNT study. *Neurology* 2010; 75(8):712–17.

Rozen TD, Oshinsky ML, Gebeline CA, et al. Open label trial of coenzyme Q10 as a migraine preventive. *Cephalagia* 2002; 22(2):137–41.

Sandor PS, Di Clemente L, Coppola G, et al. Efficacy of coenzyme Q10 in migraine prophylaxis: a randomized controlled trial. *Neurology* 2005; 64(4):713–15.

Schoenen J, Jacquy J, Lenaerts M. Effectiveness of high-dose riboflavin in migraine prophylaxis. A randomized controlled trial. *Neurology* 1998; 50(2):466–70.

Sun-Edelstein C, Mauskop A. Foods and supplements in the management of migraine headaches. *Clinical Journal of Pain* 2009; 25(5):446–52.

Varkey E, Cider A, Carlsson J, et al. A study to evaluate the feasibility of an aerobic exercise program in patients with migraine. *Headache* 2009; 49(4):563–70.

Wagner W, Nootbaar-Wagner U. Prophylactic treatment of migraine with gamma-linolenic and alpha-linolenic acids. *Cephalalgia* 1997; 17(2):127–30.

## PREMENSTRUAL SYNDROME, Chapter 15

Bendich A. The potential for dietary supplements to reduce premenstrual syndrome (PMS) symptoms. *Journal of the American College of Nutrition* 2000; 19(1):3–12.

Bertone-Johnson ER, Hankinson SE, Bendich A, et al. Calcium and vitamin D intake and risk of incident premenstrual syndrome. *Archives of Internal Medicine* 2005; 165(11):1246–52.

Bianchi-Demicheli F, Ludicke F, Lucas H, Chardonnens D. Premenstrual dysphoric disorder: current status of treatment. *Swiss Medical Weekly* 2002; 132(39-40):574–78.

Case AM, Reid RL. Menstrual cycle effects on common medical conditions. *Comprehensive Therapy* 2001; 27(1):65–71.

Daugherty JE. Treatment strategies for premenstrual syndrome. *American Family Physician* 1998; 58(1):183192,197–98.

Frackiewicz EJ, Shiovitz TM. Evaluation and management of premenstrual syndrome and premenstrual dysphoric disorder. *Journal of the American Pharmaceutical Association* 2001; 41(3):437–47.

Kljakovic M, Pullon S. Allergy and the premenstrual syndrome (PMS). *Allergy* 1997; 52(6):681–83.

Shamberger RJ. Calcium, magnesium, and other elements in the red blood cells and hair of normals and patients with premenstrual syndrome. *Biological Trace Element Research* 2003; 94(2):123–29.

Thys-Jacobs S. Micronutrients and the premenstrual syndrome: the case for calcium. *Journal of the American College of Nutrition* 2000; 19(2):220–27.

## INSOMNIA, Chapter 16

Bootzin RR, Perlis ML. Nonpharmacologic treatments of insomnia. *Journal of Clinical Psychiatry* 1992; 53(suppl):37–41.

Buscemi N, Vandermeer B, Pandya R, et al. Melatonin for treatment of sleep disorders. *Evidence Report Technology Assessment* 2004; 108:1–7.

Eddy M, Walbroehl GS. Insomnia. *American Family Physician* 1999; 59(7):1911–16, 1918.

Hadley S, Petry JJ. Valerian. *American Family Physician* 2003; 67(8):1755–58.

Hudson C, Hudson SP, Hecht T, MacKenzie J. Protein source tryptophan versus pharmaceutical grade tryptophan as an efficacious treatment for chronic insomnia. *Nutritional Neuroscience* 2005; 8(2):121–27.

Lewith GT, Godfrey AD, Prescott P. A single-blinded, randomized pilot study evaluating the aroma of *Lavandula augustifolia* as a treatment for mild insomnia. *Journal of Alternative and Complementary Medicine* 2005; 11(4):631–37.

Morin CM, Hauri PJ, Espie CA, et al. Nonpharmacologic treatment of chronic insomnia. An American Academy of Sleep Medicine review. *Sleep* 1999; 22(8):1134–56.

Rajput V, Bromley SM. Chronic insomnia: a practical review. *American Family Physician* 1999; 60(5):1431–38.

Riemersma-van der Lek RF, Swaab DF, Twisk J, et al. Effect of bright light and melatonin on cognitive and noncognitive function in elderly residents of group care facilities: a randomized controlled trial. *Journal of the American Medical Association* 2008; 299(22):2642–55.

Tworoger SS, Yasui Y, Vitiello MV, et al. Effects of a yearlong moderate-intensity exercise and a stretching intervention on sleep quality in postmenopausal women. *Sleep* 2003; 26(7):830–36.

Youngstedt SD. Effects of exercise on sleep. *Clinics in Sports Medicine* 2005; 24(2):355–65.

## IRRITABLE BOWEL SYNDROME, Chapter 17

Bach DR, Erdmann G, Schmidtmann M, Monnikes H. Emotional stress reactivity in irritable bowel syndrome. *European Journal of Gastroenterology and Hepatology* 2006; 18(6):629–36.

Barrett JS, Gibson PR. Clinical ramifications of malabsorption of fructose and other short-chain carbohydrates. *Practical Gastroenterology* [serial online] 2007; 31(8):51–65.

Bijkerk CJ, de Wit NJ, Muris JW, et al. Soluble or insoluble fibre in irritable bowel syndrome in primary care? Randomised placebo controlled trial. *British Medical Journal* 2009; 339:b3154.

Brandt LJ, Chey WD, Foxx-Orenstein AE, et al. An evidence-based systematic review on the management of irritable bowel syndrome. *American Journal of Gastroenterology* 2009; 104(suppl1):S8–S35.

Bundy R, Walker AF, Middleton RW, et al. Artichoke leaf extract reduces symptoms of irritable bowel syndrome and improves quality of life in otherwise healthy volunteers suffering from concomitant dyspepsia: a subset analysis. *Journal of Alternative and Complementary Medicine* 2004; 10(4):667–69.

Chapman CM, Gibson Gr, Rowland I. Health benefits of probiotics: are mixtures more effective than single strains? *European Journal of Nutrition* 2011; 50(1):1–17.

Creed F. How do SSRIs help patients with irritable bowel syndrome? *Gut* 2006; 55(8):1065–67.

Dapoigny M, Stockbrugger RW, Azpiroz F, et al. Role of alimentation in irritable bowel syndrome. *Digestion* 2003; 67(4):225–33.

Daley AJ, Grimmett C, Roberts L, et al. The effects of exercise upon symptoms and quality of life in patients diagnosed with irritable bowel syndrome: a randomised controlled trial. *International Journal of Sports Medicine* 2008; 29(9):778–82.

Floch MH. Use of diet and probiotic therapy in the irritable bowel syndrome: analysis of the literature. *Journal of Clinical Gastroenterology* 2005; 39(4 Suppl 3):S243–S246.

Ford AC, Talley NJ, Spiegel BMR, et al. Effect of fibre, antispasmodics, and peppermint oil in the treatment of irritable bowel syndrome: systematic review and meta-analysis. *British Medical Journal* 2008; 337:a2313.

Friedman G. Diet and the irritable bowel syndrome. *Gastroenterology Clinics of North America* 1991; 20(2):313–24.

Gerson CD, Gerson MJ. A collaborative health care model for the treatment of irritable bowel syndrome. *Clinical Gastroenterology and Hepatology* 2003; 1(6):446–52.

Grigoleit HG, Grigoleit P. Peppermint oil in irritable bowel syndrome. *Phytomedicine* 2005; 12(8):601–06.

Grundmann O, Yoon SL. Irritable bowel syndrome: epidemiology, diagnosis and treatment: an update for health-care practitioners. *Journal of Gastroenterology and Hepatology* 2010; 25(4):691–99.

Heizer WD, Southern S, McGovern S. The role of diet in symptoms of irritable bowel syndrome in adults: a narrative review. *Journal of the American Dietetic Association* 2009; 109(7):1204–14.

Johannesson E, Simren M, Strid H, et al. Physical activity improves symptoms in irritable bowel syndrome: a randomized controlled trial. *American Journal of Gastroenterology* 2011. [Epub]

Kennedy T, Jones R, Darnley S, et al. Cognitive behaviour therapy in addition to antispasmodic treatment for irritable bowel syndrome in primary care: randomized controlled trial. *British Medical Journal* 2005; 331(7514):435–40.

Levy RL, Linde JA, Feld KA, et al. The association of gastrointestinal symptoms with weight, diet, and exercise in weight-loss program participants. *Clinical Gastroenterology and Hepatology* 2005; 3(10):992–96.

Lindfors P, Unge P, Bjornsson S, et al. Effects of hypnotherapy on IBS in different clinical settings—results from two randomized, controlled trials. Presentation at Digestive Disease Week 2006 conference. Los Angeles, CA: May 20–25, 2006.

Liu JH, Chen GH, Yeh HZ, et al. Enteric-coated peppermint-oil capsules in the treatment of irritable bowel syndrome: a prospective, randomized trial. *Journal of Gastroenterology* 1997; 32(6):765–68.

Logan AC, Beaulne TM. The treatment of small intestinal bacterial overgrowth with enteric-coated peppermint oil: a case report. *Alternative Medicine Review* 2002; 7(5):410–17.

Moayyedi P, Ford AC, Talley NJ, et al. The efficacy of probiotics in the treatment of irritable bowel syndrome: a systematic review. *Gut* 2010; 59(3):325–32.

McKay DL, Blumberg JB. A review of the bioactivity and potential health benefits of peppermint tea (Mentha piperita L.). *Phytotherapy Research* [serial online] 2006; June 12.

Meier R. Probiotics in irritable bowel syndrome. *Annals of Nutrition and Metabolism* 2010; 57(suppl1):12–13.

Morcos A, Dinan T, Quigley EM. Irritable bowel syndrome: role of food in pathogenesis and management. *Journal of Digestive Diseases* 2009; 10(4):237–46.

Morgan T, Robson KM. Irritable bowel syndrome: diagnosis is based on clinical criteria. *Postgraduate Medicine* 2002; 112(5):30–32, 35–36, 39–41.

Nobaek S, Johansson ML, Molin G, et al. Alteration of intestinal microflora is associated with reduction in abdominal bloating and pain in patients with irritable bowel syndrome. *American Journal of Gastroenterology* 2000; 95(5):1231–38.

O'Mahony L, McCarthy J, Kelly P, et al. Lactobacillus and bifidobacterium in irritable bowel syndrome: symptom responses and relationship to cytokine profiles. *Gastroenterology* 2005; 128(3):541–51.

Pittler MH, Ernst E. Peppermint oil for irritable bowel syndrome: a critical review and metaanalysis. *American Journal of Gastroenterology* 1998; 93(7):1131–35.

Posserud I, Agerforz P, Ekman R, et al. Altered visceral perceptual and neuroendocrine response in patients with irritable bowel syndrome during mental stress. *Gut* 2004; 53(8):1102–08.

Posserud I, Ersryd A, Simren M. Functional findings in irritable bowel syndrome. *World Journal of Gastroenterology* 2005; 12(18):2830–38.

Roberts L, Wilson S, Singh S, et al. Gut-directed hypnotherapy for irritable bowel syndrome: piloting a primary care–based randomized controlled trial. *British Journal of General Practice* 2006; 56(523):115–21.

Santosa S, Farnworth E, Jones PJ. Probiotics and their potential health claims. *Nutrition Reviews* 2006; 64(6):265–74.

Shepard SJ, Parker FC, Muir JG, et al. Dietary triggers of abdominal symptoms in patients with irritable bowel syndrome: randomized placebo-controlled evidence. *Clinical Gastroenterology and Hepatology* 2008; 6(7):765–71.

## CELIAC DISEASE, Chapter 18

Akobeng AK, Ramanan AV, Buchan I, Heller RF. Effect of breast feeding on risk of celiac disease: a systematic review and meta-analysis of observational studies. *Archives of Disease in Childhood* 2006; 91(1): 39–43.

Alaedini A, Green PHR. Narrative review: celiac disease: understanding a complex autoimmune disorder. *Annals of Internal Medicine* 2005; 142(4):289–98.

Biagi F, Campanella J, Martucci S, et al. A milligram of gluten a day keeps the mucosal recovery away: a case report. *Nutrition Reviews* 2004; 62(9):360–63.

Dahele A, Ghosh S. Vitamin $B_{12}$ deficiency in untreated celiac disease. *American Journal of Gastroenterology* 2001; 96(3):745–50.

Fasano A. Surprises from celiac disease. *Scientific American* 2009; 301(2):54–61.

Helms S. Celiac disease and gluten-associated diseases. *Alternative Medicine Review* 2005; 10(3):172–92.

Hischenhuber C, Crevel R, Jarry B, et al. Review article: safe amounts of gluten for patients with wheat allergy or coeliac disease. *Alimentary Pharmacology & Therapeutics* 2006; 23(5):559–75.

Kupper C. Dietary guidelines and implementation for celiac disease. *Gastroenterology* 2005; 128(4 Suppl 1):S121–S127.

Lee SK, Green PH. Celiac sprue (the great modern-day imposter). *Current Opinions in Rheumatology* 2006; 18(1):101–07.

Rubio-Tapia A, Kyle RA, Kaplan EL, et al. Increased prevalence and mortality in undiagnosed celiac disease. *Gastroenterology* 2009; 137(1):88–93.

Srinivasan U, Jones E, Carolan J, Feighery C. Immunohistochemical analysis of coeliac mucosa following ingestion of oats. *Clinical and Experimental Immunology* 2006; 144(2):197–203.

Storsrud S, Olsson M, Arvidsson Lenner R, et al. Adult coeliac patients do tolerate large amounts of oats. *European Journal of Clinical Nutrition* 2003; 57(1):163–69.

Thompson T. Oats and the gluten-free diet. *Journal of the American Dietetic Association* 2003; 103(3):376–79.

Thompson T, Dennis M, Higgins LA, et al. Gluten-free diet survey: are Americans with coeliac disease consuming recommended amounts of fibre, iron, calcium and grain foods? *Journal of Human Nutrition and Dietetics* 2005; 18(3):163–69.

## CANCER PREVENTION, Chapter 19

Adamson RH, Thorgeirsson UP. Carcinogens in foods: heterocyclic amines and cancer and heart disease. *Advances in Experimental Medicine and Biology* 1995; 369:211–20.

Allen NE, Beral V, Casabonne D, et al. Moderate alcohol intake and cancer incidence in women. *Journal of the National Cancer Institute* 2009; 101(5):296–305.

Alothaimeen A, Ezzat A, Mohamed G, et al. Dietary fat and breast cancer in Saudi Arabia: a case-control study. *Eastern Mediterranean Health Journal* 2004; 10(6):8769–86.

Al Sarakbi W, Salhab M, Mokbel K. Dairy products and breast cancer risk: a review of the literature. *International Journal of Fertility and Women's Medicine* 2005; 50(6):244–49.

al-Sereiti MR, Abu-Amer KM, Sen P. Pharmacology of rosemary (Rosmarinus officinalis Linn.) and its therapeutic potentials. *Indian Journal of Experimental Biology* 1999; 37(2):124–30.

Amitabha R. Cancer preventive role of selected dietary factors. *Indian Journal of Cancer* 2005; 42(1):11–20.

Bairati I, Meyer F, Jobin E, et al. Antioxidant vitamins supplementation and mortality: a randomized trial in head and neck cancer patients. *International Journal of Cancer* 2006; 119(9):2221–24.

Bartsch H, Nair J, Owen RW. Dietary polyunsaturated fatty acids and cancers of the breast and colorectum: emerging evidence for their role as risk modifiers. *Carcinogenesis* 1999; 20(12):2209–18.

Basu A, Imrhan V. Tomatoes versus lycopene in oxidative stress and carcinogenesis: conclusions from clinical trials. *European Journal of Clinical Nutrition* 2007; 61(3):295–303.

Boehm K, Borrelli F, Ernst E, et al. Green tea (Camellia sinensis) for the prevention of cancer. *Cochrane Database of Systematic Reviews* 2009; (3):CD005004.

Boffetta P, Couto E, Wichmann J, et al. Fruit and vegetable intake and overall cancer risk in the European Prospective Investigation into Cancer and Nutrition (EPIC). *Journal of the National Cancer Institute* 2010; 102(8):529–37.

Brown AC, Shah C, Liu J, et al. Ginger's (Zingiber officinale Roscoe) inhibition of rat colonic adenocarcinoma cells proliferation and angiogenesis in vitro. *Phytotherapy Research* 2009; 23(5):640–45.

Caygill CP, Charlett A, Hill MJ. Fat, fish, fish oil and cancer. *British Journal of Cancer* 1996; 74(1):159–64.

Chan JM, Gann PH, Giovannucci EL. Role of diet in prostate cancer development and progression. *Journal of Clinical Oncology* 2005; 23(32):8152–60.

Cho E, Smith-Warner SA, Spiegelman D, et al. Dairy foods, calcium, and colorectal cancer: a pooled analysis of 10 cohort studies. *Journal of the National Cancer Institute* 2004; 96(13):1015–22.

Chung M, Balk EM, Brendel M, et al. Vitamin D and calcium: systematic review of health outcomes. Evidence Report/Technology Assessment No. 183. AHRQ Publication No. 09-E015, Rockville, MD: Agency for Healthcare Research and Quality. August 2009.

Cross AJ, Ferrucci LM, Risch A, et al. A large prospective study of meat consumption and colorectal cancer risk: an investigation of potential mechanisms underlying this association. *Cancer Research* 2010; 70(6):2406–14.

Cross AJ, Leitzmann MF, Gail MH, et al. A prospective study of red and processed meat intake in relation to cancer risk. *Public Library of Science Medicine* 2007; 4(12):e325.

Danaei G, Vander Hoorn S, Lopez AD, et al. Causes of cancer in the world: comparative risk assessment of nine behavioural and environmental risk factors. *Lancet* 2005; 366(9499):1784–93.

de Deckere EA. Possible beneficial effect of fish and fish n-3 polyunsaturated fatty acids in breast and colorectal cancer. *European Journal of Cancer Prevention* 1999; 8(3):213–21.

Duviox A, Blasius R, Delhalle S, et al. Chemopreventive and therapeutic effects of curcumin. *Cancer Letters* 2005; 223(2):181–90.

Edenharder R, Sager JW, Glatt H, et al. Protection by beverages, fruits, vegetables, herbs, and flavonoids against genotoxicity of 2-acetylaminofluorene and 2-amino-1-methyl-6-phenylimidazol[4,5-b]pyridine (PhIP) in metabolically competent V79 cells. *Mutation Research* 2002; 521(1-2):57-72.

Edinger MS, Koff WJ. Effect of the consumption of tomato paste on plasma prostate-specific antigen levels in patients with benign prostate hyperplasia. *Brazilian Journal of Medical and Biological Research* 2006; 30(8):1115-19.

Eliassen AH, Colditz GA, Rosner B, et al. Adult weight change and risk of postmenopausal breast cancer. *Journal of the American Medical Association* 2006; 296(2):193-201.

Franceschi S, Bidoli E, La Vecchia C, et al. Tomatoes and risk of digestive-tract cancers. *International Journal of Cancer* 1994; 59(2):181-84.

Freudenheim JL, Marshall JR, Vena JE, et al. Premenopausal breast cancer risk and intake of vegetables, fruits, and related nutrients. *Journal of the National Cancer Institute* 1996; 88(6):340-48.

Garland CF, Garland FC, Gorham ED, et al. The role of vitamin D in cancer prevention. *American Journal of Public Health* 2006; 96(2):252-61.

Gikas PD, Mokbel K. Phytoestrogens and the risk of breast cancer: a review of the literature. *International Journal of Fertility and Women's Medicine* 2005; 50(6):250-58.

Giovannucci E, Liu Y, Stampfer MJ, Willett WC. A prospective study of calcium intake and incident and fatal prostate cancer. *Cancer Epidemiology, Biomarkers, and Prevention* 2006; 15(2):203-10.

Giugliano D, Ceriello A, Esposito K. The effects of diet on inflammation: emphasis on the metabolic syndrome. *Journal of the American College of Cardiology* 2006; 48(4):677-85.

Gonzalez CA. The European Prospective Investigation into Cancer and Nutrition (EPIC). *Public Health Nutrition* 2006; 9(1A):124-26.

Hall MN, Chavarro JE, Lee IM, et al. A 22-year prospective study of fish, n-3 fatty acid intake, and colorectal cancer risk in men. *Cancer Epidemiology, Biomarkers and Prevention* 2008; 17(5): 1136-43.

Hanf V, Gonder U. Nutrition and primary prevention of breast cancer: foods, nutrients and breast cancer risk. *European Journal of Obstetrics, Gynecology, and Reproductive Biology* 2005; 123(2):139-49.

Hedelin M, Balter KA, Chang ET, et al. Dietary intake of phytoestrogens, estrogen receptor-beta polymorphisms and the risk of prostate cancer. *Prostate* 2006; 66(14):1512-20.

Hercberg S, Czernichow S, Galan P. Antioxidant vitamins and minerals in prevention of cancers: lessons from the SU.VI.MAX study. *British Journal of Nutrition* 2006; 96(Suppl 1):S28-S30.

Holick MF. The vitamin D epidemic and its health consequences. *Journal of Nutrition* 2005; 135(11):S2739-S2748.

Hour TC, Liang YC, Chu IS, Lin JK. Inhibition of eleven mutagens by various tea extracts, (-)epigallocate-chin-3-gallate, gallic acid and caffeine. *Food and Chemical Toxicology* 1999; 37(6):569-79.

Huang HY, Caballero B, Chang S, et al. The efficacy and safety of multivitamin and mineral supplement use to prevent cancer and chronic disease in adults: a systematic review for a National Institutes of Health State-of-the-Science conference. *Annals of Internal Medicine* 2006; 145(5):372–85.

Huxley RR, Ansary-Moghaddam A, Clifton P, et al. The impact of dietary and lifestyle risk factors on risk of colorectal cancer: a quantitative overview of the epidemiological evidence. *International Journal of Cancer* 2009; 125(1):171–80.

Johnson EJ. The role of carotenoids in human health. *Nutrition in Clinical Care* 2002; 5(2):56–65.

Korde LA, Wu AH, Fears T, et al. Childhood soy intake and breast cancer risk in Asian American women. *Cancer Epidemiology, Biomarkers, and Prevention* 2009; 18(4):1050–59.

Lappe JM, Travers-Gustafson D, Davies KM, et al. Vitamin D and calcium supplementation reduces cancer risk: results of a randomized trial. *American Journal of Clinical Nutrition* 2007; 85(6):1586–91.

Lu J, Jiang C. Antiangiogenic activity of selenium in cancer chemoprevention: metabolite-specific effects. *Nutrition and Cancer* 2001; 40(1):64–73.

MacLean CH, Newberry SJ, Jojica WA, et al. Effects of omega-3 fatty acids on cancer risk: a systematic review. *Journal of the American Medical Association* 2006; 295(4):403–15.

Maier H, Dietz A, Gewelke U, et al. Tobacco and alcohol and the risk of head and neck cancer. *Clinical Investigator* 1992; 70(3-4):320–27.

Martinez ME, Thomson CA, Smith-Warner SA. Soy and breast cancer: the controversy continues. *Journal of the National Cancer Institute* 2006; 98(7):430–31.

McTiernan A, Kooperberg C, White E, et al. Recreational physical activity and the risk of breast cancer in postmenopausal women: the Women's Health Initiative Cohort Study. *Journal of the American Medical Association* 2003; 290(10):1331–36.

Moriarty RM, Naithani R, Surve B. Organosulfur compounds in cancer chemoprevention. *Mini Reviews in Medicinal Chemistry* 2007; 7(8):827–38.

Neuhouser ML, Wassertheil-Smoller S, Thomson C, et al. Multivitamin use and risk of cancer and cardiovascular disease in the Women's Health Initiative cohorts. *Archives of Internal Medicine* 2009; 169(3):294–304.

Norat T, Bingham S, Ferrari P, et al. Meat, fish, and colorectal cancer risk: the European Prospective Investigation into Cancer and Nutrition. *Journal of the National Cancer Institute* 2005; 97(12):906–16.

Palmer S. Diet, nutrition, and cancer. *Progress in Food and Nutrition Science* 1985; 9(3-4):283–341.

Park Y, Leitzmann MF, Subar AF, et al. Dairy food, calcium, and risk of cancer in the NIH-AARP Diet and Health Study. *Archives of Internal Medicine* 2009; 169(4):391–401.

Renzulli C, Galvano F, Pierdomenico L, et al. Effects of rosmarinic acid against aflatoxin B1 and ochratoxin-A-induced cell damage in a human hepatoma cell line (Hep G2). *Journal of Applied Toxicology* 2004; 24(4):289–96.

Shu XO, Zheng Y, Cai H, et al. Soy food intake and breast cancer survival. *Journal of American Medical Association* 2009; 302(22):2437–43.

Smith JS, Ameri F, Gadgil P. Effect of marinades on the formation of heterocyclic amines in grilled beef steaks. *Journal of Food Science* 2008; 73(6):T100–05.

Smith-Warner SA, Spiegelman D, Yaun SS, et al. Alcohol and breast cancer in women: a pooled analysis of cohort studies. *Journal of the American Medical Association* 1998; 279(7):535–40.

Sharma RA, Gescher AJ, Steward WP. Curcumin: the story so far. *European Journal of Cancer* 2005; 41(13):1955–68.

Trock BJ, Hilakivi-Clarke L, Clarke R. Meta-analysis of soy intake and breast cancer risk. *Journal of the National Cancer Institute* 2006; 98(7):459–71.

Tsubura A, Uehara N, Kiyozuka Y, Shikata N. Dietary factors modifying breast cancer risk and relation to time of intake. *Journal of Mammary Gland Biology and Neoplasia* 2005; 10(1):87–100.

Usui T. Pharmaceutical prospects of phytoestrogens. *Endocrine Journal* 2006; 53(1):7–20.

Wactawski-Wende J, Kotchen JM, Anderson GL, et al. Calcium plus vitamin D supplementation and the risk of colorectal cancer. *New England Journal of Medicine* 2006; 354(7):684–96.

Weisburger JH. Comments on the history and importance of aromatic and heterocyclic amines in public health. *Mutation Research* 2002; 506-507:9–20.

Willett WC. Diet and cancer: one view at the start of the millennium. *Cancer Epidemiology, Biomarkers & Prevention* 2001; 10(1):3–8.

Wu AH, Yu MC, Tseng CC, et al. Epidemiology of soy exposures and breast cancer risk. *British Journal of Cancer* 2008; 98(1):9–14.

Yager JD, Davidson NE. Estrogen carcinogenesis in breast cancer. *New England Journal of Medicine* 2006; 254(3):270–82.

Yan L, Spitznagel EL. Soy consumption and prostate cancer risk in men: a revisit of a meta-analysis. *American Journal of Clinical Nutrition* 2009; 89(4):1155–63.

Zheng W, Lee SA. Well-done meat intake, heterocyclic amine exposure, and cancer risk. *Nutrition and Cancer* 2009; 61(4):427–46.

# INDEX

Underscored page references indicate boxed text and tables.